DATE DUE

Psychobiology and Treatment of Anorexia Nervosa and Bulimia Nervosa

AMERICAN PSYCHOPATHOLOGICAL ASSOCIATION SERIES

Psychobiology and Treatment of Anorexia Nervosa and Bulimia Nervosa

Katherine A. Halmi, M.D.

Professor of Psychiatry
Director, Eating Disorders Program
New York Hospital—Cornell Medical Center
Westchester Division
White Plains, New York

AMERICAN PSYCHOPATHOLOGICAL ASSOCIATION SERIES

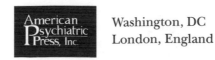

Washington, DC
London, England

Note: The authors have worked to ensure that all information in this book concerning drug dosages, schedules, and routes of administration is accurate as of the time of publication and consistent with standards set by the U.S. Food and Drug Administration and the general medical community. As medical research and practice advance, however, therapeutic standards may change. For this reason and because human and mechanical errors sometimes occur, we recommend that readers follow the advice of a physician who is directly involved in their care or the care of a member of their family.

Copyright © 1992 American Psychiatric Press, Inc.
ALL RIGHTS RESERVED
Manufactured in the United States of America on acid-free paper
First Edition
95 94 93 92   4 3 2 1

American Psychiatric Press, Inc.
1400 K Street, N.W., Washington, DC   20005

Library of Congress Cataloging-in-Publication Data

Psychobiology and treatment of anorexia nervosa and bulimia nervosa /
   [edited by] Katherine A. Halmi. — 1st ed.
      p.   cm.—(American Psychopathological Association)
   Includes bibliographical references and index.
   ISBN 0-88048-506-X (alk. paper)
   1. Anorexia nervosa—Congresses.   2. Anorexia nervosa—
Physiological aspects—Congresses.   3. Bulimia—Congresses.
4. Bulimia—Physiological aspects—Congresses.   I. Halmi,
Katherine A.
   [DNLM: 1. Eating Disorders—diagnosis.   2. Eating Disorders—
psychology.   3. Eating Disorders—therapy.   4. Psychotherapy.   WM
175 P9735]
RC552.A5P77—1993
616.85′26—dc20
DNLM/DLC
for Library of Congress   92-17984
                                           CIP

British Library Cataloguing in Publication Data
A CIP record is available from the British Library.

Contents

Section I
Epidemiology, Classification, and Diagnoses

Section II
Eating Behavior

Section III
Longitudinal and Outcome Studies

Section IV
Neuroendocrinology, Neuropeptides, and Metabolism

Section V
Family Studies

Section VI
Treatment Studies

Contributors

Arnold E. Andersen, M.D.
Professor of Psychiatry, University of Iowa, Iowa City, Iowa

Andrew Broocks, M.D.
University of Göttingen, Göttingen, Germany

Regina C. Casper, M.D.
Professor of Psychiatry and the Committee on Human Nutrition and
Nutritional Biology, University of Chicago, Chicago, Illinois

Christopher Dare, M.B.
Senior Lecturer, The Institute of Psychiatry, The Maudsley Hospital,
London, England

Ivan Eisler, B.A.
Senior Lecturer, The Institute of Psychiatry, The Maudsley Hospital,
London, England

Madelyn H. Fernstrom, Ph.D.
Associate Professor of Psychiatry and Epidemiology, University of
Pittsburgh, Pittsburgh, Pennsylvania

Manfred M. Fichter, M.D.
Professor of Psychiatry, University of Munich,
Munich, Germany

Paul Garfinkel, M.D., F.R.C.P.C.
Professor and Chair, Department of Psychiatry, University of Toronto,
Toronto, Canada

Katherine A. Halmi, M.D.
Professor of Psychiatry and Director, Eating Disorders Program, New
York Hospital—Cornell Medical Center, Westchester Division, White
Plains, New York

Hans W. Hoek, M.D., Ph.D.
Lecturer, Department of Psychiatry, Academic Hospital, University of
Utrecht, Utrecht, Netherlands

L. K. George Hsu, M.D.
Associate Professor of Psychiatry and Director, Outpatient Eating
Disorders Program, University of Pittsburgh, Pittsburgh, Pennsylvania

Laura Lynn Humphrey, Ph.D.
Associate Professor of Psychiatry and Behavioral Sciences and Director,
Program for Anorexia and Bulimia, Northwestern University Medical
School, Chicago, Illinois

Walter H. Kaye, M.D.
Associate Professor of Psychiatry and Director, Eating Disorders
Module, University of Pittsburgh, Pittsburgh, Pennsylvania

P. Daniel F. Le Grange, Ph.D.
Senior Lecturer, University of Cape Town, Cape Town, South Africa

James E. Mitchell, M.D.
Professor of Psychiatry, University of Minnesota, Minneapolis,
Minnesota

Elizabeth Philipp, M.D.
Technical University, München, München, Germany

Karl Martin Pirke, M.D.
Professor of Psychology, Department of Psychoendocrinology,
University of Trier, Trier, Germany

Nancy C. Raymond, M.D.
Assistant Professor of Psychiatry, University of Minnesota, Minneapolis,
Minnesota

Gerald F. M. Russell, M.D.
Professor of Psychiatry, The Institute of Psychiatry, The Maudsley
Hospital, London, England

Ulrich Schweiger, M.D.
Max Planck Institute for Psychiatry, München, Germany

Joseph A. Silverman, M.D.
Clinical Professor of Pediatrics, College of Physicians & Surgeons,
Columbia University, New York, New York

Michael Strober, Ph.D.
Professor of Psychiatry, University of California at Los Angeles; and
Director, Eating Disorders Program, UCLA Neuropsychiatric Institute,
Los Angeles, California

Walter Vandereycken, M.D., Ph.D.
Professor of Psychiatry, Catholic University of Leuven, Leuven, Belgium

B. Timothy Walsh, M.D.
Professor of Clinical Psychiatry, College of Physicians & Surgeons,
Columbia University, New York, New York

Theodore E. Weltzin, M.D.
Assistant Professor of Psychiatry, University of Pittsburgh, Pittsburgh,
Pennsylvania

Thomas Wilckens, M.D.
Tufts University, Boston, Massachusetts

Preface

—⸗⸝●⸜⸗—

The eating disorders anorexia nervosa and bulimia nervosa are both interrelated and distinct disorders. In the past 15 years, research on these disorders has burgeoned, providing empirical evidence for a more accurate classification schema for eating disorders. This book is the result of the proceedings of the 1991 American Psychopathological Association meeting. The aim of the program at that meeting was to bring together recent clinical research into all facets of anorexia nervosa and bulimia nervosa.

In the first sections of this book, diagnostic schemata of eating disorders are reviewed from the perspectives of cross-cultural, longitudinal, and family studies. Following this, the psychobiology of anorexia nervosa and bulimia nervosa is presented from the facets of neuroendocrinology and the psychological perceptions associated with eating behavior. Next, the contribution of the family in developing and maintaining eating disorders is examined from the perspective of family interaction studies. In the concluding section, developments in the integration of psychodynamic concepts into the psychotherapy of anorexia nervosa and bulimia nervosa, cognitive-behavioral approaches, and the pharmacological treatment of eating disorders are reviewed.

Section I

Epidemiology, Classification, and Diagnoses

Chapter 1

Historical Development

Joseph A. Silverman, M.D.

———➤●◄———

Ⅰn this chapter, I describe a few of
the more important events in the
history of eating disorders. The
data are taken from the English, French, and American literature of the
past three and one-third centuries. Because space limitations bar any
encyclopedic presentation, certain well-known cases have been deliberately omitted.

Accounts describing cases of self-starvation have occurred with great
frequency from the days of Biblical antiquity to the Middle Ages. These
tales, although interesting, are of questionable value as medical reports;
they are a curious melange of truth, hyperbole, religiosity, and, occasionally, fraud. Some of these anecdotes were spread by word of mouth; others
were recorded in written form, but were insufficiently detailed. As a result, they cannot be seriously regarded as bona fide reports of anorexia
nervosa.

The 17th Century

During the second half of the 17th century, printed pamphlets began to
appear in profusion. It was in this form that detailed case reports of
self-starvation began to surface. As the news about these patients was
disseminated, much commentary was evoked. The very thought that a
human being would deliberately starve herself for any reason provoked,
intrigued, and tantalized the public.

3

A case in point occurred in 1667, when an 18-year-old English girl named Martha Taylor developed anorexia nervosa. Before her illness, this young woman lived in utter obscurity. She was the daughter of a lead miner and resided with her family in Over-Haddon, near Bakewell in Derbyshire. Despite her lowly birth and impoverished social status, Martha was catapulted to national fame by her 15-month episode of self-starvation. As word of her illness spread, she was besieged with visitors, including the clergy, the peerage, and physicians. Shortly thereafter, three books were published in London describing her illness in detail (H.A. 1669; Reynolds 1669; Robins 1668). Furthermore, a prominent physician was dispatched by the Royal Society with orders to travel 40 miles on horseback to visit Martha, to examine her thoroughly, and to submit a written report on her true condition (Johnston 1669).

The propositus had a history of aberrant behavior. At age 11 she had been struck on the back and developed lower-extremity paralysis that lasted 2 weeks. After a full recovery, she became depressed by "religious melancholy," and her paralysis returned, in association, allegedly, with 6 months of delirium.

Once these symptoms had disappeared, she went on to develop a cough so intense that "she could be heard at 400 to 500 paces" (i.e., one-half mile). Subsequently, she occupied herself night and day reading the Holy Scriptures or other religious books. Her last menstrual period occurred on St. Michael the Archangel's Day (September 29, 1667), when she was 18 years old. Soon thereafter, she was afflicted by a siege of vomiting. She began to decrease her intake of food and by St. Thomas's Day (December 21, 1667) had stopped eating. It is alleged that she took no solid food for the ensuing 12–13 months and subsisted on a few drops of syrup or the juice of a roasted raisin. It is stated that she excreted neither urine nor stool (Bliss and Branch 1960; Johnston 1669; Reynolds 1669; Silverman 1986).

Her physical findings are described as follows:

> She is worn away so bare that she hath very small left on her but skin and
> bone, she hath no belly to be seen, for her entrailes is dryed up insomuch
> that you may see her backbone through the skin of her belly, nothing she
> can be likened to but to the picture of death all her body over. (Robins
> 1668, p. 4)

As word of Martha's fast spread about the countryside, she was "visited so plentifully by the curious of many parts, as also by the Religious of all persuasions" (Reynolds 1669). At the request of Dr. Walter Needham, physician and curator-elect of England's Royal Society, John Reynolds (master at the old grammar school of nearby King's Norton) traveled 60 miles to investigate. He published shortly thereafter a "Narrative of the Superennial Fast under all the Havocks and depredations whereof the Derby-shire Damosell hath hitherto been sustained, though emaciated into the ghostliness of a Skeleton to the great astonishment of the Vulgus" (Reynolds 1669). Learned in theology and medicine, Reynolds was not surprised that one could endure prolonged periods of abstinence. Convinced by the genuineness of Martha's illness, he subtitled his report: "Proving that without any Miracle, the Texture of Humane Bodies may be so altered that Life may be long continued without supplies of Meat and Drink."

Fasting in young women was not a new phenomenon to Reynolds (1669): "Most of these Damosells fall into this abstinence between the age of fourteen and twenty years." Unable to assign a cause for the illness, he hypothesized, "Tis probable that the feminal humours in these virgins may by a long abode in their vessels grow acid. . . . Her age confirms the probability of a ferment in the feminals" (pp. 33–34).

Some were convinced of Martha's integrity (H.A. 1669; Reynolds 1669; Robins 1668); others had doubts and suspected her of cheating. In his report to the Royal Society, Dr. Nathaniel Johnston considered Martha and her mother to be sly, secretive, and untrustworthy. He believed that Martha had fooled most of her visitors. He thought that she had duped not only the "commonfolk," but the wise. He went on to take the extreme step of asking the Royal Society to petition the king, Charles II, to appoint "some doctor (with justices of the peace and with reliable witnesses present), to examine the affected parts of the girl with his own eyes" (Johnston 1669, p. 140). The Royal Society took no action on Johnston's request.

On October 20, 1668, Thomas Hobbes, England's leading philosopher and political theorist, wrote the following letter:

The young woman at Over-Haddon hath been visited by divers persons of this house. My Lord himself (i.e., William Cavendish, third earl of Devonshire), hunting the hare one day, with other gentlemen and some of his servants, went to see her on purpose: and they all agree with the relation you say was made to yourself. They further say on their own knowledge that part of her belly touches her back-bone. She began (as her mother says) to lose her appetite in December last, and had lost it quite in March following:

insomuch as that for the last six months she has not eaten or drunk anything at all, but only wets her lips with a feather dipt in water. Some of the
neighbouring ministers visit her often: others that see her for curiosity give
her money, sixpence or a shilling, which she refuseth, but her mother
taketh. But it does not appear they gain by it so much as to breed a suspi-
cion of a cheat. The woman is manifestly sick, and 'tis thought that she
cannot last much longer. Her talk (as the gentlewoman that went from this
house told me) is most heavenly. To know the certainty there be many
things necessary which cannot honestly be pryed into by a man. Whether
any excrement pass, or none at all. For if it pass, though in small quantity,
yet it argues food proportionable, which may, being little, be given her
secretly. Whether no urine at all pass; for liquors also nourish as they go. I
think it were somewhat inhumane to examine these things too nearly,
when it so little concerneth the commonwealth: nor do I know of any law
that authoriseth a justice of peace, or other subject, to restrain the liberty
of a sick person so far as were needful for a discovery of this nature. I
cannot therefore deliver any judgement in the case. The examining
whether such a thing as this be a miracle belongs I think to the Church.
(Hobbes 1907, pp. 45–47)

In 1689, 22 years after Martha Taylor's fast, a new textbook of medicine
was published in London, *Phthisiologia, seu Exercitationes de Phthisi.* Its author was Richard Morton, a fellow of the College of Physicians. In this
seminal volume, translated into English 5 years later and subtitled *A Treatise of Consumptions,* Morton outlined in painstaking detail the many disease processes that cause wasting of body tissues. All of the material was
based on his own clinical observations, with little reference to books. The
text, which is richly descriptive, is best known for his comments on tuber-
culosis. A specialist in the treatment of this disease, he was the first physician to state that tubercles are always present in the pulmonary form.

Morton is best known today as the author of the first medical account
of anorexia nervosa, a condition that he referred to as "a Nervous Consumption," caused "by Sadness, and anxious Cares" (Bliss and Branch
1960, p. 10). The clinical description of his two cases, printed in its en-
tirety, is as follows.

Case 1

Mr. Duke's daughter in St. Mary Axe, in the year 1684, and the Eighteenth
Year of her Age, in the Month of July fell into a total suppression of her
Monthly Courses from a multitude of Cares and Passions of her Mind, but

without any Symptom of the Green-Sickness following upon it. From which time her Appetite began to abate, and her Digestion to be bad; her Flesh also began to be flaccid and loose, and her looks pale, with other Symptoms usual in an Universal Consumption of the Habit of the Body, and by the extream and memorable cold Weather which happened the Winter following, this Consumption did seem to be not a little improved; for that she was wont by her studying at Night, and continual poring upon Books, to expose her self both Day and Night to the injuries of the Air, which was at that time extreamly cold, not without some manifest Prejudice to the System of her Nerves. The Spring following, by the Prescription of some Emperick, she took a Vomit, and after that I know not what Steel Medicines, but without any Advantage. So from that time loathing all sorts of Medicaments, she wholly neglected the care of her self for two full Years, till at last being brought to the last degree of a Marasmus, or Consumption, and thereupon subject to frequent Fainting Fits, she apply'd her self to me for Advice.

I do not remember that I did ever in all my Practice see one, that was conversant with the Living so much wasted with the greatest degree of a Consumption (like a Skeleton only clad with skin), yet there was no Fever, but on the contrary a coldness of the whole Body; no Cough, or difficulty of Breathing, nor an appearance of any other Distemper of the Lungs, or of any other Entrail: No Loosness, or any other sign of a Colliquation, or Preternatural expence of the Nutritious Juices. Only her Appetite was diminished, and her Digestion uneasie, with Fainting Fits, which did frequently return upon her. Which Symptoms I did endeavour to relieve by the outward application of Aromatick Bags made to the Region of the Stomack, and by Stomack-Plaisters, as also by the internal use of bitter Medicines, Chalybeates, and Juleps made of Cephalick and Antihysterick Waters, sufficiently impregnated with Spirit of Salt Armoniack, and Tincture of Castor, and other things of that Nature. Upon the use of which she seemed to be much better, but being quickly tired with Medicines, she beg'd that the whole Affair might be committed again to Nature, whereupon consuming every day more and more, she was after three Months taken with a Fainting Fit and Dyed. (Morton 1694, pp. 8–9)

Case 2

The Son of the Reverend Minister Steele, my very good Friend, about the Sixteenth Year of his Age, fell gradually into a total want of Appetite, occasioned by his studying too hard, and the Passions of his Mind, and upon that into an Universal Atrophy, pining away more and more for the space of two Years, without any Cough, Fever, or any other Symptom of any Distemper of his Lungs, or any other Entrail; as also without a Looseness, or Diabetes, or any other sign of a Colliquation, or Preternatural Evacuation.

And therefore I judg'd this Consumption to be Nervous, and to have its seat in the whole Habit of the Body, and to arise from the System of Nerves being distemper'd. I began, and first attempted his Cure with the use of Antiscorbutick, Bitter, and Chalybeate Medicines, as well Natural as Artificial, but without any benefit; and therefore when I found that the former Method did not answer our Expectations, I advis'd him to abandon his Studies, to go into the Country Air, and to use Riding, and a Milk Diet (and especially to drink Asses Milk) for a long time. By the use of which he recover'd his Health in great measure, though he is not yet perfectly freed from a Consumptive state; and what will be the event of this Method, does not yet plainly appear. (Morton 1694, p. 10)

The 18th Century

Seventy-five years would pass before another important account of self-starvation appeared. In 1764, Robert Whytt, Professor of the Theory of Medicine at Edinburgh, published a book, *Observations on the Nature, Causes, and Cure of Those Disorders Which Have Been Commonly Called Nervous, Hypochondriac or Hysteric to Which Are Prefixed Some Remarks on the Sympathy of the Nerves*. Beneath the title, printed in Greek, was the Hippocratic epigraph, "Sympathia panda," meaning, "Emotion is everything."

In his text, Whytt (1764, pp. 253–254) wrote a description of "a nervous atrophy" and presented a case study, with the following comments:

A marasmus, or sensible wasting of the body, not attended with sweatings, any considerable increase of the excretions by urine or stool, a quick pulse, or feverish heat, may deserve the name of nervous. . . . But this kind of atrophy, tho' not, perhaps, owing to any fault in the spirits, or even in the brain or nervous system in general, may yet deserve the name of nervous, as it seems, frequently, to proceed from an unnatural or morbid state of the nerves, of the stomach, and intestines. . . . Further, the watching or want of refreshing rest, and low spirits or melancholy, which generally accompany this disease, may contribute to prevent the proper nutrition of the body.

Whytt's case report is as follows:

Another lad of 14 years of age, of a thin and delicate habit, and of quick and lively feelings, whose pulse in health used to beat 70 and 80 times in a minute; about the beginning of June 1757, was observed to be low-spirited and thoughtful, to lose his appetite, and have a bad digestion. Altho' he lost flesh daily, yet he had no nightsweats, no extraordinary discharge of urine and was costive. His tongue was clean, his skin cooler than natural, and when in bed, his pulse beat only 43 times in a minute; nay about the middle of July, when reduced almost to skin and bone, his pulse, in a horizontal posture, did not exceed 39. About the end of August, his distemper took a sudden turn; he then began to have such a craving for food, with a quick digestion, that he grew faint unless he eat almost every two hours; he had two or three stools a-day; his pulse beat from 96 to 110; his skin was warm, and his veins, which scarce could be seen before, became now turgid with blood. The strong apprehensions he formerly had of dying left him, he was sure he should recover; and accordingly, by the middle of October, he was plumper than ever he had been before. Towards the end of November, his appetite became moderate, and his pulse gradually returned to its natural state.

It was observable, that the pulse was slowest towards the evening, and generally of a proper strength and fulness.

Since, with all my attention, I neither could discover the cause of the patient's first complaints, nor of the sudden and contrary turn which they took afterwards; I shall not pretend to reason on his case; but I thought it deserved to be mentioned, as a good instance of a nervous atrophy; and of the effect of such disorders in making the pulse much slower, than ever it has been observed in a natural state. (Whytt 1764, pp. 303–305)

The 19th Century

Almost 100 years would elapse before another truly significant account of eating disorders appeared in print. When it did, in 1860, it failed to receive the attention it deserved, despite its importance. It was quickly forgotten and did not appear again for more than another century (Silverman 1989; Skrabanek 1983). This paper, perhaps the seminal report of the 19th century, was written by Dr. Louis-Victor Marcé (1860a) of Paris and was titled "Note sur une forme de délire hypochondriaque consécutive aux dyspepsies et caractérisée principalement par le refus d'aliments." Marcé's report was published in Paris. It was then almost immediately translated into English and republished in an abbreviated form in London.

Marcé was a member of both the faculty of the University of Paris and the staff of the Bicêtre. He was a prodigious writer of texts on various psychiatric subjects. In 1860, Marcé stated the following:

Amongst the numerous and varied forms of dyspepsia, there are some which should especially attract the attention of psycopathists, on account of the peculiar mental condition thereby determined. . . . We see, for instance, young girls, who at the period of puberty, and after a precocious physical development, become subject to inappetancy carried to the utmost limits. Whatever the duration of their abstinence, they experience a distaste for food, which the most pressing want is unable to overcome. . . . Deeply impressed, whether by the absence of appetite or by the uneasiness caused by digestion, these patients arrive at a delirious conviction that they cannot or ought not to eat. In one word, the gastric nervous disorder becomes cerebro-nervous. (1860b, p. 264)

Marcé (1860b) had observed several cases where the patient had lived "six months, a year, and even more, upon a few spoonfuls of soup or a few mouthfuls of sweetmeat or pastry daily" (p. 264). Another patient lived on 50 grams a day of food, which was carefully weighed. He described the emaciation, cachexia, and death in these patients.

Marcé (1860b, p. 265) further commented:

I would venture to say that the first physicians who attended the patients misunderstood the true signification of this obstinate refusal of food: far from seeing in it a delirious idea of a hypochondriacal nature, they occupied themselves solely with the state of the stomach, and prescribed, as a matter of course, bitters, tonics, iron, exercize, hydro-therapeutics with a view to stimulate the activity of the digestive functions. However apparently excellent these therapeutic measures may be, they always proved insufficient when the malady was in the advanced stage. It is then no longer the stomach that demands attention . . . it is the delirious idea which constitutes henceforth, the point of departure, and in which lies the essence of the malady; the patients are no longer dyspeptics—they are insane.

Marcé (1860b, p. 265) continued:

The hypochondriacal delirium, then, cannot be advantageously encountered so long as the subjects remain in the midst of their own family and their habitual circle. . . . It is therefore indispensable to change the habitation and surrounding circumstances, and to entrust the patients to the care of strangers.

The next important event in the history of eating disorders occurred on August 8, 1868, when the *Lancet* published the "Address in Medicine" delivered before the annual meeting of the British Medical Association at

Oxford. The speaker was Dr. William W. Gull of Guy's Hospital. In this address, Gull described the general state of medicine and the progress made in science and philosophy. In his lengthy report, there appears "one relevant, and rather confused, sentence, constituting 0.5% of the whole lecture" (Skrabanek 1983, p. 122).

Gull (1868, p. 175) stated:

> At present our diagnosis is mostly one of inference, from our knowledge of the liability of the several organs to particular lesions; thus we avoid the error of supposing the presence of mesenteric disease in young women emaciated to the last degree through hysterical apepsia, by our knowledge of the latter affliction, and by the absence of tubercular disease elsewhere.

This brief statement, seemingly unrelated to anything else in Gull's oration, deeply embedded and difficult to find, went unnoted for at least the next 5 years.

On September 6, 1873, the first of a pair of articles appeared in London's *Medical Times and Gazette.* Three weeks later, the second part was published. Both were written by Dr. Charles Lasègue, professor of clinical medicine in the Faculty of Medicine of the University of Paris. The title was "On hysterical anorexia," and the papers were a translation of Lasègue's original report in French, published in Paris 5 months earlier in April 1873, and titled, "L'anorexie hystérique." In this essay, Lasègue (1873a) described the findings in eight patients, ages 18–32.

The main thrust of the report was to emphasize the emotional etiology of this illness. Lasègue conveyed a sense of the spirit and feelings of these patients, the nuances of their disturbed relationships, and the subtleties of their intrapsychic turmoil (Bliss and Branch 1960).

Lasègue (1873b, p. 265) wrote:

> A young girl, between 15 and 20 years of age, suffers from some emotion which she avows or conceals. Generally it relates to some real or imaginary project, to a violence done to some sympathy, or to some more or less conscient desire.

Lasègue (1873b, pp. 265–266) cautioned his readers to realize the gravity of the situation:

> Woe to the physician who, misunderstanding the peril, treats as a fancy without object or duration, an obstinacy which he hopes to vanquish by medicines, friendly advice, or by the still more defective resource, intimi-

dation. With hysterical subjects, a first medical fault is never reparable. Ever on the watch for judgements concerning themselves, especially such as are approved by the family, they never pardon. At this initial period, the only prudent course is to observe, to keep silent, and to remember that when voluntary inanition dates from several weeks, it has become a pathological condition, having a long course to run.

Lasègue (1873b, p. 266) continued:

> The family has but two methods at its service which it always exhausts, . . . entreaties and menaces . . . and which both serve as a touchstone. The delicacies of the table are multiplied in the hopes of stimulating the appetite, but the more the solicitude increases, the more the appetite diminishes . . . What dominates in the mental condition of the hysterical patient is, above all, the state of quietude . . . I might almost say a condition of contentment truly pathological. Not only does she not sigh for recovery, but she is not ill-pleased with her condition, notwithstanding all the unpleasantness it is attended with. Here we have . . . an inexhaustible optimism against which supplications and menaces are alike of no avail.

Lasègue described in a general way the subsequent effects of inanition including amenorrhea, cachexia, obstipation, skin changes, fatigue, orthostatic hypotension, paleness, and heart murmurs. The effect of all these, Lasègue (1873a, 1873b, 1873c) wrote, is to redouble the anxieties of relatives and friends who now consider the case to be desperate. The patient then "begins to be anxious from the sad appearance of those who surround her, and for the first time her self-satisfied indifference receives a shock" (Lasègue 1873c, p. 368). At this point Lasègue (1873c, p. 368) wrote:

> The moment has now arrived when the physician, if he has been careful in managing the case with a prevision of the future, resumes his authority. Treatment is no longer submitted to with a mere positive condescendance, but is sought for with an eagerness that the patient tries to conceal.

On October 24, 1873, Dr. William W. Gull addressed the Clinical Society of London. He was, however, no longer simply Dr. Gull, but was now Sir William W. Gull, Baronet, having been created a peer by a grateful Queen Victoria for saving the life of the Prince of Wales. The subject of his address, which was published in 1874, was "Anorexia nervosa (apepsia hysterica, anorexia hysterica)." In the opening sentence, Gull wrote:

In an address on medicine, delivered at Oxford in the autumn of 1868, I referred to a peculiar form of disease occurring mostly in young women, and characterized by extreme emaciation, and often referred to latent tubercle and mesenteric disease. I remarked that at present our diagnosis of this affection is negative, so far as determining any positive cause from which it springs. (p. 22)

With these two sentences, Gull took the necessary steps to establish his "primacy" as the 19th century's limner of anorexia nervosa. Gull (1874, p. 22) continued: "The subjects of this affection are mostly of the female sex, and chiefly between the ages of 16 and 23. I have occasionally seen it in males at the same age."

Gull (1874) described three cases, known as Misses A, B, and C, and included their woodcut portraits both before and after illness. He stated:

After these remarks were penned, Dr. Francis Webb directed my attention to the paper of Dr. Lasègue; . . . which was published in the Archives Générales de Médecine, April 1873, and translated into the pages of the Medical Times, Sept. 6 and 27, 1873. . . . it is plain that Dr. Lasègue and I have the same malady in mind, though the forms of our illustrations are different. Dr. Lasègue does not refer to my address at Oxford, and it is most likely he knew nothing of it. There is, therefore, the more value in his paper, as our observations have been made independently. We have both selected the same expression to characterize the malady. (p. 25)

In his 1874 article, Gull emphasized the clinical findings of starvation and did not really concern himself, as did Lasègue, with the illness's emotional aspects. Thus Gull simply noted the occurrence of amenorrhea, constipation, loss of appetite, decreased vital signs, and emaciation.

Gull's recommended treatment is simple, but perhaps a bit heavy-handed and authoritarian: "The treatment required is obviously that which is fitted for persons of unsound mind. The patients should be fed at regular intervals, and surrounded by persons who would have moral control over them; relations and friends being generally the worst attendants" (Gull 1874, p. 26).

It should be noted that following the publications of Gull and Lasègue, the rather unfortunate term "anorexia nervosa" took hold.

One is forced to wonder why both Gull and Lasègue failed to acknowledge the important contribution of Louis-Victor Marcé, who published his report in 1860, 8 years before Gull's "Address in Medicine," and 13–14 years before the so-called definitive papers of Lasègue and Gull. Marcé, after all, was not an obscure French physician; he was one of France's medical and psychiatric elite. His essay was printed in the leading psychiatric journal of France; it was almost immediately republished in English in one of London's most prominent journals. Did Gull and Lasègue know of Marcé's contribution? Did they ignore it? We will never know the answers.

The 20th Century

During the 20th century, two major events occurred that led to a revolution in our understanding of eating disorders. The first came from the pen of Dr. Hilde Bruch, who was, in her lifetime, considered to be the "doyenne" of anorexia nervosa. A prodigious worker and a prolific writer, she delved into the psyche of anorectic patients in an attempt to find common threads in their emotional pathology. She discovered that three areas of disordered function can be recognized in the anorectic patient:

> 1) . . . a disturbance of delusional proportions in the body image and body concept. Cachexia is regarded with unconcern, and is defended as normal and right, and as the only possible security against the dreaded fate of being fat. The true anorexic is identified with her skeleton-like appearance, denies its abnormality, and actively maintains it.
>
> 2) . . . a disturbance in the accuracy of the perception or cognitive interpretation of stimuli arising in the body, with failure to recognize signs of nutritional need as the most pronounced deficiency. Awareness of hunger in the ordinary sense seems to be absent. The patient's sullen comment, "I do not need to eat," probably expresses what she feels and experiences most of the time.
>
> 3) . . . a paralyzing sense of ineffectiveness which pervades all thinking and activities. They experience themselves as acting only in response to demands coming from other people in situations, and not as doing things because they want to. (Bruch 1973, pp. 251–254)

Thus it was not until the end of the 20th century that we had some insight into the true psychopathology of these patients. For the preceding 300 years, this poorly understood illness had been ascribed variously to "a ferment in the feminals" (Reynolds 1669), "a nervous consumption" (Morton 1689), "a nervous atrophy" (Whytt 1764), a hypochondriacal delirium" (Marcé 1860b), "a hysteria linked to hypochondriasis" (Lasègue 1873b), and "a perversion of the ego" (Gull 1874, 1888).

The 20th century brought forth a second contribution of extreme importance. This was the seminal report of Gerald Russell (1979), "Bulimia Nervosa: An Ominous Variant of Anorexia Nervosa." Having studied 30 patients (28 females and 2 males), Russell described in detail this seemingly new illness and listed its diagnostic criteria:

1) the patients suffer from powerful and intractable urges to overeat;
2) they seek to avoid the fattening effects of food by inducing vomiting or abusing purgatives or both;
3) they have a morbid fear of becoming fat. (p. 445)

Russell reported how this group of patients, like those with anorexia nervosa, were determined to keep their weight below a self-imposed threshold. In contrast to the anorectic patient, the patient with bulimia nervosa tended to be heavier, more active sexually, and more likely to menstruate regularly and remain fertile. Russell also described the physical and metabolic effects secondary to self-induced vomiting and purging. Finally, he outlined a treatment plan.

At the end of his report, Russell (1979) stressed his concern that the prognosis in bulimia nervosa might be less favorable than in true anorexia nervosa, for the following reasons: "1) bulimia nervosa is more resistant to treatment; 2) physical complications are more frequent and dangerous; and 3) the risk of suicide is considerable" (p. 448).

Conclusion

It is not surprising that descriptions of anorexia nervosa preceded those of bulimia nervosa by more than 300 years. The anorectic patient, with her ghostly skeletal frame, is shocking to all observers and difficult to ignore. The bulimic patient, on the other hand, with her more normal weight, appearance, and activities, is able to carry out her furtive self-destructive techniques with little fear of detection.

References

Bliss EL, Branch CHH: Anorexia Nervosa: Its History, Psychology, and Biology. New York, Hoeber, 1960

Bruch H: Eating Disorders: Obesity, Anorexia Nervosa, and the Person Within. New York, Basic Books, 1973

Gull W: The address in medicine delivered before the annual meeting of the British Medical Association, at Oxford. Lancet 2:171–176, 1868

Gull W: Anorexia nervosa (apepsia hysterica, anorexia hysterica). Transactions of the Clinical Society of London 7:22–28, 1874

Gull W: Anorexia nervosa. Lancet 1:516–517, 1888

H.A.: Mirabile Pecci: or the non-such wonder of the Peak in Derbyshire. London, T Parkhurst, 1669

Hobbes T: Nervous atrophy, in Medical Lectures and Aphorisms. Edited by Gee S. London, Oxford, 1907, pp 45–47

Johnston N: Letter in Latin (dated June 29, 1669) to Dr. Timothy Clarke "concerning the young fasting woman in Derbyshire, named Martha Taylor, together with his apprehension of some imposture in the affair . . ." Journal Book of the Royal Society, London, 1667–1671 3:389–392, 1669

Lasègue C: De l'anorexie hystérique. Archives Générales de Médecine 1:385–403, 1873a

Lasègue C: On hysterical anorexia. Medical Times and Gazette 2:265–266, 1873b

Lasègue C: On hysterical anorexia. Medical Times and Gazette 2:367–369, 1873c

Marcé L-V: Note sur une forme de délire hypochondriaque consécutive aux dyspepsies et caractérisée principalement par le refu d'aliments. Annales Médico-psychologiques 6:15–28, 1860a

Marcé L-V: On a form of hypochondriacal delirium occurring consecutive to dyspepsia, and characterized by refusal of food. Journal of Psychological Medicine and Mental Pathology 13:264–266, 1860b

Morton R: Phthisiologia, seu Exercitationes de Phthisi. London, S Smith, 1689

Morton R: Phthisiologia: Or, a Treatise of Consumptions. London, Smith & Walford, 1694

Reynolds J: A Discourse Upon Prodigious Abstinence; Occasioned by the Twelve Months Fasting of Martha Taylor, the Famed Derbyshire Damosell, etc. London, R W, 1669

Robins T: Newes From Darby-shire: or the Wonder of All Wonders; Being a Perfect and True Relation of . . . one Martha Taylor . . . She Hath Fasted Forty Weeks and More, etc. London, T P, 1668

Russell G: Bulimia nervosa; an ominous variant of anorexia nervosa. Psychol Med 9:429–448, 1979

Silverman J: Anorexia nervosa in seventeenth century England as viewed by physician, philosopher, and pedagogue. International Journal of Eating Disorders 5:847–853, 1986

Silverman J: Louis-Victor Marcé, 1828–1864: anorexia nervosa's forgotten man. Psychol Med 19:833–835, 1989

Skrabanek P: Notes toward the history of anorexia nervosa. Janus 70:109–128, 1983

Whytt R: Observations on the Nature, Causes, and Cure of Those Disorders Which Have Been Commonly Called Nervous, Hypochondriac or Hysteric to Which Are Prefixed Some Remarks on the Sympathy of the Nerves. Edinburgh, Becket, DeHondt & Balfour, 1764

Chapter 2

Are Eating Disorders Culture-Bound Syndromes?

Walter Vandereycken, M.D., Ph.D.
Hans W. Hoek, M.D., Ph.D.

Psychiatric concepts, research methodologies, and even data are embedded in *social systems*. The work of the practitioner and the powers of the profession originate in the same dynamic systems of values and relationships and experiences. Through them psychiatric diagnostic categories are constrained by history and culture as much as by biology. (Kleinman 1988, pp. 3–4)

Because the body is the most potent metaphor of society, it is not surprising that disease is the most salient metaphor of structural crisis. All disease is disorder— metaphorically, literally, socially and politically. (Turner 1984, p. 114)

Looking at the social context of the psychiatric profession, as expressed in the first motto, Kleinman (1988) stressed that a psychiatric diagnosis is a semiotic act in which a person's experiences are reinterpreted as signs of particular disease states, and as such it represents a culturally constrained activity referring to a society in which human misery is "medicalized." Using a diagnostic category, such as eating disorders, we should be aware of "a tacit professional ideology that exaggerates what is universal in psychiatric disorder and de-emphasizes what is culturally particular" (Kleinman 1988, p. 22). For a long time, both clinicians and researchers have tried to decipher the enigma of anorexia nervosa as a disease entity. In recent decades both feminists and family therapists enlarged the scope by exploring the socioecological meanings of an eating disorder: the disease has been transformed into an illness experience, a human predicament, an interactional message, a sociocultural metaphor, and so on. But it looks as if medical labels have been silently replaced by sociocultural ones (McLorg and Taub 1987; Smead 1983).

In this chapter we address the often-heard question of whether eating disorders are "symptomatic" for our age and culture. The consideration of psychopathology as crystallization of culture (Bordo 1985) has been elaborated especially in the case of anorexia nervosa, in which a variety of cultural currents—axes of continuity—seem to converge. Historical studies have suggested a diachronic continuity between anorexia nervosa and other forms of self-starvation (see Silverman, Chapter 1, this volume), which seem to emerge as "anorexia multiforme—a medical chameleon that changes with the times" (DiNicola 1990a, p. 167). But a historical connection with anorexia-like illnesses is in our opinion questionable (see, e.g., Van Deth and Vandereycken 1991, 1992). We confine ourselves here, however, to another axis of converging cultural streams, the synchronic continuity (i.e., the connection with contemporary cultural practices and norms).

In the eyes of transcultural or contextually oriented psychiatrists, anorexia nervosa became the typical Western example of a culture-bound syndrome (Kleinman 1988; Littlewood and Lipsedge 1985, 1986, 1987; Prince 1983, 1985; Swartz 1985a). A *culture-bound syndrome* is a constellation of signs or symptoms, categorized as a dysfunction or disease, that is restricted to certain cultures primarily by reason of distinctive psychosocial features of those cultures. This definition (adapted from Prince 1985) implies that the disorder cannot be understood apart from its specific cultural context (Ritenbaugh 1982). According to this view, it is the cultural meanings of thinness and eating (tied up with contemporary Western orientations to the female body) that constitute eating disorders like anorexia nervosa and bulimia nervosa, although psychobiological and family vulnerability factors place certain persons at higher risk for this affliction.

> Where the body is valued differently and eating conveys meanings other than personal control, obesity will not signify a moral offense or aesthetic

blemish; starvation will not be a voluntary choice, but rather an unavoidable fact of life. In such a cultural context, anorexia nervosa does not possess coherence as a local category. (Kleinman 1988, p. 71)

Hence, Kleinman found it reasonable to speculate that this culture-bound syndrome will increase in prevalence in rapidly industrializing non-Western societies, especially among the elite class assimilating the Western values of female slenderness as an expression of sexual attraction and social prestige.

Supporting Data for the Sociocultural Approach

DiNicola (1990b) gave an excellent and detailed overview of the many clinical and epidemiological studies that support a sociocultural approach to anorexia nervosa (Table 2–1). We confine ourselves here to a brief summary of the available data (for sources and technical discussion refer to DiNicola's article).

There is ample evidence that anorexia nervosa is a "Western" illness: it shows a development gradient across cultures, with predominance in industrialized, developed countries, linking the disorder to an affluent society. Except for some rather anecdotal accounts, anorexia nervosa appears to be uncommon outside the Western world and in Western countries of less affluence. Most interesting from a transcultural point of view is the finding that, compared with their peers in the homeland, immigrants (e.g., Greek girls in Germany and Arab college students in London) are more likely to develop an eating disorder. Together with the similarly striking fact that, since World War II, Japanese health care is facing increasing numbers of patients with anorexia nervosa, this type of evidence points to the important impact of acculturation pressures or rapid sociocultural changes. In these instances, DiNicola (1990b) considered anorexia nervosa as a "culture-change syndrome," where for most cases in the West it is a culture-bound syndrome.

Anorexia nervosa and bulimia nervosa are also viewed as relatively "modern" illnesses. The historiography of morbid self-starvation is discussed elsewhere in this volume (see Silverman, Chapter 1). If eating disorders are culture-bound syndromes, we would expect that their incidence would change over time. In the case of bulimia nervosa, we lack sufficient research data to examine trends in its occurrence (Fairburn and Beglin 1990). Its nosographic history is too young and still in debate, but we will be forced in the future to explain the fact that its recent (re)discovery—made official in a DSM category—has stirred up such an unusual curiosity from both the lay public and the scientific world. The recent history of anorexia nervosa is better documented. Studies on its incidence over extended time intervals may allow us to examine a possible trend (Table 2–2, Figure 2–1). These epidemiological data, over the last decades, show a substantial increase in incidence of the disorder, particularly among women between the ages of 15 and 25 years. But case registers and hospital records give us only an idea about the number of patients who enter the official health care system, leaving us with guesses about the proportion of "dark numbers," or number of undetected cases. Hence, these data may just reflect trends in medical consumption or changing awareness (recognition) of the disorder. But even then it may be a culturally relevant indication.

All studies show that eating disorders are rare among males. In clinical samples, the male-to-female ratio for anorexia nervosa lies consistently between 1 in 10 and 1 in 20. This strikingly unequal sex ratio has raised many questions (Hsu 1989) and became the cornerstone of feminist explanations, especially because no clear-cut biological factor seems to account for this fundamental sex difference. Moreover, which biological mechanism will explain the particular age distribution (ranging mainly from puberty to early adulthood)? How do we interpret the marked race

Table 2–1.   Supporting data for the sociocultural approach to eating disorders

Culture	Development gradient across cultures ("Western" illness)
History	Increasing incidence ("modern" illness)
Sex	Females predominate
Race	Caucasians predominate
Social class	Middle and upper classes

Occupation at risk	With emphasis on weight or body shape
	    Valued for bodily appearance (actors, models)
	    Valued for physical performance (dancers, athletes)
	    Involved in food and weight management (dietitians)

Predisposing factors	Developmental, family, sociocultural factors No known biological cause
Precipitating factors	Life events (family and environmental changes) Distressing sexual experiences

Source.   Adapted from DiNicola 1990b.

difference, with a conspicuous rarity of eating disorders among nonwhite females within multiracial Western societies? This factor may be associated with the ethnocentric attitude of the dominant society, including its health care services. Ethnic differences may then reflect "how the prevailing attitudes of the social system in which the clinician/researcher works are linked inexorably to how cases are presented, researched, described, and diagnosed" (Dolan 1991, p. 76).

Although eating disorders occur across the social class spectrum, a significantly greater incidence is found in the middle and upper classes. But, as with ethnicity, the social class bias might be connected with the struc-

Table 2–2. Studies on the incidence of anorexia nervosa

Study	Source	Region	Incidence[a]
Theander 1970	Hospital records	South Sweden	
1931–1940			0.1
1941–1950			0.2
1951–1960			0.5
Kendell et al. 1973			
1965–1971	Case register	Camberwell (London)	0.66
1966–1969	Case register	Northeast Scotland	1.6
Szmukler et al.			
1986	Case register	Northeast Scotland	
1978–1982			4.06
Jones et al. 1980	Hospital records	Monroe County	
1960–1969	+ case register	(New York)	0.4
1970–1976			0.6
Willi and Grossman			
1983	Hospital records	Zürich (Switzerland)	
1956–1958			0.4
1963–1965			0.6
1973–1975			1.1
Hoek and Brook			
1985	Case register	Assen (Holland)	
1974–1982			5.0
Lucas et al. 1988	Hospital records	Rochester (Minnesota)	
1935–1949	+ case register		2.8 (11.5)[b]
1950–1964			2.6 (7.5)[b]
1965–1979			4.0 (10.9)[b]

[a]Incidence per 100,000 per year. [b]Incidence rates represent the definite cases. (In parentheses are the total incidence rates of definite, probable, and possible cases.)

tures, norms, and thresholds of the health care system. Indeed, in European countries like Belgium and the Netherlands, with rather generous state health insurance, those class differences seem to have less impact on the presentation and recognition of eating disorders. Nevertheless, in the rather egalitarian society of Norway, the skewed distribution of anorexia nervosa in the higher socioeconomic classes is unusual when compared with other psychosomatic disorders (Askevold 1982).

Some occupations appear to have a greater potential risk for being linked to the development of an eating disorder. A typical example is the fashion and ballet world, in which the combination of thin body ideal and competitiveness or high performance expectation may play a significant role as a psychosocial stressor. However, it is impossible to say at this point if those individuals displaying anorectic attitudes or behavior "tend to gravitate selectively into areas of culture where there is greater emphasis on body image or if actual demands of these subsets of culture lead to the psychopathological setting necessary to develop this disorder" (Joseph et al. 1982, p. 57). In other words, are "pre-anorectic" persons more easily attracted by the ballet world, or are ballet dancers more prone to anorexia nervosa? This issue also applies to the other professions at risk. "It

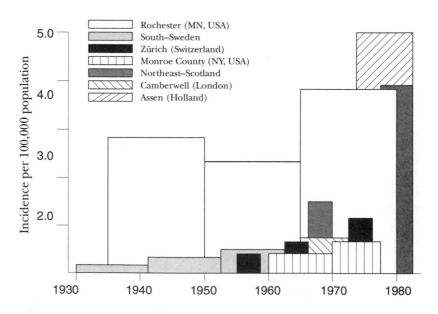

Figure 2–1. Registered incidence of anorexia nervosa per year per 100,000 population in different regions.

would be interesting to know if specialists in eating disorders have personal or family histories of eating disorders" (DiNicola 1990b, p. 255).

A final argument for the sociocultural approach is the fact that no biological process, marker, or event has yet been demonstrated to be the primary cause of an eating disorder. Biological factors may have a predispositional significance and seem to play an important role in the aggravation and perpetuation of eating disorders, whereas most of the predisposing and precipitating factors are psychosocial in nature. As with the vulnerability-stress model of many mental disorders, the relative importance ascribed to biological versus psychosocial influences will depend on the conceptualization of the disorder. In the medical disease model, biological processes are viewed as the central engine directing the behavioral disorder; the psychosocial predicament model emphasizes that the biological engine is only working under the command of the interaction between person and environment. This is an age-old discussion that lies beyond our scope.

Even if several of the previously presented arguments are still open to discussion, the combination of these probably interrelated data highlights an undeniable dimension in the presentation, recognition, and interpretation of a phenomenon we call eating disorder. A discussion of the sociocultural approach usually stresses the linkage between body culture (dieting, fitness) and eating disorders. This issue has been elaborated in great detail by many authors (e.g., Bennett and Gurin 1982; Chernin 1981; Gordon 1990; Nasser 1988a, 1988b; Schwartz 1986; Swartz 1985b). Although unmistakably a very valuable perspective, we believe it should be placed within a larger sociocultural analysis.

Decoding the Sociocultural Meanings

The Government of the Body

According to Bynum (1988), fasting women in medieval Italy and modern Portuguese peasant society do not just have an "anorectic" behavior in common, but represent the exponents of cultures in which the female is associated with body and sexuality (food and fertility). They share a symbolic view of non-eating as a form of sanctity or empowerment: fasting symbolizes purity through suffering (restraint from food and sex). It is the spiritual purification and domination of the flesh that brings these Christian women closer to God. One could interpret their fasting also as a way to develop a sense of identity, a "self." But it concerns an inner self completely different from the public self modern females are shaping by means of dieting and physical exercises in pursuit of an aesthetic ideal: in the former the denial of food is aimed at serving the soul; in the latter the concern with diet and ideal weight becomes a project in service of the body (Bordo 1990).

In his book *Discipline and Punish*, the French philosopher Michel Foucault (1979) made the distinction between two social constructions of the modern body: the "intelligible body" represents the wider cultural arena of social control, whereas the "useful body" is the practical and direct locus of social control through which culture is converted into habitual bodily activity. The former includes scientific, philosophic, and aesthetic representations of the body, which are translated in a set of practical rules and regulations (norms of beauty, models of health): by obeying these sociocultural prescriptions, for example through the "discipline" of diet and exercise, the living body is shaped into a socially adapted and useful body, regulated in the interest of public health, economy, and political order. Or in the words of the anthropologist Mary Douglas (1982), the images of the physical body may reflect or reproduce (in "natural symbols") the categories and concerns of the society at large, the "social body." When modern women "discipline" their bodies, they comply with or obey societal norms; hence a "diagnosis" of their behavior should include the "decoding" of cultural images, because their bodies may be "read" as the surface on which culture has "written" dominant meanings (Bordo 1990).

The sociologist Bryan S. Turner (1984) explored the meaning of the body in urban, secular, capitalist society in which the body became an object of exact calculation. Dietary practices, for example, shifted "away from an eighteenth-century concern for long life as a religious value to the nineteenth-century concern for the efficient quantification of the body" (Turner 1984, pp. 36–37). Capitalism and industrialization are linked to the rise of consumerism incorporating an inevitable contradiction: it required asceticism at the place of (mass) production, "but at the point of consumption it required a new life-style, embodied in the ethic of calculating hedonism, and a new personality type, the narcissistic person" (Turner 1984, p. 102). Dietary practices are now aids to self-presentation, because consumerism and the mass market have blurred the exterior marks of social distinction (status) and personal difference (identity). To be a successful "self" in competitive social relations requires a successful body, disciplined to enhance personal value with the help of a growing sector of "body-work professions" (dietitians, cosmetologists, plastic surgeons) and a powerful "keep-fit industry." The beauty culture became scientific, and medical sciences promoted the rise of disciplined and useful bodies. The medical diet seeks to preserve the inner body, the "body-machinery" (health, youth), whereas the consumer diet is aimed at enhancing the surface of the body, the "face-work" (beauty, distinction); keeping the body "in good shape" then means to make it both productive and attractive, competitive and distinctive, successful and desirable, a rational tool and a vehicle of pleasure. Controlled eating or dietary regimens refer to the imposed government of the body and the embodiment of calculating hedonism (Turner 1984).

In this ongoing contradiction between ascetic production and hedonistic consumption, we are repeating the old dialectics between mind and body, reason and emotion, will and desire, restraint and passion, self-control and self-indulgence. The agonistic structure of advanced consumer capitalism has produced an unstable construction of personality (Crawford 1985): as "producer-selves," cultivating the work ethic, we must repress desires for immediate gratification; but as "consumer-selves," complying with hedonism, we must hunger for immediate satisfaction. This sociocultural contradiction inscribes itself in our bodies, with eating and dieting as the central arenas for its expression (Bordo 1990). In an extreme but characteristic way, eating disorders translate the agonistic and unstable construction of modern personality: the hunger for unrestrained consumption or "letting go" is exhibited in the bulimic person's uncontrollable food binges, but it clashes with the performance principle of "getting in firm control" as expressed in the bulimic person's necessity for vomiting, compulsive exercising, or laxative purges. In the same sense,

> the coexistence of anorexia and obesity reveals the instability of the contemporary personality construction, the difficulty of finding homeostasis between the "producer" and "consumer" aspects of the self. While bulimia embodies the unstable "double-bind" of consumer capitalism, anorexia and obesity embody an attempted "resolution" of that double-bind. (Bordo 1990, pp. 98–99)

But neither the extreme repression of desire (anorexia) nor the total submission (obesity) is accepted by the culture as appropriate responses, probably because their face-work is reflecting a personality type beyond the limits of what consumer society can tolerate. The emaciated represents too rigid (almost inhuman) self-control and the overweight refers to disgusting (animal-like) self-indulgence.

Narcissism, Rebellion, and the Control Paradox

Sociologists describe modern consumer society as dominated by a culture of narcissism (Lasch 1979). Striving for self-fulfillment—the magic credo of our times—individuals depend on validation from others. In this quest for validation, the self is expected to be transparent through its physical appearance. Looking in the mirror is the daily judgment of my (lack of) success: what does my body (self) look like (success) in the mirror (society)? Following the performance ethic and assisted by scientific "disciplines," the "successful self" can also be calculated using weight charts, calorie tables, and fitness schemes. "Looking good," as advertised in consumer society, reflects the hedonistic narcissism of visible performance: "enjoy your being successful!"

> To the extent that modern culture can be described as narcissistic in encouraging pseudo-liberation through consumption, therapy groups, the health cult and the norm of happiness, anorectic self-obsession with appearance may be simply an extreme version of modern narcissism. Anorexia is thus a neurotic version of a widespread "mode of living" which is centered on jogging, keep-fit, healthy diets, weight-watching and calculating hedonism. (Turner 1984, p. 203)

But, although denied by those who are anorectic, it is a painful narcissism.

Anorexia nervosa cannot escape, however, from a triple "control paradox" (Lawrence 1979). Basically, controlling weight is used by many women as a substitute for controlling the real issues in their lives over which they have no control (Orbach 1978). Anorexia nervosa may then be viewed, first, as an act of rebellion both in the private and the public domain. In the overprotective (mostly middle-class) family, food refusal is a powerful form of protest against both patriarchal authority (with emphasis on performance and competition, requiring independence) and matriarchal control (stressing obedience and compliance as exponents of dependency), as well as an attempt to escape from these inherently contradictory expectations. But the refusal to mature, clearly reflected in the psychobiological growth retardation resulting from the self-starvation, will convince the parents of the necessity to ask for medical help to bring their child under control again, because she is lacking autonomy and docility at the same time: her "sick" body is endangering her future (which looked to be very promising), and her "sick" mind is making her a disobedient and naughty child (where she used to be "the best little girl in the world").

A second expression of a control paradox is to be found in the anorectic person's self-experience. Having a low self-esteem—eventually compensated for or masked by a perfectionistic achievement orientation—and searching for autonomy and identity, the self-starvation gives the anorectic person an enormous sense of self-mastery (the victory of mind over body, the dominance of culture over nature). In accordance with the 19th century German philosopher Ludwig Feuerbach's famous aphorism, "Man is what he eats," anorectic persons gain the feeling that

> they are what they eat and what they do not eat. However, in choosing anorexia they become involved in a paradoxical dialectic which is both social and physiological. Through an act of disobedience, they reproduce the norm of female beauty. Their search for autonomy is fateful, resulting in the dominance of nature over culture. (Turner 1984, p. 201)

Indeed, very soon the anorectic person looses control over biological processes (e.g., weight loss, hunger and satiety regulation, restlessness, insomnia), and often the ascetic governing of the body turns into enslavement by an anarchical body imposing uncontrollable urges to binge on food. The quest for self-control over both the internal (body) and external (family, society) environment ends up in a loss of control.

A final paradox concerns the link between anorexia nervosa and the culture of slenderness prevailing in Western societies. The feministic explanations are somewhat contradictory in this respect (see, e.g., Boskind-Lodahl 1976; Chernin 1981; Lawrence 1987). Is the anorectic behavior a symptom of or a protest against the contemporary female "beauty myth" (Wolf 1990)? Comparing 19th century tight-laced corsets with 20th century anorexia nervosa, Turner (1984) pointed to a similarity in contradictory symbolism of the corset and the self-starvation: it is simultaneously an affirmation of female beauty or sexual attractiveness and a denial of sexuality or more specifically of fertility. The anorectic person claims that her weight loss is necessary to become more acceptable or attractive (for herself or others?), but it produces a socially unattractive body. So what is she striving for or what is she avoiding? Does she comply with fashion rules—the "politics of beauty" (Lakoff and Scherr 1984)—or does she rebel? "Women's magazines tell women they *can* control their bodies; but women's experiences of sexual harassment make them feel they *cannot* control what their bodies are said to provoke" (Wolf 1990, p. 163). Perhaps the anorexia nervosa is meant to achieve a basic self-security in both ways. But the paradoxical end product of the compulsive pursuit of beauty through slenderness should be situated within a larger sociocultural context, in which

> . . . it represents a sexualization of society by which we are forced to be sexually acceptable in order to be socially acceptable. However, by becoming desirable we also suppress desire. . . . The consumer regime of the modern period simultaneously stimulates and suppresses desire in the interest of increased consumption; the asceticism of diet is harnessed to the hedonism of consumption. (Turner 1984, p. 200)

The fundamental question is not whether the anorectic woman is a conforming victim or a rebelling heroine, but should be translated as: What do eating disorders express about the position of women in a male-ruled world? Turner (1984) convincingly argued "that we should not see anorexia nervosa as an isolated epidemic of modern society, but rather treat it as part of a complex collection of female disorders in the context of changes within Western society over at least the last hundred years" (p. 192). Young women especially seem to be faced with confusing role expectations (at home and in the public domain), which may increase their insecurity and intensify their striving for perfection and control (Barnett 1986; Bemporad et al. 1988). But using weight control as a substitute for effective control of their lives "is symptomatic of the desperate situation it seeks to rectify" (Lawrence 1979, p. 100). From a psychodynamic viewpoint it is often assumed that the anorectic patient is afraid of growing up and accepting the traditional female role. But from a feminist perspective, rather than a "rejection of femininity," anorectic and bulimic women are considered to be trying desperately to fit themselves into a stereotyped feminine role (imposed by a sexist society). This is reflected both in the relentless pursuit of thinness and in a passive, accommodating, and helpless attitude toward life. In almost classic feminist terms, these women feel trapped between two opposing tensions: the strong desire for recognition from a man and an inordinate fear of men and their power to reject. The matter, however, is more complex than that.

Anorexia like other "women's complaints" is part of a symbolic struggle against forms of authority and an attempt to resolve the contradictions of the female self, fractured by the dichotomies of reason and desire, public and private, body and self. (Turner 1984, p. 202)

Conclusion

Few people will question the assumption that the current culture of slenderness is linked to the (increasing?) occurrence of eating disorders in females. When connecting anorexia nervosa and bulimia nervosa to culture, one can interpret the relationship in three ways (DiNicola 1990b). First, the strong thesis of this connection is that culture acts as a cause by providing a blueprint for anorectic behavior. Second, the moderate thesis states that specific cultural factors trigger the eating disorder, which is further determined by many other factors (including family and psychobiological mechanisms). Third, the weak thesis considers culture as an envelope or context for the expression of the eating disorder. Comparing the disorder to a morbid play, where do we put culture in this theater: on stage directing the actor with a script (cause), in the audience or the rest of the cast expecting the actor to tune in (trigger), or just in the scenery or lighting accentuating the actor's performance (context or background)?

The data supporting a sociocultural approach are mainly correlational in nature and do not provide specific evidence for a causal model. We have to keep in mind

that cultural influences do not in a precise sense *cause* serious eating disorders like bulimia and anorexia nervosa. Culture is mediated by the psychology of the individual as well as the more immediate social context of the family. Both individual and family characteristics may be either predisposing or protecting for any particular disorder. (Garner et al. 1983, p. 81)

If environmental factors play a role in the development of eating disorders, it remains unclear in which way and to what extent they act as "pathogenic" or "pathoplastic" influences. They may be looked on as predisposing, precipitating, or perpetuating factors, or some combination of the three (interaction between vulnerability, risk, and stress).

What are the implications of the sociocultural approach? We have discussed some hermeneutic attempts to decipher the cultural messages of an eating disorder. What can culture help us learn about the disorder and vice versa? If one uses the sociocultural viewpoint as the optical tube through which the disorder is analyzed, anorexia nervosa can be observed as a kaleidoscopic picture reflecting, for example, "the living image of an unfortunate encounter between economic well-being and relational malaise" (Selvini-Palazzoli 1985, p. 204). Looking through the prism of the eating disorder, the cultural light may be dispersed in a meaningful spectrum of contrasting colors, such as

> contradictory social pressures on women of affluent families and an anxiety directed at the surface of the body in a system organized around narcissistic consumption. Only a social system based on mass consumption can afford the luxury of slimming. (Turner 1984, p. 93)

Extrapolating global theories to concrete approaches in everyday practice is what pragmatic clinicians expect. But the practical implications of the sociocultural viewpoint for the prevention and treatment of eating disorders are still waiting further elaboration. The approach is difficult to translate into therapeutic strategies, although mainly feminist therapists have tried to incorporate elements of sociopolitical criticism and self-reflection into their treatment models (e.g., Lawrence 1987; Orbach 1986). With regard to prevention (Crisp 1988; Frankenburg et al. 1982; Vandereycken and Meermann 1984), one would expect important implications as to intervention at the primary level (i.e., altering possible predisposing or precipitating factors in the community at large). But apart from some nice wishful slogans about the necessity of changing people's attitudes toward body shape and beauty norms (e.g., through education), and of detecting and guiding those specifically at risk for developing an eating disorder, realistic preventive measures seem to be restricted to the secondary level. This means that one attempts to improve (e.g., by means of popular and professional information) the early detection of the disorder so that its development can be stopped or reversed by adequate interventions.

Finally, the culture-bound occurrence of eating disorders should question present-day nosological thinking according to the medical model whose use of disease entities tends to overaccentuate static and universal elements of human behavior (nature) at the cost of the more dynamic and particular aspects (nurture, culture). Even if one can delineate diagnostically a coherent constellation of features, its labeling—be it in DSM terms or political metaphors—can be viewed as part of the same cultural process that is shaping the disorder. Each clinician inevitably reproduces ideologies. Diagnostic, explanatory, and therapeutic models imply the professional's own constructs about normality and hence about nature and nurture. Professional practice may encourage or modify illness behavior, and this also applies to our interest in eating disorders demonstrated by the proliferation of conferences and publications (Swartz 1987). We consider it exaggerated to speak about anorexia nervosa and bulimia nervosa as a "social epidemic" (Gordon 1990). Instead, both the striking sensation-guided popular curiosity and the unusually growing attention from various professional circles appear to reach epidemic-like proportions. We suspect that eating disorders may tell us something about the linkage between medicalization and commercialization in present-day consumer society. We cannot escape the paradox, however, that it requires sufficient distance to examine closely one's own position. Therefore, what role we are playing today in this health care market of supply and demand is up to future social historians to reconstruct.

References

Askevold F: Social class and psychosomatic illness. Psychother Psychosom 38:256–259, 1982

Barnett LR: Bulimarexia as symptom of sex-role strain in professional women. Psychotherapy 23:311–315, 1986

Bemporad JR, Ratey JJ, O'Driscoll G, et al: Hysteria, anorexia and the culture of self-denial. Psychiatry 51:96–103, 1988

Bennett W, Gurin J: The Dieter's Dilemma: Eating Less and Weighing More. New York, Basic Books, 1982

Bordo S: Anorexia nervosa: psychopathology as the crystallization of culture. Philosophical Forum 17:73–104, 1985

Bordo S: Reading the slender body, in Body/Politics: Women and the Discourses of Science. Edited by Jacobus M, Fox Keller E, Shuttlewood S. New York, Routledge, 1990, pp 83–112

Boskind-Lodahl M: Cinderella's stepsisters: a feminist perspective on anorexia nervosa and bulimia. Signs: Journal of Women in Culture and Society 2:342–356, 1976

Bynum CW: Holy anorexia in modern Portugal. Cult Med Psychiatry 12:239–248, 1988

Chernin K: The Obsession: Reflections on the Tyranny of Slenderness. New York, Harper & Row, 1981

Crawford R: A cultural account of 'health': self-control, release, and the social body, in Issues in the Political Economy of Health Care. Edited by McKinlay J. New York, Methuen, 1985, pp 60–103

Crisp AH: Some possible approaches to prevention of eating and body weight/shape disorders, with particular reference to anorexia nervosa. International Journal of Eating Disorders 7:1–17, 1988

DiNicola VF: Anorexia multiforme: self-starvation in historical and cultural context, part 1: self-starvation as a historical chameleon. Transcultural Psychiatry Research Review 27:165–196, 1990a

DiNicola VF: Anorexia multiforme: self-starvation in historical and cultural context, part 2: anorexia nervosa as a culture-reactive syndrome. Transcultural Psychiatry Research Review 27:245–286, 1990b

Dolan B: Cross-cultural aspects of anorexia nervosa and bulimia: a review. International Journal of Eating Disorders 10:67–79, 1991

Douglas M: Natural Symbols. New York, Pantheon, 1982

Fairburn CG, Beglin SJ: Studies of the epidemiology of bulimia nervosa. Am J Psychiatry 147:401–408, 1990

Foucault M: Discipline and Punish. New York, Vintage, 1979

Frankenburg F, Garfinkel PE, Garner DM: Anorexia nervosa: issues in prevention. Journal of Preventive Psychiatry 1:469–483, 1982

Garner DM, Garfinkel PE, Olmsted MP: An overview of sociocultural factors in the development of anorexia nervosa, in Anorexia Nervosa: Recent Developments in Research. Edited by Darby PL, Garfinkel PE, Garner DM, et al. New York, Alan R Liss, 1983, pp 65–82

Gordon RA: Anorexia and Bulimia: Anatomy of a Social Epidemic. Cambridge, MA, Basil Blackwell, 1990

Hoek HW, Brook FG: Patterns of care of anorexia nervosa. J Psychiatr Res 19:155–160, 1985

Hsu LKG: The gender gap in eating disorders: why are eating disorders more common among women? Clinical Psychology Review 9:393–407, 1989

Jones DJ, Fox MM, Babigian HM, et al: Epidemiology of anorexia nervosa in Monroe County, New York: 1960–1976. Psychosom Med 42:551–558, 1980

Joseph A, Wood IK, Goldberg SC: Determining populations at risk for developing anorexia nervosa based on selection of college major. Psychiatry Res 7:53–58, 1982

Kendell RE, Hall DJ, Hailey A, et al: The epidemiology of anorexia nervosa. Psychol Med 3:200–203, 1973

Kleinman A: Rethinking Psychiatry: From Cultural Category to Personal Experience. New York, Free Press, 1988

Lakoff RT, Scherr RL: Face Value: The Politics of Beauty. Boston, MA, Routledge & Kegan Paul, 1984

Lasch C: The Culture of Narcissism. New York, WW Norton, 1979

Lawrence M: Anorexia nervosa—the control paradox. Women's Studies International Quarterly 2:93–101, 1979

Lawrence M (ed): Fed Up and Hungry: Women, Oppression, and Food. New York, Peter Bedrick Books, 1987

Littlewood R, Lipsedge M: Culture-bound syndromes, in Recent Advances in Psychiatry, Vol 5. Edited by Granville-Grossman K. Edinburgh, Churchill Livingstone, 1985, pp 105–144

Littlewood R, Lipsedge M: The 'culture-bound syndromes' of the dominant culture, in Transcultural Psychiatry. Edited by Cox JL. London, Croom Helm, 1986, pp 253–273

Littlewood R, Lipsedge M: The butterfly and the serpent: culture, psychopathology and biomedicine. Cult Med Psychiatry 11:289–335, 1987

Lucas AR, Beard CM, O'Fallon WM, et al: Anorexia nervosa in Rochester, Minnesota: a 45-year study. Mayo Clin Proc 63:433–442, 1988

McLorg PA, Taub DE: Anorexia nervosa and bulimia: the development of deviant identities. Deviant Behavior 8:177–189, 1987

Nasser M: Culture and weight consciousness. J Psychosom Res 32:573–577, 1988a

Nasser M: Eating disorders: the cultural dimension. Soc Psychiatry 23:184–187, 1988b

Orbach S: Fat Is a Feminist Issue. London, Paddington Press, 1978

Orbach S: Hunger Strike: The Anorectic's Struggle as a Metaphor for Our Age. New York, WW Norton, 1986

Prince R: Is anorexia nervosa a culture-bound syndrome? Transcultural Psychiatry Research Review 20:299–300, 1983

Prince R: The concept of culture-bound syndromes: anorexia nervosa and brain-fag. Soc Sci Med 21:197–203, 1985

Ritenbaugh C: Obesity as a culture-bound syndrome. Cult Med Psychiatry 6:347–361, 1982

Schwartz H: Never Satisfied: A Cultural History of Diets, Fantasies, and Fat. New York, Free Press, 1986

Selvini-Palazzoli M: Anorexia nervosa: a syndrome of the affluent society. Transcultural Psychiatry Research Review 22:199–205, 1985

Smead VS: Anorexia nervosa, buliminarexia and bulimia: labelled pathology and the Western female. Women and Therapy: A Feminist Quarterly 2:19–35, 1983

Swartz L: Anorexia nervosa as a culture-bound syndrome. Soc Sci Med 20:725–730, 1985a

Swartz L: Is thin a feminist issue? Women's Studies International Forum 8:429–437, 1985b

Swartz L: Illness negotiation: the case of eating disorders. Soc Sci Med 24:613–618, 1987

Szmukler G, McCance C, McCrone L, et al: Anorexia nervosa: a psychiatric case register study from Aberdeen. Psychol Med 16:49–58, 1986

Theander S: Anorexia nervosa: a psychiatric investigation of 94 female patients. Acta Psychiatr Scand Suppl 214:1–94, 1970

Turner BS: The Body and Society: Explorations in Social Theory. Oxford, Basil Blackwell, 1984

Vandereycken W, Meermann R: Anorexia nervosa: is prevention possible? Int J Psychiatry Med 14:191–205, 1984

Van Deth R, Vandereycken W: Was nervous consumption a precursor of anorexia nervosa? Journal of the History of Medicine 46:3–19, 1991

Van Deth R, Vandereycken W: What happened to the 'fasting girls'? a follow-up in retrospect, in The Course of Eating Disorders. Edited by Herzog W, Deter HC, Vandereycken W. Berlin, Springer, 1992, pp 348–366

Willi J, Grossman S: Epidemiology of anorexia nervosa in a defined region of Switzerland. Am J Psychiatry 140:564–567, 1983

Wolf N: The Beauty Myth. London, Chatto & Windus, 1990

Chapter 3

Classification and Diagnosis

Paul Garfinkel, M.D., F.R.C.P.C.

⟶⊰⊱⟵

The eating disorders anorexia nervosa and bulimia nervosa have assumed an increased importance over the past two decades, as clinicians and investigators have recognized their frequency and the difficulties associated with their treatment and course. Diagnostic considerations have received more attention as they have in psychiatry in general and, for anorexia nervosa, have passed through several phases. In the 20th century, these phases included the view that anorexia nervosa was entirely a form of pituitary disease, or a nonspecific variant of many other psychiatric disorders, and the more current view of its being a specific syndrome with core clinical features that distinguish it from other states. In the late 1970s, recognition of the frequency of the symptom bulimia gave rise to awareness of both its frequency within the anorexia nervosa syndrome and within a large group of people who had many of the features of anorexia nervosa, but without achieving such low body weight. Since then, patients with bulimia nervosa have been the subject of much study, and classification of the syndrome has been refined.

In this chapter, I review the current view of the core clinical features of these syndromes, highlight some possible new developments that could affect future plans for classification, and contrast the viewpoint that anorexia nervosa and bulimia nervosa represent distinct syndromes with the various nonspecific classifications.

Criteria for Anorexia Nervosa

Various methods of classification have been suggested for anorexia nervosa. Some have concentrated on psychopathology alone (Bruch 1973; Norris 1979; Rollins and Piazza 1978); however, these criteria have often been difficult to determine objectively. Since 1969, a variety of operational criteria have been developed; these criteria emphasize signs and symptoms and usually include the psychopathology, the behavior, and disturbed endocrine function. In 1970, Russell suggested three criteria for the diagnosis of anorexia nervosa: 1) behavior that is designed to produce marked weight loss; 2) the characteristic psychopathology of a morbid fear of becoming fat; and 3) evidence of an endocrine disorder—in females, amenorrhea, and in males, loss of sexual potency and interest. Although others have since suggested diagnostic criteria (American Psychiatric Association 1987; Feighner et al. 1972; Garrow et al. 1975; Norris 1979; Rollins and Piazza 1978), they generally involve aspects of Russell's original criteria. The DSM-III-R (American Psychiatric Association 1987) diagnostic criteria are provided in Table 3–1. These criteria are discussed in greater detail below.

Behavior Designed to Produce Marked Weight Loss

The criterion of behavior designed to produce marked weight loss in Russell's (1970) classification corresponds with DSM-III-R criterion A: "refusal to maintain body weight over a minimal normal weight for age and height, e.g., weight loss leading to maintenance of body weight 15% below that expected; or failure to make expected weight gain during a period of growth, leading to body weight 15% below that expected" (American Psychiatric Association 1987, p. 67).

There has been general agreement that a drive for thinness is necessary for the diagnosis of anorexia nervosa. Different investigators have described this in somewhat differing terms. Bruch (1973) wrote of the "relentless pursuit of thinness." Theander (1970) emphasized the changed attitude toward food and eating that results from "the pursuit of thinness." Selvini-Palazzoli (1974) referred to this as "the deliberate wish to be slim." Ziegler and Sours (1968) stated that "the pursuit of thinness as a pleasure in itself" is a necessary diagnostic criterion. Crisp (1977) described the weight phobia in which there is the preoccupation to maintain a subpubertal body weight and to avoid weight gain. The DSM-III-R criteria added a degree of precision by describing "the refusal to maintain body weight over a minimal normal weight for age and height" (American Psychiatric Association 1987, p. 67), including both weight loss and a failure to make expected weight—the latter to account for younger patients who would be expected to continue growing.

Although there has been agreement on the presence of the drive for thinness and the need for weight loss, the amount of weight loss that is necessary for the diagnosis has varied. This is not surprising because there have been no studies to determine when the symptoms of starvation actually supervene or when physiological consequences are first evident. Some criteria have not specified an amount of weight loss (Norris 1979; Russell 1970); for others the weight lost from premorbid levels has ranged from 10% (Dally 1969) to 25% (Feighner et al. 1972). The DSM-III-R criterion of 15% of expected weight is useful because it permits the diagnosis of definite cases early in their course, and, as noted above, it takes into account the younger patient who is still growing.

Psychopathology Characterized by a Morbid Fear of Becoming Fat

The criterion of psychopathology characterized by a morbid fear of becoming fat in Russell's (1970) classification corresponds with the cri-

---

Table 3–1.   DSM-III-R diagnostic criteria for anorexia nervosa

---

A. Refusal to maintain body weight over a minimal normal weight for age and height, e.g., weight loss leading to maintenance of body weight 15% below that expected; or failure to make expected weight gain during period of growth, leading to body weight 15% below that expected.

B. Intense fear of gaining weight or becoming fat, even though underweight.

C. Disturbance in the way in which one's body weight, size, or shape is experienced, e.g., the person claims to "feel fat" even when emaciated, believes that one area of the body is "too fat" even when obviously underweight.

D. In females, absence of at least three consecutive menstrual cycles when otherwise expected to occur (primary or secondary amenorrhea). (A woman is considered to have amenorrhea if her periods occur only following hormone, e.g., estrogen administration.)

Source.   Reprinted from American Psychiatric Association: *Diagnostic and Statistical Manual of Mental Disorders,* 3rd Edition, Revised. Washington, DC, American Psychiatric Association, 1987, p. 67. Used with permission.

teria B and C in DSM-III-R—it involves both the intense fear of becoming fat and the weight and shape concerns, related to the person's attitudes and feelings about her body as a whole, or particular body parts. The presence of this core psychopathology has been demonstrated in empirical studies using self-report instruments (Garner and Garfinkel 1979; Garner et al. 1983) and structured interviews (Cooper and Fairburn 1987). This morbid fear of becoming fat is a feature that distinguishes anorexia nervosa from other psychiatric syndromes.

The earlier DSM-III (American Psychiatric Association 1980) criteria described this feature in terms of "body image disturbance." Many studies of body image in anorexia nervosa have focused on a narrow definition, related to visual self-perception, and data here show that many people with anorexia nervosa do not overestimate their sizes and that overestimation is not unique to those with the disorder (Touyz and Beumont 1988). Given these data, it was appropriate to change this criterion in DSM-III-R to focus on the attitudinal and affective dimensions of body image.

People with anorexia nervosa do demonstrate high levels of body dissatisfaction both clinically and in empirical studies (Garner et al. 1983). However, there can be a significant overlap in levels of body dissatisfaction between people with anorexia nervosa and the general female population. For example, Lindholm and Wilson (1988) found levels of body dissatisfaction in dieting subjects to equal those of patients with anorexia nervosa. Garner et al. (1984) found body dissatisfaction, as measured by self-report, to be as high in weight-preoccupied college students as in patients with anorexia nervosa.

It is desirable to link anorexia nervosa and bulimia nervosa in terms of the core psychopathology of attitudes toward weight. The word *overconcern* with weight and shape in the DSM-III-R description of bulimia nervosa is vague and hard to determine reliably. It is also possibly confusing to use the term *overconcern* for a group of people with such low body weight as that occurring in anorexia nervosa. Because of this, there is a desire to change the criterion in DSM-IV slightly—to emphasize the central concern of weight and shape in the evaluation of the self, which is more clearly differentiable from that in nonclinical populations. Also, reference must be made to the denial of the serious consequences of the weight loss, a phenomenon frequently observed in anorexia nervosa and, although poorly understood, noted by Lasègue (1873) more than 100 years ago. By emphasizing the disturbance in the way in which one's body weight or shape is experienced in terms of 1) reference to extremes of self-evaluation and 2) denial, overlap with the general population can be reduced. Even if there is some overlap on this criterion with the general population, false positives are greatly reduced when this criterion is coupled with the first criterion—the low body weight and desire for thinness.

Evidence of an Endocrine Disorder

The criterion of evidence of an endocrine disorder in Russell's (1970) classification—in females, amenorrhea, and in males, loss of sexual potency and interest—corresponds with the criterion D in DSM-III-R: "absence of at least three consecutive menstrual cycles when otherwise expected to occur" (American Psychiatric Association 1987, p. 67). Dally (1969), Russell (1970), and DSM-III-R included amenorrhea as a diagnostic criterion; others, including DSM-III, did not. There is no doubt that amenorrhea is a common feature in anorexia nervosa, and that in part it is based on loss of body weight and fat. But the presence of amenorrhea is incompletely understood and can occur in a significant minority of women with anorexia nervosa before there is any real weight loss (Theander 1970).

There is value in retaining the criterion for amenorrhea, because it is seen so regularly in anorexia nervosa and because it provides emphasis for the hypothalamic dysfunction that occurs in this syndrome. Whether it is included as a diagnostic criterion or not, however, has little bearing on the definition of a case.

Bulimic and Restricting Subtypes of Anorexia Nervosa

A number of studies have documented important and reliable differences between anorectic patients who are periodically bulimic (anorexia nervosa, bulimic subtype) and those who are consistent dietary "restricters" (anorexia nervosa, restricting subtype) (Casper et al. 1980; Garfinkel et al. 1980; Michalide and Andersen 1985; Strober et al. 1982; Vandereycken and Pierloot 1983; Yellowlees 1985). Bulimic anorectic people differ from restricting anorectic people on a number of parameters. Bulimic anorectic people have generally weighed more before the illness and more commonly have been obese. They also come from families in which obesity is more common. They are also much more likely to induce vomiting and misuse laxatives in their attempts to control their weight. They are an impulsive group, evident not only in their eating behavior but in other areas as well. They frequently have problems with alcohol or street drugs; they may steal; and, compared with restricting anorectic people, they more frequently attempt self-mutilation and suicide. An impulsive cognitive style has been demonstrated in this group (Toner et al. 1987). Bulimic anorectic people also differ in personality characteristics. They are frequently borderline, narcissistic, or antisocial—discharging impulse through action—in contrast to the far more inhibited restricting anorectic group (Piran et al. 1988). On all these dimensions, bulimic anorectic people resemble people with bulimia nervosa (Garner et al. 1985). Because of this resemblance, some have recommended that the two groups of bulimic people be classified together. However, there must be important differences between bulimic people who lose large amounts of weight and meet criteria for anorexia nervosa and those who never do. For this reason, and because of the important differences between the two anorexia nervosa groups, it is recommended that in DSM-IV anorexia nervosa be subclassified by the presence or absence of bulimia.

Criteria for Bulimia Nervosa

When Russell (1979) first proposed diagnostic criteria for bulimia nervosa, he suggested three components: 1) the patients suffer from powerful and intractable urges to overeat; 2) they seek to avoid the fattening effects of food by inducing vomiting, abusing purgatives, or both; and 3) they have a morbid fear of becoming fat. These criteria, which are discussed in greater detail below, have undergone various modifications. The DSM-III-R diagnostic criteria for bulimia nervosa are provided in Table 3–2. The DSM-III criteria did not include reference to the shape and weight concerns and did not include a frequency criterion, both present in DSM-III-R. These modifications have resulted in the diagnosis becoming much more restrictive. Ben-Tovim (1988) found a greater than 10-fold reduction in the frequency of the syndrome when the more restrictive DSM-III-R criteria were applied.

Patients Suffer From Powerful and Intractable Urges to Overeat

The Russell (1979) criterion that patients suffer from powerful and intractable urges to overeat corresponds to DSM-III-R criterion A: "recurrent episodes of binge eating (rapid consumption of a large amount of food in a discrete period of time)"; criterion B: "a feeling of lack of control over eating behavior during the eating binges"; and criterion D: "a minimum average of two binge eating episodes a week for at least 3 months" (American Psychiatric Association 1987, pp. 68–69).

Although there has been a consensus on the need for the presence of binge eating as a diagnostic criterion for bulimia nervosa, there has not been agreement on the definition of what constitutes a binge and on the minimum binge frequency for the syndrome. With regard to what constitutes a binge, some have focused on the quantity of food eaten, others on the subjective state of the person, and others on the need for discrete episodes of overeating or on the rapid rate of eating. This last component should be removed from DSM-IV because many patients report a slow or moderate rate of eating, and it is difficult to determine reliably the speed of such eating.

The other three components—quantity of food eaten, subjective state, and the need for discrete episodes of overeating—should be specified in determining the presence of a binge. With regard to quantity of food eaten, some have recommended that if the amount is greater than the patient feels is allowed, it is considered a binge. This definition, however, can lead to the rather strange situation of some patients "bingeing" on two cookies. Much more appropriate is having the quantity be excessive by objective standards. Although some have specified actual quantities—for example, greater than 1,200 (Katzman and Wolchik 1984) or 1,000

Table 3–2. DSM-III-R diagnostic criteria for bulimia nervosa

A. Recurrent episodes of binge eating (rapid consumption of a large amount of food in a discrete period of time).

B. A feeling of lack of control over eating during the eating binges.

C. The person regularly engages in either self-induced vomiting, use of laxatives or diuretics, strict dieting or fasting, or vigorous exercise in order to prevent weight gain.

D. A minimum average of two binge eating episodes a week for at least 3 months.

E. Persistent overconcern with body weight and shape.

Source. Reprinted from American Psychiatric Association: *Diagnostic and Statistical Manual of Mental Disorders,* 3rd Edition, Revised. Washington, DC, American Psychiatric Association, 1987, pp. 68–69. Used with permission.

(Fairburn 1987) calories—what is most relevant is that the person is eating more than is normal, given what other people eat, the time of the person's last meal, and the social circumstances (Fairburn 1987). This approach to quantity of food eaten permits its objective definition and takes into account the great individual variation in food consumption that has been documented in bulimia nervosa (R. Davis et al. 1988; Mitchell et al. 1988b).

Binge eating episodes are characterized by a subjective sense of loss of control; that is, the sense that the person cannot prevent the occurrence of the binge or terminate it once it has started (Fairburn 1987). Various dysphoric mood states precede the binge and precipitate it; the binge itself has the immediate effect of reducing the unpleasant mood (Abraham and Beumont 1982), but this effect is then followed by physical discomfort and fear of gaining weight.

The third criterion of the binge, that the eating occurs in a discrete period of time, refers to a definite time-limited period that is not necessarily limited to a single setting. It is included to remove continual snacking or "grazing" from qualifying as a binge.

Far less clear is the frequency of bingeing necessary for the syndrome. In DSM-III-R, a minimum of two binges per week was specified, and, as noted above, this does have a significant impact on the definition of a case. There is definite value in setting a minimum frequency to exclude the person who binge eats who is infrequently bulimic and who does not display the full syndrome. However, the problem here is the arbitrary nature of setting the frequency of binge eating at twice per week. When investigators have tried to study this issue by relating frequency of binge eating to coexisting psychopathology, the results have been mixed, with some finding increasing psychopathology as frequency of binge eating increases (Williamson et al. 1987) and others finding no such relationship (Fairburn and Cooper 1984). G. T. Wilson and R. Eldredge (personal communication, January 1981) were also unable to relate frequency of pretreatment binge episodes to posttreatment outcome. Others have noted the predictive value of such frequent behaviors (Mitchell et al. 1989).

Although including a minimum frequency for binge episodes in the criteria for bulimia nervosa is necessary, further research must be conducted to determine the most appropriate cutting point. It is also necessary to take into account the fluctuating nature of the symptoms in bulimia nervosa, and thus determine the frequency of binge episodes as an average over a period of time.

Patients Seek to Avoid the Fattening Effects of Food by Inducing Vomiting, Abusing Purgatives, or Both

Russell's (1979) criterion that patients seek to avoid the fattening effects of food by inducing vomiting, abusing purgatives, or both corresponds with DSM-III-R criterion C: the person regularly engages in self-induced vomiting, use of laxatives or diuretics, strict dieting or fasting, or vigorous exercise to prevent weight gain.

This criterion refers to the presence of purging behavior in Russell's classification and to purging or other means to control weight in DSM-III-R. Although the DSM-III-R criteria are much less restrictive than those of Russell, DSM-III-R is a great improvement over DSM-III, which did not include reference to these behaviors.

There are good reasons to include purging behaviors as a diagnostic criterion. First, as Fairburn (1987) and Garner et al. (1992) noted, the presence of vomiting and laxative abuse is often an indication of the intensity of the concern with weight and shape. Second, although dieting and vigorous exercising are not seen to be especially unusual, self-induced vomiting and laxative misuse are thought to be pathological behaviors in our society (Huon et al. 1988). Third, purging behaviors are discrete and easily defined and quantified, thus obviating some of the problems associated with defining a binge. Fourth, evidence suggests that bulimic people who purge differ from binge eaters who do not purge in terms of psychopathology. Bulimic people who do not purge tend to have less body image disturbance and less anxiety concerning eating relative to bulimic people who purge (C. J. Davis et al. 1986; Duchman et al. 1986). A significant problem in these studies is that bulimic people who do not purge tend to be obese and it is therefore not clear what role obesity plays in accounting for these differences. However, Willmuth et al. (1988) found that bulimic people who purge displayed greater general psychopathology and attitudes toward eating and weight, even though those who were bulimic and did not purge were at a normal weight. J. E. Mitchell (personal communication, September 1991) found that bulimic people who did not purge binged less often and were less likely to engage in impulsive self-harming behaviors. A final argument in favor of restricting the diagnosis of bulimia nervosa to those who purge relates to prediction of course. The serious physiological complications of this disorder are often directly related to the various pathological weight-control methods (Mitchell et al. 1988a).

The above argument points strongly to limiting the diagnosis of bulimia nervosa to those who induce vomiting or misuse laxatives. This limitation raises two concerns. First, what about binge eaters who do not purge? These people constitute a relatively small sample of patients presenting to eating disorders clinics: 6% of bulimic patients at the University of Minnesota (J. E. Mitchell, personal communication, September 1991). As noted above, they tend to be obese and may frequent weight-control groups for obesity. Some would likely meet the recommended criteria for binge eating disorder, as suggested later in this chapter. However, more research is required to understand their course of illness and the psychopathological differences and similarities to bulimia nervosa.

Second, what about binge eaters who engage in behavior other than vomiting or laxative misuse to control weight? As noted above, dieting and exercise are considered to be much more "normal" by our society. But there are many bulimic patients with diabetes who omit insulin to control weight; other bulimic patients take thyroxine, diuretics, or amphetamines in efforts to control weight. While Fornari et al. (1990) suggested that medication manipulation be included as part of this diagnostic criterion, until future research is able to delineate how these patients resemble or differ from those with typical bulimia nervosa, there is merit in the more restrictive diagnosis.

Patients Have a Morbid Fear of Becoming Fat

The Russell (1979) criterion for bulimia nervosa that patients have a morbid fear of becoming fat corresponds to DSM-III-R criterion E: "persistent overconcern with body shape and weight" (American Psychiatric Association 1987, p. 69).

The earlier DSM-III criteria for bulimia did not include the shape and weight concerns. There are several advantages to the inclusion of this criterion. First, it covers what many view to be the central psychopathology in bulimia nervosa—the morbid fear of becoming fat or of body fat—and it is this that leads to behaviors to control body weight (Fairburn and Garner 1988). This distinguishes bulimia nervosa from binge eating, which may occur independent of such weight concerns.

Second, this criterion makes the diagnosis much more restrictive. DSM-III, by focusing primarily on overeating, defined a group of people who have in common the symptom of bulimia rather than the full syndrome (Fairburn and Garner 1988). An example of the differentiation would be the diagnostic consideration of people who overeat and gain weight while displaying features of a major depression but without the shape and weight concerns and behavior to control weight. Most clinicians would find it useful to distinguish such patients from those with a primary eating disorder, and, according to the older DSM-III criteria, these patients would be considered as a single group.

Third, inclusion of the shape and weight concerns draws the syndrome closer to its related disorder, anorexia nervosa. Shared psychopathologies have been noted in empirical studies of the two syndromes (Garner and Fairburn 1988), excluding the distinguishing features previously found to be characteristic of people with bulimia (Garfinkel et al. 1980; Garner et al. 1985).

Fourth, inclusion of the shape and weight concerns draws the DSM classification closer to the ICD-10 (World Health Organization 1992) classification. In ICD-10, the psychopathology of bulimia nervosa is characterized by a morbid fear of fatness and the patient setting for herself a sharply defined weight threshold, well below her premorbid weight.

Excessive weight and shape concerns are regularly seen in bulimia nervosa. For example, Garfinkel et al. (1992) reported that 97% of 104 patients with bulimia nervosa displayed overconcern with either shape or weight or both, when assessed by a structured interview, the Eating Disorder Examination. Cooper et al. (1989) found that patients with anorexia nervosa and bulimia nervosa demonstrated significantly higher levels of weight and shape concerns than did control women, using the Eating Disorder Examination. Wilson and Smith (1989) administered the Eating Disorder Examination to patients with bulimia nervosa and to psychology students who scored as restrained eaters on the Revised Restraint Scale. The results strongly supported the finding of elevated weight and shape concerns among the bulimic subjects. In a related study, Rosen et al. (1990) reported that women with bulimia nervosa could be differentiated from restrained-eating control subjects on the basis of a self-report scale, the Body Shape Questionnaire.

These data suggest that although concerns with weight and shape are common in the general female population, they differ in people with bulimia nervosa by virtue of their intensity and in people with anorexia nervosa by their central role in governing the person's evaluation of her sense of self-esteem. Although there is some overlap with the normal female population on this criterion alone, false positives are minimized when criteria A–D of DSM-III-R are required for the diagnosis. The presence of this last criterion—DSM-III-R criterion E—however, eliminates people who binge and vomit but do not have these weight and shape concerns from being diagnosed with bulimia nervosa.

Body Dissatisfaction in Relation
to Weight and Shape Concerns

As noted earlier in the chapter, the concept of body image involves both a self-perceptual component and an attitudinal and affective dimension. Until recently, empirical studies have concentrated on the self-perceptual component alone. Attitudes and feelings about one's body have received far less attention in the literature on eating disorders, although this is now changing, in part because of recent emphasis given to increasing body dissatisfaction in young women in contemporary society (Kirkley and Burge 1989).

Garfinkel et al. (1992) reported on the high degrees of body dissatisfaction in a large sample of women with bulimia nervosa. Using the body dissatisfaction subscale of the Eating Disorders Inventory (Garner et al. 1983), they found that almost one-half the bulimic women scored at or above the 90th percentile for normal women, and less than one-fifth of the patients scored at the median level of the comparison sample. Not surprisingly, levels of body dissatisfaction were correlated with weight and shape concerns, as measured by the Eating Disorder Examination. Patients with the highest degree of self-loathing displayed the greatest "feelings of fatness," dietary restraint, and feelings of ineffectiveness and the most psychopathology on general measures. This group had often been overweight, and they displayed a strong desire for thinness and a thinner ideal image on a distorting photograph technique. Garfinkel et al. (1992) recommended that consideration be given to altering the criterion for "overconcern with weight and shape" to include the closely linked concept of body dissatisfaction, because it taps the neglected affective dimension of body image and because abnormalities in body image more closely reflect the deficits in self-esteem regulation that may underlie the morbid fear of fat and excessive governance of self-worth by concerns with weight and shape.

Need to Establish Binge Eating
Disorder as a Diagnostic Entity

Stunkard (1959) originally described a binge eating syndrome among those who are obese, in which large amounts of food were consumed in a relatively short period, followed by severe discomfort and feelings of self-denigration. There was little interest in this syndrome until several studies demonstrated that between 20% and 50% of obese people binge eat (Loro and Orleans 1981; Marcus et al. 1985).

Spitzer et al. (1992) recently suggested criteria for this syndrome, which they have termed *binge eating disorder* (Table 3–3). This term is preferred over *compulsive overeating,* because the term *compulsive* is misleading in this context (Garner et al. 1992). People with this syndrome fail to meet diagnostic criteria for bulimia nervosa because they lack the compensatory weight-control behaviors and the overconcern with weight and shape. The initial field trials of this topic found that 30% of people attending weight-control programs and 1.7% of a community sample met criteria for binge eating disorder.

Table 3–3.   Diagnostic criteria for binge eating disorder

A. Recurrent episodes of binge eating. An episode of binge eating is characterized by both of the following:
   (1) eating, in a discrete period of time (e.g., within any 2-hour period), an amount of food that is definitely larger than most people would eat in a similar period of time
   (2) a sense of lack of control over eating during the episode (e.g., a feeling that one cannot stop eating or control what or how much one is eating)

B. During most binge episodes, at least three of the following behavioral indicators of loss of control are present:
   (1) eating much more rapidly than usual
   (2) eating until feeling uncomfortably full
   (3) eating large amounts of food when not feeling physically hungry
   (4) eating large amounts of food throughout the day with no planned mealtimes
   (5) eating alone because of being embarrassed by how much one is eating
   (6) feeling disgusted with oneself, depressed, or feeling very guilty after overeating

C. The binge eating occurs, on average, at least twice a week for a 6-month period.

D. The binge eating causes marked distress.

E. Does not occur exclusively during the course of Bulimia Nervosa and the individual does not abuse medication (e.g., diet pills, thyroid medication) in an attempt to avoid weight gain.

Source.   Reprinted from American Psychiatric Association: *DSM-IV Options Book: Work in Progress 9/1/91.* Washington, DC, American Psychiatric Association, 1991. Used with permission.

Binge eating among obese people is associated with psychopathology and with resistance to change in weight-control programs. Marcus et al. (1988b) found that obese binge eaters had higher scores of depression and general psychopathology, in comparison with obese people who did not binge. They have also found a higher frequency of psychiatric disorders, especially major depression, in obese binge eaters (Marcus et al. 1988a). Several studies have shown that obese binge eaters do less well in behavioral weight-control programs for obese people, suggesting a somewhat different course for the binge eating group (Gormally et al. 1980; Keefe et al. 1984).

The initial studies of epidemiology and comparative psychopathologies indicate the need for this diagnostic category. A specific diagnostic category will probably be required, rather than submerging these people in the "not otherwise specified" category of DSM-III-R or as atypical eating disorders, but this must await further studies of epidemiology, comparative psychopathology, and course.

Other Views of the Classification of Eating Disorders

The foregoing discussion focused on the diagnostic criteria for anorexia nervosa and bulimia nervosa, with a view that these are distinct psychiatric syndromes with characteristic features that distinguish them from other disorders and that are reliable over time. However, there have been other points of view—including whether anorexia nervosa and bulimia nervosa are variants of other illnesses, whether anorexia nervosa represents a nonspecific syndrome that can occur in many emotional disorders, and whether anorexia nervosa represents the end point on a continuum of dieting.

Eating Disorders as Variants of Other Illnesses

The earliest writers, such as Gull (1868), Gilles de la Tourette (1895), and Dejerine and Gauckler (1911), considered anorexia nervosa a distinct disorder; others have considered it a variant of affective disorder, schizophrenia, obsessional disorder, and hysteria. Table 3–4 presents a comparison of weight-loss features among these disorders.

Table 3–4. Comparison of clinical features of anorexia nervosa, conversion disorder, schizophrenia, and depression

Clinical feature	Anorexia nervosa	Conversion disorder	Schizophrenia	Depression
Intense drive for thinness	Marked	None	None	None
Self-imposed starvation	Marked (due to fear of body size)	None	Marked (due to delusions about food)	None
Disturbance in body image	Present (lack of awareness of change in body size and lack of satisfaction or pleasure in the body)	None	None	None
Appetite	Maintained (but with fear of giving in to impulse)	Variable	Maintained	True anorexia
Satiety	Usually bloating, nausea, early satiety	Variable	Variable	Variable
Avoidance of specific foods	Present (for carbohydrates or foods presumed to be high in "calories")	None	Present (of foods that are thought to be poisoned)	Loss of interest in all food
Bulimia	Present in about 50%	May occur	Rare	Rare
Vomiting	Present (to prevent weight gain)	Present (expresses some symbolic meaning)	Rare (to prevent undesirable effects on the body)	None
Laxative abuse	Present (to prevent weight gain)	Infrequently present (expresses some symbolic meaning)	None	None
Activity level	Increased	Reduced or no change	No change	Reduced
Amenorrhea	Present	May occur	May occur	May occur

Source. Reprinted from Garfinkel PE, Kaplan AS, Garner DM, et al: "The differentiation of vomiting and weight loss as a conversion disorder from anorexia nervosa." *Am J Psychiatry* 140:1019–1022, 1983. Used with permission.

Depression.   Clinically, eating disorders and depression may be difficult to distinguish from one another because of shared signs and symptoms, familial tendencies, natural history, similar neuroendocrine abnormalities, and responses to medications. These similarities have caused some to suggest that eating disorders are variants of affective illness (Cantwell et al. 1977). However, close examination suggests that these arguments are not strong and that although there is an association between these disorders—in terms of risk and course—there are also features that distinguish them.

A depressed mood is frequently seen in patients with anorexia nervosa and bulimia nervosa. Vegetative features of a major depression are common (40%) in patients with these eating disorders (Piran et al. 1985). However, such depressive syndromes are common in people with a variety of illnesses, and starvation itself may produce cognitive, affective, and social changes resembling major depression.

Most compelling are the familial and natural history data. An increased risk of depression in first-degree relatives of both anorexia nervosa and bulimia nervosa patients has regularly been reported (Altshuler and Weiner 1985; Piran et al. 1985). Toner et al. (1986) found a sixfold increase in the frequency of affective disorder among women with anorexia nervosa treated 4–8 years earlier, a finding that held even for those who had completely recovered from the eating disorder.

Others have inferred links between bulimia nervosa and affective disorder based on shared neurohumoral abnormalities or responses to medications. However, the actual degree of similarity on neuroendocrine parameters is unclear. The Toronto group found patients with bulimia nervosa to have an overproduction of cortisol, as is seen in depression; but bulimia nervosa patients had normal growth hormone and 3-methoxy-4-hydroxyphenylglycol (MHPG) responses to clonidine (Kaplan et al. 1989a) and normal thyroid-stimulating hormone responses to thyrotropin-releasing hormone (Kaplan et al. 1989b), unlike the situation in depression. Furthermore, circadian melatonin responses were not blunted, unless patients displayed a concomitant major depression (Kennedy et al. 1989). Furthermore, although patients with bulimia nervosa and patients with depression respond to short-term tricyclic or other antidepressant medications (Garfinkel and Garner 1987), one cannot infer a common syndrome because the mechanisms producing the responses may differ.

In both eating disorders and depression, self-esteem is reduced. In patients with eating disorders, loss of self-esteem is specifically linked to the fear of fat and of body weight and to loss of control over eating, whereas with primary depression the sense of worthlessness is more generalized. The familial risk data and the data on the course of anorexia nervosa suggest a shared association; the other data that have been suggested to provide a link, however, are not strong.

Schizophrenia. R. Dubois (1913) first described anorexia nervosa as occurring in an adolescent girl with signs of schizophrenia. Since that time, several writers have felt that anorexia nervosa is a variant of schizophrenia (Binswanger 1944; Nicolle 1939). Some features of schizophrenia appear to be present in patients with anorexia nervosa. Volitional defects seen in schizophrenia may seem present in patients with anorexia nervosa because of their general negativism, indecisiveness, and social withdrawal. The body-image distortion may reach delusional proportions and resemble psychotic perceptions and delusions. However, the fundamental schizophrenic disturbances in affect, thought processes, and volition are not found in anorexia nervosa. Several studies have shown no increased risk for schizophrenia in anorectic patients or in their families (Dally 1969; Theander 1970).

Obsessional disorder. Many patients with anorexia nervosa display obsessional symptomatology, leading some to conclude that it is a form of obsessive-compulsive neurosis (F. S. DuBois 1949; Palmer and Jones 1939). Smart et al. (1976) and Solyom et al. (1982) confirmed the obsessive nature of a group of patients with anorexia nervosa with psychometric testing. However, the obsessional symptomatology in some patients is magnified by the severe starvation state. Although some patients have obsessional character traits, this does not signify an obsessive-compulsive disorder. Anorectic patients do not view many of their obsessional-like symptoms as ego-alien, as they would true symptoms of an obsessive-compulsive disorder. Only the anorectic patient's preoccupation with food is seen as ego-alien; her preoccupations with weight, body shape, and drive for thinness are not.

Hysteria (conversion disorder). At several points in the last 100 years, investigators have felt that anorexia nervosa was a hysterical symptom. Lasègue (1873) termed this disorder *anorexie hysterique* after observing hysterical symptoms in a patient with anorexia nervosa. Gilles de la Tourette (1895) considered anorexia nervosa to be a manifestation of hysteria and different from what he termed *anorexie gastrique,* which was due to gastrointestinal symptoms. Both Janet (1919) and Dally (1969) felt that there was a subgroup of patients with anorexia nervosa who also had hysteria. Hysterical personality disorder, somatization disorder, and conversion disorder have all been linked to hysterical phenomena, but anorexia nervosa does not clearly resemble any of these. Garfinkel et al. (1983) reported significant differences between patients who they feel have a conversion disorder and those who have anorexia nervosa.

Anorexia nervosa as a nonspecific symptom.   Bliss and Branch (1960) introduced the concept that anorexia nervosa was a nonspecific symptom that occurred in many emotional disorders that presented with significant weight loss and that it was virtually impossible to distinguish it from other forms of emaciation. Anorexia nervosa then became an umbrella diagnosis that encompassed illnesses such as schizophrenia, depression, conversion disorder, and other emotional states in which there was significant weight loss. According to Bliss and Branch, "anorexia nervosa is a symptom found at times in almost all psychiatric categories" (p. 18). This view is not accepted today. Many investigators view anorexia nervosa as distinct from other causes of weight loss. The distinguishing features center around the fundamental drive for thinness and associated behaviors as described above.

Anorexia Nervosa and the Continuum of Weight-Preoccupied Women

Some investigators have regarded anorexia nervosa as qualitatively distinct, and others support its existence along a continuum (Berkman 1948; Nylander 1971). Crisp (1977) argued that the disorder represents a psychobiological regression to a prepubertal state that is distinct and different from other forms of dieting behavior. Diagnostically, Crisp emphasized the need for a specific degree of weight loss below a critical menstrual weight threshold. Bruch (1973) considered the psychopathology that she felt is responsible for the development of the disorder to distinguish it from other forms of dieting. She described ego deficits that are manifest as an overwhelming sense of ineffectiveness and disturbances in body image and affective and visceral perceptions.

A study by Garner et al. (1984) supports this view. Using psychometric instruments, they compared patients with anorexia nervosa with extremely weight-preoccupied women selected from college and ballet students. They found a continuum of weight concerns that did not parallel the continua of psychopathology that were observed in patients with anorexia nervosa. The weight-preoccupied, nonclinical sample had disturbances in dieting, perfectionism, and attitudes about shape that were similar to the anorexia nervosa group. Other disturbances in psychological functioning, such as feeling ineffective, lack of interoceptive awareness, and interpersonal distrust, were much less common in the nonclinical group. These findings support Bruch's contention that patients with anorexia nervosa are distinct in underlying psychopathology as well as in the intensity of the desire for thinness and associated behaviors.

References

Abraham SF, Beumont PJV: How patients describe bulimia or binge eating. Psychol Med 12:625–635, 1982

Altshuler KZ, Weiner MF: Anorexia nervosa and depression: a dissenting view. Am J Psychiatry 142:328–332, 1985

American Psychiatric Association: Diagnostic and Statistical Manual of Mental Disorders, 3rd Edition. Washington, DC, American Psychiatric Association, 1980

American Psychiatric Association: Diagnostic and Statistical Manual of Mental Disorders, 3rd Edition, Revised. Washington, DC, American Psychiatric Association, 1987

Ben-Tovim DI: DSM-III, draft DSM-IIIR, and the diagnosis and prevalence of bulimia in Australia. Am J Psychiatry 145:1000–1002, 1988

Berkman JM: Anorexia nervosa, anterior pituitary insufficiency, Simmonds' cachexia, and Sheehan's disease, including some observation on disturbances in water metabolism associated with starvation. Postgrad Med 3:237–246, 1948

Binswanger L: Der fall Ellen West. Schweiz Arch Neurol Psychiatr 54:69–117, 1944

Bliss EL, Branch CHH: Anorexia Nervosa: Its History, Psychology and Biology. New York, Paul B Hoeber, 1960

Bruch H: Eating Disorders. New York, Basic Books, 1973

Cantwell DP, Sturzenberger S, Burrows J, et al: Anorexia nervosa: an affective disorder? Arch Gen Psychiatry 34:1087–1093, 1977

Casper RC, Eckert ED, Halmi KA, et al: Bulimia: its incidence and clinical importance in patients with anorexia nervosa. Arch Gen Psychiatry 37:1030–1035, 1980

Cooper Z, Fairburn CG: The Eating Disorders Examination: a semi-structured interview for the assessment of the specific psychopathology of eating disorders. International Journal of Eating Disorders 6:1–8, 1987

Cooper Z, Cooper PJ, Fairburn CG: The validity of the Eating Disorder Examination. Br J Psychiatry 154:807–812, 1989

Crisp AH: Diagnosis and outcome of anorexia nervosa: the St. George's view. Proceedings of the Royal Society of Medicine 70:464–470, 1977

Dally P: Anorexia Nervosa. New York, Grune & Stratton, 1969

Davis CJ, Williamson DA, Goreczny T: Body image distortion in bulimia: an important distinction between binge-purgers and binge eaters. Paper presented at the annual convention of the Association for the Advancement of Behavior Therapy, Chicago, IL, March 1986

Davis R, Freeman RJ, Garner DM: A naturalistic investigation of eating behavior in bulimia nervosa. J Consult Clin Psychol 56:273–279, 1988

Dejerine J, Gauckler E: Les manifestations fonctionelles des psychoneuroses, leur traitment par la psychotherapie. Paris, Masson, 1911

DuBois FS: Compulsion neurosis with cachexia (anorexia nervosa). Am J Psychiatry 106:107–115, 1949

Dubois R: De L'anorectic mentale conume prodrome de la demence precoce. Ann Med Psychol (Paris) 10:431–438, 1913

Duchman EG, Williamson DA, Strickler PM: Dietary restraint and bulimia. Paper presented at the Annual Convention of the Association for the Advancement of Behavior Therapy, Chicago, IL, March 1986

Fairburn CG: The definition of bulimia nervosa: guidelines for clinicians and research workers. Annals of Behavioral Medicine 9:3–7, 1987

Fairburn CG, Cooper PJ: Binge-eating, self-induced vomiting and laxative abuse: a community study. Psychol Med 14:401–410, 1984

Fairburn CG, Garner DM: Diagnostic criteria for anorexia nervosa and bulimia nervosa: the importance of attitude to shape and weight, in Diagnostic Issues in Anorexia Nervosa and Bulimia Nervosa. Edited by Garner DM, Garfinkel PE. New York, Brunner Mazel, 1988, pp 36–65

Feighner JP, Robins E, Guze SB, et al: Diagnostic criteria for use in psychiatric research. Arch Gen Psychiatry 26:57–63, 1972

Fornari V, Edelman R, Katz JC: Medication manipulation in bulimia nervosa: an additional diagnostic criterion? International Journal of Eating Disorders 9:585–588, 1990

Garfinkel PE, Garner DM: The Role of Drug Treatments for the Eating Disorders. New York, Brunner/Mazel, 1987

Garfinkel PE, Moldofsky H, Garner DM: The heterogeneity of anorexia nervosa: bulimia as a distinct subgroup. Arch Gen Psychiatry 37:1036–1040, 1980

Garfinkel PE, Kaplan AS, Garner DM, et al: The differentiation of vomiting and weight loss as a conversion disorder from anorexia nervosa. Am J Psychiatry 140:1019–1022, 1983

Garfinkel PE, Goldbloom DS, Olmsted MP, et al: Body dissatisfaction in bulimia nervosa: relationship to weight and shape concerns and psychological functioning. International Journal of Eating Disorders 11:151–161, 1992

Garner DM, Fairburn CG: Relationship between anorexia nervosa and bulimia nervosa: diagnostic implications, in Diagnostic Issues in Anorexia Nervosa and Bulimia Nervosa. Edited by Garner DM, Garfinkel PE. New York, Brunner/Mazel, 1988, pp 56–79

Garner DM, Garfinkel PE: The Eating Attitudes Test: an index of the symptoms of anorexia nervosa. Psychol Med 9:273–279, 1979

Garner DM, Olmsted MP, Polivy J: The Eating Disorder Inventory: a measure of cognitive-behavioral dimensions of anorexia nervosa and bulimia, in Anorexia Nervosa: Recent Developments in Research. Edited by Darby PL, Garfinkel PE, Garner DM, et al. New York, Allan R Liss, 1983, pp 173–184

Garner DM, Olmsted MP, Polivy J, et al: Comparison between weight-preoccupied women and anorexia nervosa. Psychosom Med 46:255–260, 1984

Garner DM, Garfinkel PE, O'Shaughnessy M: The validity of the distinction between bulimia with and without anorexia nervosa. Am J Psychiatry 142:581–587, 1985

Garner DM, Shafer CL, Rosen LW: Diagnostic issues in eating disorders, in Assessment and Diagnosis of Child and Adolescent Psychiatric Disorders: Current Issues and Procedures. Edited by Hooper SR, Hynd GW, Mattison RE. Hillsdale, NJ, Lawrence Erlbaum, 1992, pp 261–303

Garrow JS, Crisp AH, Jordan HA, et al: Pathology of eating group report. Dahlem Konferenzen, Life Sciences Research Report. Edited by Silverstone T. Berlin, 1975

Gormally J, Rardin D, Black S: Correlates of successful response to a behavioral weight control clinic. Journal of Counseling Psychology 27:179–191, 1980

Gull WW: The address in medicine delivered before the annual meeting of the BMA at Oxford. Lancet 2:171, 1868

Huon GF, Brown L, Morris S: Lay beliefs about disordered eating. International Journal of Eating Disorders 7:133–138, 1988

Janet P: Des Obsessions et la Psychasthenie. Paris, Felix Alcan, 1919

Kaplan AS, Garfinkel PE, Warsh JJ, et al: Clonidine challenge test in bulimia nervosa. International Journal of Eating Disorders 8:425–435, 1989a

Kaplan AS, Garfinkel PE, Brown GM: The DST and TRH test in bulimia nervosa. Br J Psychiatry 154:86–92, 1989b

Katzman MA, Wolchik SA: Bulimia and binge eating in college women: a comparison of personality and behavioral characteristics. J Consult Clin Psychol 52:423–428, 1984

Keefe PH, Wyshogrod D, Weinberger E, et al: Binge eating and outcome of behavioral treatment of obesity: a preliminary report. Behav Res Ther 22:319–321, 1984

Kennedy S, Garfinkel PE, Parienti V, et al: Changes in melatonin but not cortisol are associated with depression in eating disorder patients. Arch Gen Psychiatry 46:73–78, 1989

Kirkley BG, Burge JC: Dietary restriction in young women: issues and concerns. Annals of Behavioral Medicine 11:66–72, 1989

Lasègue C: De l'anorexie hysterique. Arch Gen de Med 385, 1873. Reprinted in Kaufman RM, Heiman M (eds): Evolution of Psychosomatic Concepts. Anorexia Nervosa: A Paradigm. New York, International Universities Press, 1964

Lindholm L, Wilson GT: Body image assessment in patients with bulimia nervosa and normal controls. International Journal of Eating Disorders 7:527–539, 1988

Loro AD, Orleans CS: Binge eating in obesity: preliminary findings and guidelines for behavioral analysis and treatment. Addict Behav 6:155–166, 1981

Marcus MD, Wing RR, Lamparski DM: Binge eating and dietary restraint in obese patients. Addict Behav 10:163–168, 1985

Marcus MD, Wing RR, Ewing L, et al: Lifetime prevalence of psychiatric disorder in obese binge eaters compared to non-binge eaters. Paper presented at the 9th annual meeting of the Society of Behavioral Medicine, Boston, MA, April 1988a

Marcus MD, Wing RR, Hopkins J: Obese binge eaters: affect, cognitions and response to behavioral weight control. J Consult Clin Psychol 53:433–439, 1988b

Michalide A, Andersen A: Subgroups of anorexia nervosa and bulimia: validity and utility. J Psychiatr Res 19:121–128, 1985

Mitchell JE, Pomeroy C, Huber M: A clinician's guide to the eating disorders medicine cabinet. International Journal of Eating Disorders 7:211–233, 1988a

Mitchell JE, Morley J, Laine D, et al: Monitored eating behavior in women with bulimia nervosa, in Eating Behavior in Eating Disorders. Edited by Walsh BT. Washington, DC, American Psychiatric Press, 1988b, pp 189–197

Mitchell JE, Pyle PL, Hatsukami D, et al: A 2–5 year follow-up study of patients treated for bulimia. International Journal of Eating Disorders 8:157–165, 1989

Nicolle G: Prepsychotic anorexia. Proceedings of the Royal Society of Medicine 32:153–162, 1939

Norris D: Clinical diagnostic criteria for primary anorexia nervosa. South African Medical Journal 56:987–992, 1979

Nylander I: The feeling of being fat and dieting in a school population: an epidemiologic interview investigation. Acta Sociomedica Scandinavica 3:17–26, 1971

Palmer HD, Jones MS: Anorexia nervosa as a manifestation of compulsion neurosis. Archives of Neurology and Psychiatry 41:856–860, 1939

Piran NP, Kennedy S, Owens M, et al: Anorexia nervosa, bulimia and affective disorder. J Nerv Ment Dis 173:395–400, 1985

Piran N, Lerner P, Garfinkel PE, et al: Personality disorders in restricting and bulimic forms of anorexia nervosa. International Journal of Eating Disorders 7:589–599, 1988

Rollins N, Piazza E: Diagnosis of anorexia nervosa: a critical appraisal. Journal of the American Academy of Child Psychiatry 17:126–137, 1978

Rosen JC, Vara L, Wendt S, et al: Validity studies of the Eating Disorder Examination. International Journal of Eating Disorders 9:519–528, 1990

Russell GFM: Anorexia nervosa: its identity as an illness and its treatment, in Modern Trends in Psychological Medicine. Edited by Price JK. London, Butterworth, 1970, pp 131–164

Russell GFM: Bulimia nervosa: an ominous variant of anorexia nervosa. Psychol Med 9:429–449, 1979

Selvini-Palazzoli M: Self Starvation. London, Chaucer, 1974

Smart DE, Beumont PJV, George GCW: Some personality characteristics of patients with anorexia nervosa. Br J Psychiatry 128:57–60, 1976

Solyom L, Miles JE, O'Kane J: A comparative psychometric study of anorexia nervosa and obsessive neurosis. Can J Psychiatry 27:282–286, 1982

Spitzer RL, Devlin M, Walsh BT, et al: A multisite field trial of diagnostic criteria for binge eating disorder. International Journal of Eating Disorders 11:191–203, 1992

Strober M, Salkin B, Burroughs J, et al: Validity of the bulimia-restricter distinctions in anorexia nervosa: parental personality characteristics and familial psychiatric morbidity. J Nerv Ment Dis 170:345–351, 1982

Stunkard AJ: Eating patterns and obesity. J Behav Ther Exp Psychiatry 12:333–336, 1959

Theander S: Anorexia nervosa: a psychiatric investigation of 94 female patients. Acta Psychiatr Scand Suppl 214:1–94, 1970

Toner BB, Garfinkel PE, Garner DM: Long-term follow-up of anorexia nervosa. Psychosom Med 48:520–529, 1986

Toner BB, Garfinkel PE, Garner DM: Cognitive style in bulimic and dietary restricting anorexia nervosa. Am J Psychiatry 144:510–512, 1987

Tourette G de la: Traite clinique et therapeutique de l'hysterie. Paris, Plou, Nourit, 1895

Touyz SW, Beumont PJV: Body image and its disturbance, in Handbook of Eating Disorders. Edited by Beumont PJV, Burrows GD, Casper RC. Amsterdam, Elsevier, 1988, pp 171–188

Vandereycken W, Pierloot R: The significance of subclassification in anorexia nervosa: a comparative study of clinical features in 141 patients. Psychol Med 13:543–549, 1983

Williamson DA, Prather RC, Upton L, et al: Severity of bulimia: relationship with depression and other psychopathology. International Journal of Eating Disorders 6:39–47, 1987

Willmuth ME, Leitenberg H, Rosen JC, et al: A comparison of purging and non-purging normal weight bulimics. International Journal of Eating Disorders 7:825–835, 1988

Wilson GT, Smith D: Assessment of bulimia nervosa: an evaluation of the Eating Disorders Examination. International Journal of Eating Disorders 8:173–179, 1989

World Health Organization: The ICD-10 Classification of Mental and Behavioural Disorders: Clinical Descriptions and Diagnostic Guidelines. Geneva, World Health Organization, 1992

Yellowlees AJ: Anorexia and bulimia in anorexia nervosa: a study of psychosocial functioning and associated psychiatric symptomatology. Br J Psychiatry 146:648–652, 1985

Ziegler R, Sours JA: A naturalistic study of patients with anorexia nervosa. Compr Psychiatry 9:644–651, 1968

Chapter 4

Family-Genetic Studies

Michael Strober, Ph.D.

———⟫●⟪———

Current interest in the role of family-genetic factors in eating disorders stems from expanding knowledge of the role of inherited and environment-based factors in risk and vulnerability to psychiatric disorders. Hypotheses linking both abnormal heredity and pathogenic family influences to eating disturbance have a long history. In his seminal 1873 account of anorexia nervosa, Lasègue wrote:

> It must not cause surprise to find me thus always placing in parallel the morbid condition of the hysterical subject and the preoccupations of those who surround her. These two circumstances are intimately connected and we should acquire an erroneous idea of the disease by confining ourselves to an examination of the patient . . . the moral medium amidst which the patient lives exercises an influence which it would be equally regrettable to overlook or misunderstand. (p. 368)

Indeed, following Lasègue's publication, and William Gull's (1874) simultaneous report to the Clinical Society of London, the notion that family environment was fertile ground for the development of anorexia nervosa was accepted by many as an indisputable fact (Vandereycken and van Deth 1990).

By the same token, in a rarely cited paper published more than a decade before those of Lasègue and Gull, Louis Victor-Marcé (1860) speculated that "hereditary antecedents" played a formative role in predisposing certain young people to a form of hypochondriacal insanity, the description of which is identical to the entity anorexia nervosa (see Silverman 1989). Still, Marcé believed, as did Gull and Lasègue, that certain deviant elements of the family's behavior loomed large in perpetuating the illness and in impeding proper and effective treatment.

The etiology of the eating disorders is widely assumed to be complexly determined by multifactorial processes. Even so, highly polarized viewpoints continue. To some, it is simply improbable that genetics or biology is the core etiology, considering the apparently willful character of the symptoms and their connection to prevailing cultural attitudes governing weight and shape. Yet, others contend with equal conviction that eating disorders are not merely the invariable consequences of extreme dieting behavior. The fact remains that anorexia nervosa is an uncommon illness—its morbid risk among females being in the range of 0.1%–0.7% (Crisp et al. 1976; Cullberg and Engstrom-Lindberg 1988; Lucas et al. 1988). Bulimia nervosa, although relatively common by genetic-epidemiological standards, affects no more than 2% of females (Fairburn and Beglin 1990). Taking this into account, the idea that genetics may influence individual differences in the psychopathology and pathophysiology of food intake regulation is plausible and need not be considered alien to theories that focus on nongenetic familial processes.

Studies of the Familiality of Eating Disorders

Several uncontrolled studies are notable for reports of increased parental and sibling resemblance for eating disorders, anorexia nervosa in particular. Theander (1970) studied a Swedish sample of 94 anorectic people and found a risk of anorexia nervosa of 6.6% for their female siblings. Similar figures have been reported in studies of English (Dally and Gomez 1979), Canadian (Garfinkel et al. 1980), and American (Halmi et al. 1977) samples. A history of low adolescent weight, peculiar dietary habits, or frank anorexia nervosa was reported in 27% of mothers of 56 anorectic persons studied by Kalucy et al. (1977), and in 14% of mothers of 102 consecutively hospitalized anorectic patients studied by Crisp et al. (1980). Hudson et al. (1983) studied 420 first-degree relatives of 89 eating disorders probands: 14 with anorexia nervosa, restricting subtype; 20 with anorexia nervosa, bulimic subtype; and 55 with bulimia nervosa alone. Diagnoses were by DSM-III (American Psychiatric Association 1980) criteria based mainly on family history information obtained from proband interviews. Anorexia nervosa was diagnosed among 4.3% of the relatives of restricting anorectic probands and 4.0% of relatives of mixed bulimic anorectic probands, as compared to only 0.8% among relatives of bulimic probands. The lifetime prevalence rate of bulimia nervosa among relatives was lower: 1.4% among relatives of restricting anorectic probands, 2.1% among relatives of bulimic anorectic probands, and 2.8% among relatives of bulimic probands.

The inferences to be drawn from these accounts are, of course, ambiguous. Methodological limitations such as lack of predesignated, operationally defined diagnostic criteria, lack of blindness of relative assessments, and reliance on family history data are possible contaminating influences. Nonetheless, the observations suggest that female relatives of anorectic people are more likely to develop anorexia nervosa than the general population.

As of this writing, only a handful of studies have employed a case-control design and more rigorous methods of diagnostic assessment to investigate the transmissibility of eating disorders. These are listed in Table 4–1.

The studies vary considerably in the level of detail of methodological information provided and employ different approaches to the assessment and diagnosis of relatives. The study by Gershon et al. (1983) is notable as the first rigorously conducted family study that assessed familial aggregation of anorexia nervosa. The authors examined 99 first-degree relatives of 24 anorectic probands and 265 first-degree relatives of 44 nonpsychiatrically ill control subjects using the Schedule for Affective Disorders and Schizophrenia, Lifetime Version (Spitzer and Endicott 1978) and the Family History–Research Diagnostic Criteria (Andreasen et al. 1977). Roughly 75% of interviews were conducted blind to proband diagnosis, and 54% of relatives were personally interviewed.

In the Hudson et al. (1987) study, assessments were conducted on 283 first-degree relatives of 69 bulimic probands, in comparison to 149 relatives of community control subjects screened for eating disorders and 104 relatives of 24 probands with major depression. All diagnoses were by DSM-III criteria and were based solely on family history information obtained from structured interviews of probands.

The sample reported by Logue et al. (1989) included 30 eating disorder probands (6 with anorexia nervosa; 11 with anorexia nervosa, bulimic subtype; and 13 with bulimia nervosa) and their 132 adult first-degree relatives, who were compared with 107 relatives of screened nonpsychiatrically ill control subjects and 75 relatives of depressed control subjects. The majority (80%) of relatives were personally interviewed, but the diagnostic assessment of relatives was not blind to status of the proband.

In a well-controlled study, Kassett et al. (1989) examined risk of eating disorders among 185 first-degree relatives of 40 probands with bulimia nervosa, per DSM-III-R (American Psychiatric Association 1987) criteria, and 118 relatives of 24 screened nonpsychiatrically ill control subjects. Diagnoses of relatives were made blind to status of the proband and were based on a combination of direct interview (62% of relatives) and family history information.

The study by Strober et al. (1990), the largest of the family studies published as of this writing, examined 387 first-degree relatives over age 12 years of 97 anorectic probands and 738 relatives of 66 affective disorder probands and 117 nonaffectively psychiatrically ill probands. Although interviewers were not fully blind to proband diagnosis, all diagnostic information for relatives was assessed blindly, and personal interviews were conducted with 80% of relatives.

Despite these methodological differences, the results are fairly consistent. In four of five studies, secondary cases of anorexia nervosa were found exclusively among relatives of eating disorder probands. The lifetime risk of anorexia nervosa among relatives of eating disorder probands ranges from 1.7% to 2.2%, roughly 3–20 times that in the general population. The risk of anorexia nervosa for female relatives alone is given in only one study (Strober et al. 1990) and is in the range of 4%. The only exception to this trend is the study by Logue et al. (1989), in which no secondary familial cases of eating disorder were identified among anorectic or bulimic probands; however, these results are mitigated by the small number of probands, which may have precluded detection of familiality.

Results concerning the transmissibility of bulimia nervosa are more limited in scope. As shown in Table 4–1, only three studies have included normal-weight bulimic probands, and in only one (Kassett et al. 1989) is familial aggregation apparent. However, as already noted, the Logue et al. (1989) sample is too small for a meaningful analysis of familial risk, and the Hudson et al. (1987) study is constrained by exclusive reliance on family history data supplied by the proband. In this latter case, it is reasonable to assume that the risk estimates are spuriously low considering that bulimia nervosa is often shrouded in secrecy and deception.

Also noteworthy in this regard is a subsequent reanalysis of the Gershon et al. (1983) findings, which showed that only restricting (i.e.,

Table 4–1. Controlled studies of lifetime risk of eating disorders among first-degree relatives of eating disorder probands

Study	Probands (N)		Diagnosis in relatives (%)			Diagnosis in control relatives (%)		
	Anorexia nervosa	Bulimia nervosa	Anorexia nervosa	Bulimia nervosa	Total	Anorexia nervosa	Bulimia nervosa	Total
Gershon et al. 1983	24	—	2.0[a]	4.4[a]	6.4[a]	0.0	1.3	1.3[b]
Hudson et al. 1987	—	69	1.7	1.7	3.4	0.0	0.0	0.0[c,d]
Logue et al. 1989	17	13	0.0	0.0	0.0	0.0	0.0	0.0[b,d]
Kassett et al. 1989	—	40	2.2[a]	9.6[a]	11.8[a]	0.0	3.5	3.5[b]
Strober et al. 1990	97	—	2.1[e]	1.3[e]	3.4[e]	0.0	1.1	1.1[f]

[a]With age control. [b]Screened control subjects, no psychiatric illness. [c]Control subjects screened only for eating disorders. [d]Results on relatives of nonpsychiatrically ill control subjects only. [e]Risks to female relatives only = 4.1% for anorexia nervosa, 2.6% for bulimia nervosa, 6.7% for anorexia nervosa plus bulimia nervosa. [f]Control subjects with pathology.

not bulimic) anorectic probands conferred risk of anorexia nervosa to relatives (3.9% versus 0% among relatives of bulimic anorectic probands), whereas risk of bulimia nervosa was 3.5 times higher among relatives of bulimic anorectic probands as compared with relatives of restricting anorectic probands (Gershon et al. 1984). Clearly, whether these two phenotypes coaggregate in families, or whether there is specificity in their familial transmission, as the Gershon et al. (1984) findings suggest, is an interesting question meriting further investigation.

Twin Studies

As of this writing, there have been five studies in which differential concordance between monozygotic (MZ) and dizygotic (DZ) twin pairs has been assessed. Holland et al. (1984) identified 16 MZ and 14 DZ female pairs in which the proband suffered from anorexia nervosa. Twins were ascertained through three independent sources: referrals to the specialized eating disorders treatment program at St. George's Hospital in London, the Maudsley Hospital Twin Registry, and voluntary referral based on knowledge of the project. Zygosity was established by blood group in 10 of the 14 DZ pairs and in 15 of the 16 MZ pairs. The majority of diagnoses were based on personal interviews conducted with the twins and one or both parents. Among the 30 pairs, 9 of 16 (56%) MZ pairs were concordant for anorexia nervosa, compared to only 1 of 14 (7%) DZ pairs (MZ:DZ pair-wise ratio = 7.9:1, $P < .006$), resulting in a Smith heritability estimate of 0.54.

Two subsequent reports from this group have provided updated analyses on larger, partially overlapping samples. Holland et al. (1988) reported on a series of 45 twin pairs (25 MZ, 20 DZ), including 10 pairs who were part of the earlier study. Of the 45 pairs, 27 were voluntary referrals and 18 were identified through local hospital clinics; no further details on the exact methods of ascertainment are provided. The two ascertainment groups were not found to differ on relevant clinical or demographic variables; however, MZ twins and concordant pairs were overrepresented among volunteers. All diagnoses were by structured interview, and further information was obtained from twins and parents on eating disorders among first-degree and second-degree relatives (diagnostic methods unspecified). The respective pair-wise concordance rates for MZ and DZ twins are 56% and 5%, resulting in a heritability estimate of 0.98. Among 121 female first-degree relatives, 6 (4.9%) were given a diagnosis of anorexia nervosa, which is in line with the risk to female relatives reported by Strober et al. (1990).

In the report by Treasure and Holland (1989), a series of 67 twin probands who had received hospital treatment were studied, representing 59 pairs and an unspecified number of probands who were included in the prior two analyses. A total of 8 co-twins (7 MZ and 1 DZ) had also received hospital care and were treated as double probands. Proband-wise concordance for restricting anorexia nervosa was found to be markedly higher for MZ twins (66%) than for DZ twins (0%). In contrast, there is no evidence of differential concordance among MZ and DZ pairs for bulimia nervosa, the proband-wise rates being 35% and 29%, respectively. On the basis of these findings, the authors suggested that familiality of eating disorders results from heterogeneous mechanisms of transmissibility, with environmental factors predominating in bulimia nervosa and genetic effects being more robust in the restricting form of anorexia nervosa.

Differential concordance among MZ and DZ twins for bulimia nervosa has been the subject of two other reports. The German series of Fichter and Noegel (1990) was drawn from respondents to a press survey on bulimia nervosa, from hospital cases at a specialty clinic, and from hospitalized cases at a university psychiatric facility. A total of 21 female twin pairs were identified, including 6 female MZ pairs and 15 female DZ pairs. Zygosity was determined mainly by physical similarity. Diagnosis was based on responses to self-administered questionnaires that allowed classification by DSM-III-R criteria. Pair-wise concordance was 83.3% (5 of 6) in MZ twins and 26.7% (4 of 15) in DZ twins.

The series reported by Hsu et al. (1990) consisted of 11 twin pairs (6 MZ, 2 female DZ, and 3 opposite-sex DZ) referred over a 3-year period to the University of Pittsburgh Eating Disorders Clinic. Zygosity was based on physical similarity, and diagnoses were by direct interview. Two of the 6 MZ pairs were concordant for bulimia nervosa, compared to 0% concordance among the DZ pairs.

Familial Aggregation of Mood Disorders

Numerous studies suggest that depression is prominent in the clinical presentation of both anorexia nervosa and bulimia nervosa and that affective disturbances sometimes arise subsequent to the resolution of eating- and weight-related concerns (see Hudson and Pope 1988; Strober and Katz 1988). Accordingly, a third line of inquiry pursued in family-genetic studies has followed on the hypothesis that eating disorders and major affective disorders share transmissible etiologic factors. Family studies of major affective disorder with anorectic probands are listed in Table 4–2.

Methodological differences across studies are notable. In the study by Winokur et al. (1980), nonblind diagnoses were obtained using mainly family history data on first-degree and second-degree relatives of anorectic probands and relatives of age-matched nonpsychiatrically ill control subjects; however, the procedures used to screen control subjects are unstated. Hudson et al. (1983) relied mainly on nonblind family history information to diagnose first-degree relatives of anorectic probands, whereas relatives of nonaffectively ill psychiatric control subjects were diagnosed in blind fashion based on family history data recorded in the proband's hospital chart. In the Gershon et al. (1983) study, diagnoses of relatives were made blind to proband status, and more than 50% of the first-degree relatives of the anorectic and screened nonpsychiatrically ill control probands were personally interviewed. In both the Rivinus et al. (1984) and Logue et al. (1989) studies, control probands were screened for psychiatric illness; however, diagnoses in relatives were not established in blind fashion. In the Strober et al. (1990) study, all diagnostic information obtained on relatives was assessed without knowledge of the proband's clinical status, although interviewers themselves were not always blind; nearly 80% of relatives received face-to-face interviews.

The range of age-adjusted and unadjusted familial risk estimates for unipolar depression across the six studies is 7.2%–20.4%, with risks for bipolar illness ranging from 0% to 8.3%. For unipolar and bipolar illness combined, relative risks are in the range of 2.1–3.4 in five of six studies. The highest relative risk estimate, 25.6, comes from the Hudson et al. (1983) study; however, this figure may be spuriously inflated because the scrutiny of hospital charts is relatively insensitive to familial psychopathology and in this case may have underestimated the true risk among relatives of control probands. Still, the studies suggest that biological relatives of anorexia nervosa probands are several times more likely to develop affective disorder than relatives of control subjects.

Similar results were noted in studies of bulimic probands. Representative studies are listed in Table 4–3. Variations in methodology are similar to those in the previously discussed studies of anorectic probands.

Once again, the relative risk estimates of 0.9–23.3 suggest a significantly increased risk of affective disorders in relatives of bulimic pro-

Table 4–2. Controlled studies of lifetime risk of major affective disorders among first-degree relatives of anorexia nervosa probands

Study	Anorectic probands (N)	Diagnosis in relatives (%)			Relative risk[a]
		Unipolar depression	Bipolar illness	Total	
Winokur et al. 1980	25	20.4	6.8	27.2	2.1[b]
Gershon et al. 1983	24	13.3[c]	8.3[c,d]	21.6[c]	3.2[e]
Hudson et al. 1983	34	14.2	3.0	17.2	25.6[f]
Rivinus et al. 1984	40	16.1[c]	0.0[c]	16.1[c]	3.4[e]
Logue et al. 1989	17	14.7	—[g]	14.7	2.9[e]
Strober et al. 1990	97	7.2	1.6	8.8	2.1[h]

[a]Rate of illness in relatives of anorectic probands divided by rate of illness in relatives of control subjects. [b]Normal control subjects, nature of screening unclear. [c]With age correction. [d]Includes bipolar I, bipolar II, and schizoaffective illness. [e]Screened control subjects, no psychiatric illness. [f]Personality disorder and schizophrenic control subjects, screened for mood and eating disorders. [g]No reference to bipolar illness in text. [h]Control subjects with pathology screened for mood and eating disorders.

Table 4–3. Controlled studies of lifetime risk of major affective disorders among first-degree relatives of bulimia nervosa probands

Study	Bulimic probands (N)	Unipolar depression	Bipolar illness	Total	Relative risk[a]
Hudson et al. 1983	55	15.1	1.2	16.3	23.3[b]
Stern et al. 1984	27	—[c]	—[c]	9.0	0.9[d]
Hudson et al. 1987	69	15.5	4.2	19.8	4.2[d]
Logue et al. 1989	13	10.5	—[e]	10.5	2.1[f]
Kassett et al. 1989	40	22.0[g]	5.9	27.9[g]	3.2[f]

[a]Rate of illness in relatives of bulimic probands divided by rate of illness in relatives of control subjects. [b]Personality disorder and schizophrenic control subjects. [c]Unipolar-bipolar breakdown not stated. [d]Unscreened community control subjects. [e]No reference to bipolar illness in text. [f]Screened control subjects. [g]With age correction.

bands, the one exception being in the Stern et al. (1984) study. However, this latter result is an artifact of the investigators' failure to screen control subjects for mood disorder, thereby confounding the assessment of differential familial risk.

Whether this increased aggregation of affective disorders in families is predicted by depressive comorbidity in probands has been addressed in six studies, listed in Table 4–4.

In these studies, probands were subdivided by the presence or absence of coexisting major depression. In four of the studies (Biederman et al. 1985; Hudson et al. 1987; Kassett et al. 1989; Strober et al. 1990), relatives of probands with coexisting affective disorder had nearly twice to more than five times the risk for major affective disorder than relatives of non-affectively ill probands (relative risk range = 1.8–5.2). In two studies (Gershon et al. 1983; Logue et al. 1989), increased affective morbidity among relatives was independent of comorbidity in probands. However, it is notable that Strober et al. (1990) found no evidence of cross-transmission of eating disorders among relatives of either unipolar or bipolar probands. In short, although some results are inconsistent, the weight of evidence to date suggests that individuals with eating disorders are more likely to transmit affective illness to relatives in the presence of concomitant affective disturbance. By the same token, families of pure affectively ill probands do not seem to have any greater rate of eating disorders than expected for the general population, indicating that although eating disorders and affective disorders frequently coexist within individuals, they do not seem to share a single common familial etiology.

Eating Disorders and Alcoholism

Clinical experience also reveals that alcohol abuse or dependence is not an uncommon occurrence in patients with bulimia nervosa. Hence, it is not surprising that several studies (Bulik 1987; Halmi and Loney 1973; Hudson et al. 1983, 1987; Kassett et al. 1989; Strober et al. 1982) suggest that risk of substance use disorders is higher among relatives of probands with bulimia nervosa and probands with bulimic anorexia nervosa, compared with risk to relatives of control subjects and to the general population. Whether this implies the existence of a common familial substrate underlying certain forms of bulimia nervosa and substance abuse is unknown at present, but the possibility is intriguing and deserves further investigation.

Table 4-4. Risk of affective illness in first-degree relatives by affective status of probands

Study	Probands Affective status	n	Risk to relatives (%) Unipolar depression	Bipolar illness	Total
Gershon et al. 1983	AN with MAD	13	13.4[a]	10.1[a]	23.5[a]
	AN without MAD	11	13.1[a]	5.3[a]	18.4[a]
Biederman et al. 1985	AN with MAD	17	17.3	0.0	17.3
	AN without MAD	21	3.3	0.0	3.3
Hudson et al. 1987	BN with MAD	46	—	—	36.2[a,b]
	BN without MAD	23	—	—	18.7[a,b]
Logue et al. 1989	ED with MAD	10	13.0	—[c]	13.0
	ED without MAD	20	12.0	—[c]	12.0
Kassett et al. 1989	BN with MAD	23	29.5[a]	5.3[a]	34.8[a]
	BN without MAD	17	12.5[a]	6.6[a]	19.1[a]
Strober et al. 1990	AN with MAD	28	14.4	3.6	18.0
	AN without MAD	69	4.3	0.7	5.1

Note. AN = anorexia nervosa. MAD = major affective disorder. BN = bulimia nervosa. ED = eating disorder (anorexia nervosa and bulimia nervosa combined).
[a]With age correction. [b]Unipolar, bipolar breakdown not specified. [c]No reference to bipolar illness in text.

Summary

The evidence at hand for familial aggregation of the eating disorders appears suggestive. However, empirically firm conclusions remain limited by the scarcity of large-scale, methodologically sound investigations. Results of the twin studies are intriguing at first glance, but are especially problematic considering that these samples contain recruited cases who may be overselected for MZ and concordant pair status. There has been one association study (Biederman et al. 1984) demonstrating a higher frequency of human leukocyte antigens A26, Bw16, and B51 in anorectic patients than in nonpsychiatrically ill control subjects; however, the implications of this finding for our knowledge of genetic factors is uncertain given that patients were not stratified by presence versus absence of concomitant mood disorder and considering that available evidence concerning associations between mood disorder and human leukocyte antigens remains unconvincing (Tsuang and Faraone 1990).

By the same token, it does not appear, as once hypothesized, that the increased loading of major affective disorders in relatives of patients with anorexia nervosa and bulimia nervosa indicates that the two conditions are phenotypically variable expressions of a common etiologic factor.

Thus, our best evidence, limited though it is, is that the familial pathogenesis of eating disorders is a unique process comprising transmissible elements whose nature remains poorly understood. Strober et al. (1990) hypothesized that clustering of anorexia nervosa in families may involve inherited variations in personality traits that underlie rigid obsessionality and avoidance tendencies, characteristics that figure prominently in the behavior of anorectic persons. A further speculation in this regard is that such genotypic traits underlie, and give shape to, more pathologically extreme avoidance mechanisms in response to stressful events, and that these tendencies are linked to, or associated with, pathogenic biologic factors that facilitate metabolic adaptation to extreme calorie deprivation.

The transmissibility of bulimia nervosa is, likewise, a matter for ongoing speculation. The association of bulimia nervosa with risk for substance use disorders has emerged as a new, potentially fruitful line of inquiry that could benefit by the application of family study methods. Here, the genetic-epidemiologic framework may be especially informative in addressing important etiologic questions; specifically whether bulimic individuals, alcoholic individuals, and comorbidly affected individuals have similar or highly distinctive patterns of familial aggregation.

References

American Psychiatric Association: Diagnostic and Statistical Manual of Mental Disorders, 3rd Edition. Washington, DC, American Psychiatric Association, 1980

American Psychiatric Association: Diagnostic and Statistical Manual of Mental Disorders, 3rd Edition, Revised. Washington, DC, American Psychiatric Association, 1987

Andreasen NC, Endicott J, Spitzer RL, et al: The family history method using diagnostic criteria. Arch Gen Psychiatry 34:1229–1235, 1977

Biederman J, Rivinus T, Herzog DB, et al: High frequency of HLA-Bw16 in patients with anorexia nervosa. Am J Psychiatry 141:1109–1110, 1984

Biederman J, Rivinus T, Kemper K, et al: Depressive disorders in relatives of anorexia nervosa patients with and without a current episode of nonbipolar major depression. Am J Psychiatry 142:1495–1496, 1985

Bulik CM: Drug and alcohol abuse by bulimic women and their families. Am J Psychiatry 144:1604–1606, 1987

Crisp AH, Palmer RL, Kalucy RS: How common is anorexia nervosa? a prevalence study. Br J Psychiatry 128:549–554, 1976

Crisp AH, Hsu LKG, Harding B, et al: Clinical features of anorexia nervosa: a study of a consecutive series of 102 female patients. J Psychosom Res 24:179–191, 1980

Cullberg J, Engstrom-Lindberg M: Prevalence and incidence of eating disorders in a suburban population. Acta Psychiatr Scand 78:314–319, 1988

Dally P, Gomez J: Anorexia Nervosa. London, William Heinemann, 1979

Fairburn CG, Beglin SJ: Studies of the epidemiology of bulimia nervosa. Am J Psychiatry 147:401–408, 1990

Fichter MM, Noegel R: Concordance for bulimia nervosa in twins. International Journal of Eating Disorders 9:255–263, 1990

Garfinkel PE, Moldofsky H, Garner D: The heterogeneity of anorexia nervosa. Arch Gen Psychiatry 37:1036–1040, 1980

Gershon ES, Schreiber JL, Hamovit JR, et al: Anorexia nervosa and major affective disorders associated in families: a preliminary report, in Childhood Psychopathology and Development. Edited by Guze SB, Earls FG, Barrett JE. New York, Raven, 1983, pp 279–284

Gershon ES, Schreiber JL, Hamovit JR, et al: Clinical findings in patients with anorexia nervosa and affective illness in their relatives. Am J Psychiatry 141:1419–1422, 1984

Gull WW: Anorexia nervosa (apepsia hysterica, anorexia hysterica. Transactions of the Clinical Society of London 7:22–28, 1874

Halmi KA, Loney J: Familial alcoholism in patients with anorexia nervosa. Br J Psychiatry 123:53–54, 1973

Halmi KA, Goldberg SC, Eckert E, et al: Pretreatment evaluation in anorexia nervosa, in Anorexia Nervosa. Edited by Vigersky RA. New York, Raven, 1977

Holland AJ, Hall A, Murray R, et al: Anorexia nervosa: a study of 34 twin pairs. Br J Psychiatry 145:414–419, 1984

Holland AJ, Sicotte N, Treasure J: Anorexia nervosa: evidence for a genetic basis. J Psychosom Res 32:561–571, 1988

Hsu LKG, Chesler BE, Santhouse R: Bulimia nervosa in eleven sets of twins: a clinical report. International Journal of Eating Disorders 9:275–282, 1990

Hudson JI, Pope HG: Depression and eating disorders, in Presentations of Depression. Edited by Cameron OG. New York, Wiley, 1988, pp 1–54

Hudson JI, Pope HG, Jonas JM, et al: A family history study of anorexia nervosa and bulimia. Br J Psychiatry 142:133–138, 1983

Hudson JI, Pope HG, Jonas JM, et al: A controlled family history study of bulimia. Psychol Med 17:883–890, 1987

Kalucy RS, Crisp AH, Harding B: A study of 56 families with anorexia nervosa. Br J Med Psychol 50:381–395, 1977

Kassett JA, Gershon ES, Maxwell ME, et al: Psychiatric disorders in the first-degree relatives of probands with bulimia nervosa. Am J Psychiatry 146:1468–1471, 1989

Lasègue C: On hysterical anorexia. Medical Times and Gazette, September 27, 1873, pp 367–369

Logue CM, Crowe RR, Bean JA: A family study of anorexia nervosa and bulimia. Compr Psychiatry 30:179–188, 1989

Lucas AR, Beard CM, O'Fallon WM, et al: Anorexia nervosa in Rochester, Minnesota: a 45 year study. Mayo Clin Proc 63:433–442, 1988

Marcé LV: On a form of hypochondriacal delirium occurring consecutive to dyspepsia and characterized by refusal of food. J Psychol Med Ment Pathology 13:264–266, 1860

Rivinus TM, Biederman J, Herzog DB, et al: Anorexia nervosa and affective disorders: a controlled family history study. Am J Psychiatry 141:1414–1418, 1984

Silverman JA: Louis Victor-Marcé, 1828–1864: anorexia nervosa's forgotten man. Psychol Med 19:833–835, 1989

Spitzer RL, Endicott J: Schedule for Affective Disorders and Schizophrenia (Lifetime Version), 3rd Edition. New York, New York State Psychiatric Institute, 1978

Stern SL, Dixon KN, Nemzer E, et al: Affective disorder in the families of women with normal weight bulimia. Am J Psychiatry 141:1224–1227, 1984

Strober M, Katz JL: Depression in the eating disorders: a review and analysis of descriptive, family, and biological studies, in Diagnostic Issues in Anorexia Nervosa and Bulimia Nervosa. Edited by Garner DM, Garfinkel PE. New York, Brunner/Mazel, 1988, pp 80–111

Strober M, Salkin B, Burroughs J, et al: Validity of the bulimia-restricter distinction in anorexia nervosa. J Nerv Ment Dis 170:345–351, 1982

Strober M, Lampert C, Morrell W, et al: A controlled family study of anorexia nervosa: evidence of familial aggregation and lack of shared transmission with affective disorders. International Journal of Eating Disorders 9:239–253, 1990

Theander S: Anorexia nervosa: a psychiatric investigation of 94 female cases. Acta Psychiatr Scand Suppl 214:1–94, 1970

Treasure J, Holland AJ: Genetic vulnerability to eating disorders: evidence from twin and family studies, in Child and Youth Psychiatry: European Perspectives. Edited by Remschmidt H, Schmidt MH. New York, Hogrefe & Huber, 1989, pp 59–68

Tsuang MT, Faraone SV: The Genetics of Mood Disorders. Baltimore, MD, Johns Hopkins University Press, 1990

'Winokur A, March V, Mendels J: Primary affective disorder in relatives of patients with anorexia nervosa. Am J Psychiatry 137:695–698, 1980

Vandereycken W, van Deth R: A tribute to Lasègue's description of anorexia nervosa (1873), with completion of its English translation. Br J Psychiatry 157:902–908, 1990

Section II

Eating Behavior

Chapter 5

Psychobiology of Eating Behavior

Katherine A. Halmi, M.D.

———◦◦◦———

The unique abnormality of both anorexia nervosa and bulimia nervosa is disturbed eating behavior. Dieting has long been recognized as a necessary stimulus to the development of anorexia nervosa (Halmi 1974). In a survey done by Fairburn and Cooper (1984), the most frequent antecedent of bingeing behavior was severe dieting. The chronicity and relapse rate of aberrant eating behavior are serious problems in anorexia nervosa and bulimia nervosa (Halmi et al. 1991). Factors such as biological vulnerability, psychological disposition, family influences, and societal expectations—all of which influence dieting behavior in persons who go on to develop anorexia nervosa and bulimia nervosa—are thoroughly discussed in other chapters in this volume.

Eating behavior is not an isolated event, but rather an interaction between an organism's physiological state and environmental condition (Blundell and Hill 1986). According to Blundell and Hill's (1986) theory, the capacity to control nutrient intake to meet bodily needs requires specialized mechanisms to harmonize physiological information from the internal milieu with nutritional information in the external environment. Two essential features are perceptual capacities to identify the characteristics of food materials in the environment and a mechanism to link the biochemical consequences of ingested food with the consumed structured form. Thus, control over selection of foods must involve conditioned and unconditioned responses (Blundell and Hill 1987).

Booth (1977, 1981) emphasized that culturally derived attitudes influence food intake. He proposed that the conceptual identity of a food is the result of nutritional hedonic conditioning, which is the process whereby the nutritional functions of a food are related to its sensory characteristics. Immediate determinants of actual food intake include the influences of sensory input and somatic physiology. For example, satiation cues from the neurotransmitter serotonin are part of this conditioning process.

The chronicity of disturbed eating behavior in both anorectic and bulimic patients, the high percentage of relapse in eating disorder patients who have been treated, and the resistance of maladaptive eating behavior to change (treatment) indicate dysfunctions in perceptual capacities, internal physiology, or integrating mechanisms regulating eating behavior. Studies presented in this chapter are directly concerned with two of these areas: perceptual capacities and integrating mechanisms.

Integrating Mechanisms
Regulating Eating Behavior

Hunger and satiety perceptions are integrating processes for internal physiology and cognitive sets (attitudes toward food and conceptual identity of food). The study of hunger and satiety perceptions can show whether disturbed eating behavior is related to faulty integrating mechanisms. The first systematic tracking of hunger and satiety responses was done by Hill et al. (1984) in a study in which healthy persons recorded hunger and fullness ratings for the consumption of a highly preferred food and a less preferred food. These healthy subjects tracked hunger and fullness ratings in curves that were inversely proportional and that were similar to the ratings by control subjects in a study by Owen et al. (1985).

In the study by Owen et al. (1985), a liquid meal paradigm was used. All subjects received Sustacal, a liquid nutritionally balanced food containing 1 calorie per ml. Subjects fasted after midnight until the following morning tests, which occurred at 10:00 A.M. They controlled the rate of intake by pressing a button that controlled a small peristaltic pump. The food was delivered to the subject's mouth via a straw. The subject also controlled the length of the meal and told the examiner when she was finished. Every 2 minutes the subject made ratings on 10-cm visual analogue scales for hunger and fullness. These ratings began 8 minutes before the meal and continued during the meal and for 14 minutes after the completion of the meal. Eating disorder patients were tested on admission to an inpatient eating disorders unit, and the anorectic patients were tested again several weeks after weight restoration. Control subjects and normal-weight bulimic patients were tested at a similar time interval. All patients were within a normal weight range, were eating normally, and were free of any bingeing or purging behavior for at least 4 weeks at the time of the second examination. On both pre- and posttreatment testing occasions, two pairs of experimental meals were conducted. On one presentation the reservoir of food was hidden from the subject's view; on the other it was uncovered, and the subject could view the amount of food she was taking. The order of presentations was randomized for each pair. Owen et al. (1985) found that anorectic patients with bulimia had a "rapid rebound" of hunger shortly after the end of the meal. Although these patients were full, they were also hungry and were not satiated.

Using the same experimental meal paradigm, Halmi et al. (1989) studied 32 anorectic patients, restricting subtype; 28 anorectic patients, bulimic subtype; 30 normal-weight bulimic patients; and 19 normal-weight control subjects. There were no differences in the amount consumed in the covered (no visual cues) and uncovered (visual cues) conditions. Restricting anorectic patients had significantly lower hunger and higher fullness ratings than control subjects throughout the entire testing session. Bulimic anorectic patients had lower hunger and higher fullness ratings than control subjects before and during the meal. There was no effect of treatment on these ratings.

Hunger and fullness ratings were significantly less correlated for eating disorder subjects than for control subjects. The predominant pattern of hunger-fullness curves was a single intersection of hunger and fullness occurring during the meal. The control subjects would start out the meal not at all full and, as the meal progressed, would rapidly become more full and would end the meal when they were recording ratings of extremely full. The control subjects would remain extremely full for 20 minutes after the meal. Their hunger curves were inversely proportional to their fullness curves. In contrast, the predominant hunger-fullness curve pattern among the restricting anorectic patients was one of no intersections. They started the meal not at all hungry and remained not at all hungry throughout the meal and after. They started the meal extremely full and remained extremely full throughout the meal and after. The bulimic patients had multiple intersections of hunger and fullness occurring throughout the meal study. After treatment, both restricting anorectic patients and bulimic anorectic patients had fewer "abnormal" curve patterns.

In the study by Halmi et al. (1989), hierarchical regression analyses were used to determine the effect of palatability, amount consumed, rate of eating, body mass index, and cognitions related to ending a meal (urge to eat, preoccupation with food, willpower needed to stop eating, and satisfaction) on hunger and satiety levels. Across all subjects, palatability influenced mainly before-meal levels of hunger and satiety. Amount of meal consumed was significantly related to both before-meal levels of hunger and satiety and after-meal levels of satiety. Rate of eating was significantly related to before-meal hunger pretreatment and before- and after-meal satiety levels posttreatment. Body mass index was related only to before-meal hunger and satiety levels, which in turn strongly affected after-meal hunger and satiety levels. Satiety levels after the meal were predominantly affected by before-meal satiety levels, amount consumed, and rate of eating.

Only after treatment did the groups differ in their palatability rating. Restricting anorectic subjects gave lower ratings for palatability than control subjects, whereas bulimic subjects—both bulimic anorectic subjects and normal-weight bulimic subjects—gave higher ratings than control subjects. Most of the differences in cognitions related to ending a meal occurred before treatment, because after treatment, the patients responded similarly to control subjects. The pretreatment differences were as follows: bulimic subjects had a greater urge to eat after meals than control subjects; all three eating disorder groups were more preoccupied with thoughts of food and felt more uncomfortable after meals than control subjects; and both groups of bulimic subjects (as compared with control subjects) reported that greater willpower was needed to stop eating. At the end of a meal, bulimic subjects said they could eat more than control subjects. Eating made all eating disorder groups feel "unhappy" as compared with control subjects. Both groups of bulimic subjects felt good when they avoided eating, and all eating disorder groups had a greater fear of getting fat and of not being able to stop eating than control subjects. All of these differences disappeared with treatment.

Treatment altered most of the psychological variables assessed but had less effect on the more direct eating-related variables. As mentioned earlier, the psychological variables of preoccupation with thoughts of food and willpower needed to stop eating approximated those of control subjects after treatment. The more physiological or direct eating-related variables of satiety, hunger, palatability, amount eaten, and rate of eating continued to differ among some of the eating disorder subgroups after treatment. After treatment, all patients with anorexia nervosa continued to have lower hunger ratings compared with the other groups, and restricting anorectic patients continued to have higher levels of satiety compared with the other groups. An interesting difference emerged with those patients who had a history of bingeing and purging. They had significantly higher palatability ratings after treatment compared with the restricting anorectic patients and control subjects. These patients should be tested at least a year after maintaining a normal weight and after abstinence from bingeing and purging to determine whether these eating-related characteristics represent a state or trait phenomenon.

In a later study Halmi and Sunday (1991) showed that postmeal cognitions were most interrelated for normal-weight bulimic patients. An increase in the urge to eat was related to an increase in preoccupation with thoughts of food and a lack of satisfaction after the meal. An increase in the preoccupational thoughts of food was related to an increase in the level of willpower needed to stop eating. Urge to eat was positively correlated with monthly binge frequency for the bulimic patients. Bulimic patients who had binged the most were also the most depressed.

The disturbances in hunger and satiety perceptions in eating disorder patients seem to be sui generis. In the Halmi and Sunday (1991) study, these perceptions were not related to other areas of perceptual confusion, such as the interoceptive awareness scale on the Eating Disorders Inventory (Garner et al. 1983) or denial as measured by the L, F, and K scales of the Minnesota Multiphasic Personality Inventory (Hathaway and McKinley 1970). Thus, accumulating evidence suggests that aberrant eating behavior is directly influenced by disturbance of the integrating processes of hunger and satiety perceptions, which are based on cognitive sets and external and internal cues, all of which can be measured and subjected to experimental perturbations for characterization. Disturbed eating in eating disorder patients cannot be dismissed as merely reflecting an underlying psychodynamic turmoil.

Several other studies have indicated that anorectic patients and bulimic patients have disturbances of satiety. Garfinkel et al. (1978) showed that, in contrast to healthy subjects, patients with anorexia nervosa had an absence of satiety aversion to sucrose or "sweet taste" using a Cabanac testing method (Cabanac and Duclaux 1970). This absence of satiety aversion to sucrose was stable at 1-year follow-up and was not affected by significant weight gain to normal levels. Kissileff et al. (1986) successfully conducted laboratory studies of eating behavior in eight women with normal-weight bulimia. When they were requested to eat normally, five of these women ate "excessively" both during the liquid meal and the mixed meal. All patients ate to excess when asked, and all vomited after the meal.

Two other studies, by Mitchell and Laine (1985) and Kaye et al. (1986), investigated the composition of binges in bulimic patients in laboratory settings. The macronutrient composition of the binges was surprisingly similar in all three of the above studies and was similar to the average American diet (46% carbohydrate, 42% fat, and 12% protein). All of these studies indicated that the bulimic patients seemed to consume more as they ate rather than less, producing an increased consumption rate. This suggests that bulimic patients may have a disorder of satiety.

Perceptual Capacities: Sensory Characteristics, Conceptual Identity, and Cognitive Sets Relating to Food

The contextual dimension of the sensory and hedonic aspects of eating is sparsely studied in patients with eating disorders. Because bulimic patients tend to binge on calorie-dense foods and anorectic patients frequently hoard foods with high sugar levels, it was reasonable to suspect that the perception and preferences toward sweet- and fat-containing stimuli in anorectic patients and bulimic patients might differ from that of healthy control subjects. Drewnowski et al. (1987) tested the oral perception of sweetness and fat content using a model system that was palatable and bore a resemblance to real foods. Test stimuli included commercially available skim milk, whole milk, half-and-half, heavy cream, and heavy cream blended with safflower oil, which provided increasing levels of fat content (0.1, 3.5, 10.5, 37.6, and 52.6 g fat per 100 g fluid, respectively).

These five products were combined with sucrose added at levels of 0%, 5%, 10%, and 20% weight/weight to give a total of 20 taste samples. The samples were served chilled at 5°C and were presented to the subjects in 10-ml plastic cups for taste and hedonic evaluation. For the scaling of pleasantness, the subjects used a standard 9-point hedonic preference scale ranging from "dislike extremely" to "like extremely." For the scaling of perceived sweetness and fat content, the subjects used two unipolar 9-point category scales, sweet and fat, with each quality ranging from "absent" to "extreme." The order of stimuli was randomized to reduce potential loss of taste discrimination or taste fatigue.

In this study there were no significant differences in the perceived sweetness or fat content among the three eating disorder groups either before or after treatment. Restricting anorectic patients showed an aversion to fat solutions without sugar at all concentrations (low- and high-fat solutions). Bulimic anorectic patients showed an aversion to high-fat solutions. There were no effects of treatment except that bulimic patients showed a tendency to prefer moderately sweet solutions after treatment. Posttreatment bulimic patients had a significantly higher preference for the 10% sugar solution than did the control subjects. When optimally preferred sucrose and fat levels were determined with the response surface model, both normal-weight bulimic patients and anorectic patients preferred sweeter stimuli compared with control subjects. The anorectic patients and the bulimic patients did not differ in their optima for sucrose. Underweight anorectic patients preferred stimuli of lower fat content compared with control subjects. There were no differences in the optimal preferred fat preferences between normal-weight bulimic patients and control subjects. In the pretreatment condition, body mass index was negatively correlated with the optimally preferred sugar-to-fat ratio. The most underweight subjects expressed greater taste preferences for sweetness over fat, whereas subjects in the normal-weight range showed relatively greater preferences for fat over sugar.

This taste study showed that patients with eating disorders have no deficits in sensory perception of increasing sweetness and fatty stimuli. Underweight restricting anorectic patients and bulimic anorectic patients dislike intense "fat" taste, measured by the magnitude of their preference for the high-fat stimuli relative to that of control subjects. Restricting anorectic patients and bulimic anorectic patients showed significantly larger sweet-to-fat ratios than did control subjects, reflecting elevated preferences for sweetness relative to fat stimuli. No significant differences in taste response profiles or hedonic optimal were obtained, even following an average gain of 10.6 kg after treatment, suggesting that taste responsiveness may not be tied directly to acute changes in body weight. This study indicates that taste profiles could be a highly enduring characteristic of individuals with eating disorders. It also suggests that the pattern of sensory responsiveness to sweetness and fat during childhood or early adolescence may predate changes in body weight and serve as a psychobiological early marker for eating disorders.

Using the same taste-testing methodology, Sunday and Halmi (1991) found again that anorectic subjects disliked high-fat solutions compared with the other groups. The restricting anorectic patients also disliked solutions containing no sugar. Again in the groups with eating disorders, there were no differences in the ability to assess sweetness. Bulimic subjects showed an elevation in intensity ratings of the low-fat solutions. Although each ascending fat level was perceived as "fattier," the greatest perceived difference was between 10.5% and 37.6% fat. In general, solutions with equivalent fat levels were perceived as being fattier with increasing sucrose concentration. For all three of the eating disorder groups, the relationship between preference and perceived fattiness was negative. For control subjects, the correlations between preference and fattiness ratings were positive for 13 of the 20 solutions.

The assessment of fats in the solutions was far more difficult for all subjects. All subjects were able to discern easily the low-fat solutions from the high-fat solutions. However, the intermediate differences were less pronounced. The fat content seemed to be judged on textural qualities. Fat is not a taste, and the ability to assess fat content is learned. The ability to taste sweetness is innate and unambiguous. This may explain the more precise ability of all subjects to determine increasing intensity of sweetness compared with increasing intensity of fatness.

It could be that vomiting-induced oral changes affected the bulimic subjects' ability to assess the fatty texture of dairy solutions, and, once the vomiting ceased, this ability returned to normal. Anorectic subjects were more likely to use low preference ratings for the high-fat concentrations and bulimic anorectic subjects were more likely to use low preference ratings for the highest-fat solutions. Normal-weight bulimic subjects were less likely to use low ratings for the solutions containing the three lowest levels of fat.

Sunday and Halmi (1990) were unsuccessful in characterizing individual preference patterns across fat and sucrose concentrations mathematically, using a response surface analysis. The optimal solution for a diagnostic group yielded few individual hedonic maxima; of those subjects showing a maximum hedonic rating, the majority did not have significant total regressions, thus indicating that their responses were not well represented by this model. Drewnowski et al. (1987) studied the preferences to increasing sweet and fattiness present in semisolid cheese mixtures. In this study, conducted in France, the results were somewhat different when compared with the milk-sugar solutions. Anorectic patients disliked the high-sugar mixtures. One explanation for the difference in hedonic preferences in French anorectic subjects is that they tend to associate high-calorie food with high sweet taste.

The above studies suggest that patients with eating disorders may have different attitudes about food and eating compared with control subjects. Using multidimensional scaling procedures, Drewnowski et al. (1988) revealed that eating disorder patients associated calories with fat content to a greater extent than did control subjects and tended to dislike high-fat foods. In contrast, no differences in perceptions or preferences for carbohydrate foods were observed. This study showed that eating disorder patients associated calories with fat content to a greater degree than did control subjects. Eating disorder patients tended to dislike high-fat foods. Restricting anorectic patients showed the most rigid attitude structure, expressing preferences only for the lowest-calorie and most-nutritious foods.

Blundell and Rogers (1980) showed that the hedonic aspects of the presence of the food itself can override the previously expressed reluctance. Subjective preferences for carbohydrates marked on a preference list were considerably lower than the amount of carbohydrates actually eaten when the foods were presented. Wardle (1987) showed that the response of healthy subjects in the consumption of a meal following a preload (a defined amount of food given at a defined time prior to a meal) was related to the actual calorie content of the preload and not to the subjects' beliefs about the calorie content of the preload. Both "cognitive sets" and macronutrient content (fats, carbohydrates, proteins) are likely to influence the responses of eating disorder patients to foods.

Macronutrient content affects the attitudes and eating behavior differently in restrained (dieting) and unrestrained (nondieting) healthy subjects. One study (King et al. 1987) found that restrained subjects associated the concept of guilt more readily with foods than did unrestrained subjects. Restrained subjects associated guilt with sweet and salty snacks and high-calorie foods. These foods tend to be high in fat. Subjects who were unrestrained considered foods that were low in protein and overall nutritional value to be guilt producing.

In another study examining counterregulation (Knight and Boland 1989), the calorie content of foods was found to be less important to restrained persons than whether the foods were considered to be forbidden (desserts, candy, and high-fat foods). These restrained persons consumed larger quantities of crackers than did control persons when they anticipated either high- or low-calorie forbidden foods (milkshake or ice cream bar) but not when they anticipated isocaloric high- or low-calorie foods that were not forbidden (chef or vegetable salads).

Sunday et al. (1992) studied cognitive sets concerning food in 95 female eating disorder patients admitted to an inpatient treatment program. They also studied restrained and unrestrained healthy control subjects. All subjects rated 38 common foods for preference; presence or absence of guilt and danger; preferred monthly frequency of intake; and calorie, fat, and carbohydrate content. Cognitive ratings were examined based on the individual's perceived amounts of calories and macronutrients. The eating disorder patients were more accurate than either restrained or unrestrained control subjects in their ratings of the calorie, fat, and carbohydrate content of foods. For all subjects, estimates of calorie and fat levels were more accurate than were carbohydrate estimates. Carbohydrate content is a more confusing concept than the concept of fat or calorie content. Hedonic ratings of foods perceived as high in fat or calories were different in patients with current or past anorexia nervosa compared with restrained and unrestrained subjects.

The anorectic patients disliked the foods they perceived to be high in fat or high in calories as compared with low-fat and low-calorie foods. These attitudes did not change with treatment. The fat and calorie aversions seen in these patients appear to be stable characteristics of this disorder. Guilt and danger were perceived as separate constructs by unrestrained and restrained control subjects but not by patients. Perceived high amounts of calories or fat triggered stronger feelings of guilt and danger for restrained control subjects and patients (especially bulimic patients) as compared with unrestrained control subjects.

The above studies demonstrate that, for patients with eating disorders, cognitive sets toward food strongly influence eating behavior.

Conclusion

Eating disorder patients have differences in the integrating mechanisms of hunger and satiety and in their cognitive sets toward food compared with healthy persons. Some of these differences are affected by treatment, whereas others remain unchanged, indicating stable trait characteristics. Careful examination of control subjects showed different cognitive-emotional responses to food based on subjects' classification as restrained or unrestrained eaters. These findings indicate the need to

classify control subjects into restrained and unrestrained categories and the need to test patients before and after treatment to determine the unique eating and food-related cognitions associated with the eating disorders. Analyses of the processes of hunger and satiation during manipulation of contextual variables, such as the macronutrient content of food, should reveal distinguishing differences between eating disorder subgroups and control groups. Likewise, these differences in the perceptions of hunger and satiation should reflect underlying physiological mechanisms (e.g., neurotransmitters and hormones) that are involved in regulating eating.

References

Blundell JE, Hill AJ: Behavioral pharmacology of feeding: relevance of animal experiments for study in man, in Pharmacology of Eating Disorders. Edited by Carruba M, Blundell JE. New York, Raven, 1986, pp 51–70

Blundell JE, Hill AJ: Nutrition, serotonin and appetite: case study in the evolution of a scientific idea. Appetite 8:183–194, 1987

Blundell JE, Rogers PE: Effects of anorectic drugs on food intake, food selections and preferences, hunger motivation and subjective experiences. Appetite 1:151–165, 1980

Booth DA: Appetite and satiety as metabolic expectations, in Food Intake and Chemical Senses. Edited by Katsuki Y, Soto M, Jakagi J, et al. Tokyo, Japan, University of Tokyo Press, 1977, pp 105–110

Booth DA: How should questions about satiation be asked. Appetite 2:237–244, 1981

Cabanac M, Duclaux R: Specificity of internal signals in producing satiety for taste stimuli. Nature 227:966–976, 1970

Drewnowski A, Halmi KA, Pierce B, et al: Taste and eating disorders. Am J Clin Nutr 46:442–450, 1987

Drewnowski A, Pierce B, Halmi KA: Fat aversion in eating disorders. Appetite 10:119–131, 1988

Fairburn C, Cooper PJ: Binge eating, self-induced vomiting and laxative abuse: a community study. Psychol Med 14:401–410, 1984

Garfinkel PE, Moldefsky H, Garner D, et al: Body awareness in anorexia nervosa: disturbances in body image and satiety. Psychosom Med 40:487–497, 1978

Garner DM, Olmstead MP, Polivy J: Development and validation of a multidimensional eating disorder inventory for anorexia nervosa and bulimia. International Journal of Eating Disorders 2:15–34, 1983

Halmi KA: Anorexia nervosa: demographic and clinical features in 94 cases. Psychosom Med 36:18–26, 1974

Halmi KA, Sunday SR: Temporal patterns of hunger and satiety ratings and related cognitions in anorexia and bulimia. Appetite 16:219–237, 1991

Halmi KA, Sunday SR, Puglisi A, et al: Hunger and satiety in anorexia and bulimia nervosa. Ann N Y Acad Sci 575:431–445, 1989

Halmi KA, Eckert E, Marchi P, et al: Comorbidity of psychiatric diagnoses in anorexia nervosa. Arch Gen Psychiatry 48:712–718, 1991

Hathaway SR, McKinley JC: Minnesota Multiphasic Personality Inventory, Revised. Minneapolis, MN, University of Minnesota, 1970

Hill AJ, Magson LD, Blundell JE: Hunger and palatability: tracking ratings of subjective experience before, during, and after the consumption of preferred and less preferred foods. Appetite 5:361–371, 1984

Kaye WH, Gwirtsman HE, George DT, et al: Relationship of mood alterations to bingeing behaviour in bulimia. Br J Psychiatry 149:479–485, 1986

King GA, Hermans CP, Polivy J: Food perception in dieters and non dieters. Appetite 8:147–158, 1987

Kissileff H, Walsh T, Krall J, et al: Laboratory studies of eating behavior in women with bulimia. Physiol Behav 38:563–570, 1986

Knight LJ, Boland FJ: Restrained eating: an experimental disentanglement of the disinhibiting variables of perceived calories and food type. J Abnorm Psychol 98:412–420, 1989

Mitchell JE, Laine D: Monitored binge-eating behavior in patients with bulimia. International Journal of Eating Disorders 4:177–184, 1985

Owen WP, Halmi KA, Gibbs J, et al: Satiety responses in eating disorders. J Psychiatr Res 19:279–284, 1985

Sunday SR, Halmi KA: Taste perceptions and hedonics in eating disorders. Physiol Behav 48:587–594, 1990

Sunday SR, Halmi KA: Taste hedonics in anorexia nervosa and bulimia nervosa, in The Hedonics of Taste. Edited by Bolles R. Hillsdale, NJ, Lawrence Erlbaum, 1991, pp 185–196

Sunday SR, Einhorn A, Halmi KA: The relationship of perceived macronutrient and calorie content to affective cognitions about food. Am J Clin Nutr 55:362–371, 1992

Wardle J: Hunger and satiety: a multidimensional assessment of responses to calorie loads. Physiol Behav 40:577–582, 1987

Section III

Longitudinal and Outcome Studies

Chapter 6

Analysis of Treatment Experience and Outcome From the Johns Hopkins Eating Disorders Program: 1975-1990

Arnold E. Andersen, M.D.

—————⟶≫●≪⟵—————

Analysis of treatment outcome for a program in eating disorders, as for other psychiatric disorders, requires a stable, clearly defined treatment program, as well as a multi-dimensional analysis of both short-term and long-term results. The Eating Disorders Program at the Johns Hopkins Medical Institutions spans 15 years, involving more than 650 inpatients and close to 1,000 outpatients. But, as with a standing wave, the appearance of stability from a distance dissolves into a more impressionistic-like view of constantly moving particles when closely examined. The program has constant features, similar to the shape of the wave, but also changing features, analogous to the molecules of the water. In addition, and here the analogy

I am grateful to the Karen Carpenter Foundation for its generous support of the Johns Hopkins Eating Disorders Program for research and education.

breaks down, there are unresolved issues.

Despite the features of change (a shortcoming from a strict research viewpoint, but necessitated because of the program's clinical focus and the changing demands from third-party payers), an examination of a large, relatively homogeneous clinical population treated with some thematic consistency may provide helpful observations from its dual function as both a local community hospital and a national referral hospital, thereby representing the two major types of eating disorders programs prevalent across the United States.

The inception of the Johns Hopkins Eating Disorders Program in 1975—prior to public awareness of eating disorders and before awareness by the medical community of anorexia nervosa as more than an obscure textbook entity (bulimia nervosa was yet to be described)—was based on three factors. First was my experience with endocrinological evaluation of patients with anorexia nervosa at the National Institutes of Health. Second was the crucial and clear teaching by Professor Gerald Russell as visiting professor. Third, and a necessary component, was the appearance of a patient presenting with severe and chronic anorexia nervosa. Since that time, the program has evolved and has been enlarged, specialized, and transplanted, as well as described in a number of publications (see Andersen 1985).

The following overview is divided into four categories: patient population, program principles, program practices, and psychiatric financing. This is followed by an analysis of outcome. As agreements among clinicians and researchers are made to promote valid and reliable ratings of the severity and stage of a patient's illness (Andersen 1990), comparison of short-term and long-term outcome from distinctly different but thematically consistent long-term treatment programs will be possible and may yield definitive information concerning optimal treatments.

Patient Population

Table 6–1 provides an overview of the patient population in the Johns Hopkins Eating Disorders program.

Diagnostic Categories

Anorexia nervosa as a diagnostic category has been recognized by clinicians since the time of Morton (1694), and especially since Gull (1874)

Table 6–1. Johns Hopkins Eating Disorders Program: patient population 1975–1990

	Constant features	Changed features	Unresolved issues
Diagnostic categories	Anorexia nervosa = anorexia nervosa	1. Subdivision of anorexia nervosa into anorexia nervosa, restricting subtype, and anorexia nervosa, bulimic subtype 2. Bulimia nervosa emerges and consolidates as a syndrome	Is there a continuous spectrum (fingerprint pattern) or are there multiple discrete categories of eating disorders?
Diagnostic criteria and psychopathology	Central psychopathology continues to be irrational (morbid) fear of fatness/relentless pursuit of excessive thinness	1. Diagnosis by inclusion, not exclusion, by nonpsychiatrists 2. Diagnosis more rapid, more accurate, with added specific criteria: progression of Feighner,[a] DSM-III,[b] and DSM-III-R[c]	1. How is a binge defined? 2. Are the endocrine changes essential to diagnosis, and if so, what is the male equivalent of the amenorrhea criterion?
Gender disparity	Cases in males are rare but do occur	Males constitute 1:10 ratio in clinics and general population	Why are there so few males and why those males? Is there a nonspecific dose-response relationship or are gender-specific factors involved?
At-risk individuals	Some individuals are more at risk: white, young females, with avoidant personality features	1. Lower socioeconomic status not protective 2. Risk can be quantitated in specific groups (e.g., ballet dancers, wrestlers)	1. Can at-risk individuals be prospectively identified with valid and reliable psychological instruments? 2. Do males differ in their risk factors?
Severity of illness	Patients are often very ill on admission, and some die of their eating disorder	1. Patients are more ill on admission but fewer die than would be predicted by early follow-up studies 2. Severity of illness can be staged	1. Does early admission for adequate length of treatment lead to improved long-term outcome? 2. Are males more severely ill? 3. Is preventive intervention possible?
Prevailing sociocultural norms	Overvalued belief in thinness	Fit, muscular "tubes" replace "fried chicken wings" (tanned, bony)	1. What will be the next abnormal, abusive demand on body size and shape? 2. Role of AIDS in decreasing value of thinness?

Note. AIDS = acquired immunodeficiency syndrome.
[a]Feighner (Feighner et al. 1972). [b]DSM-III (American Psychiatric Association 1980). [c]DSM-III-R (American Psychiatric Association 1987).

and Lasègue (1873). Anorexia nervosa has remained a clinically homogeneous and recognizable entity, such that a clinician from a century ago would probably make the same diagnosis on a patient today. The subdivision of anorexia nervosa into restricting and bulimic subtypes is of more than academic importance. Several studies completed at Johns Hopkins have found that, relative to all the other subgroups of patients with eating disorders, patients with the bulimic subtype of anorexia nervosa suffer the most both psychologically and physically (Andersen and Mickalide 1985).

The other dramatic change regarding diagnostic categories has been the emergence of bulimia nervosa, not simply as a subdivision of anorexia nervosa, but as a diagnostic category at normal weight. Bulimia nervosa emerged from the population as a substantial and distinct entity, statistically overpowering its predecessor of the bulimic subtype of anorexia nervosa. Professor Gerald Russell (1979) provided the definitive description of the essential characteristics of bulimia nervosa and firmly tied it psychopathologically, through its shared motif of morbid fear of fatness, to anorexia nervosa. How such a substantial and widespread entity as bulimia nervosa could have been submerged from general view and recognition remains a mystery and a challenge.

Regarding diagnostic categories, however, the question of whether there is a continuous ("fingerprint") pattern of endlessly and subtly different categories of eating disorders, or whether there is a relatively small number of discrete categories, is unresolved. In the absence of a firm psychobiological or other pathognomonic method for diagnosis of the eating disorders, these divisions remain clinically based and, therefore, open to the various theoretical persuasions and perspicacities of different clinicians who see the same universe in different sets of clumps and clusters.

Diagnostic Criteria
and Psychopathology

The morbid fear of fatness and the relentless pursuit of excessive thinness remain the central and twin sides of the coinage of the psychopathology of eating disorders. Diagnosis of eating disorders, especially by nonpsychiatrists and also by many psychiatrists, has evolved from a process of exclusion of other disorders to one of inclusion by recognizing the defining features of these disorders.

Despite this progress, however, the definition of what constitutes a binge remains open to discussion and dispute. This is a vital definition because the term *bulimia nervosa* means "ox-hunger" and requires binge eating, but not necessarily purging, to be present. Whether to use objective criteria involving a certain number of calories of a particular nutritional density, or whether to emphasize the subjective sense of loss of control, remains undecided (Ortega et al. 1987). Also, regarding diagnostic criteria and psychopathology, it is unsettled whether endocrine changes are essential to diagnosis or are simply nonspecific consequences of weight loss. Finally, there is an implicit bias present in the criteria by having an endocrine criterion for females (amenorrhea) but no equivalent in males.

Gender Disparity

The first description of anorexia nervosa widely accepted in the English language, that of Morton, interestingly reported one male and one female. With implications to be discussed later, it was the male who did better in outcome. The fact that cases in males are uncommon but do occur has been part of the early literature of anorexia nervosa, but was submerged for some time in the first 60 years of the 20th century because of inherent biases in the diagnostic criteria.

Population samples from referral clinics do not necessarily constitute, qualitatively or quantitatively, an accurate representation of the general population. The finding of an almost precise 1:10 ratio of males to females over a period of 15 years at the Johns Hopkins Eating Disorders Program must be viewed with some caution. Having recognized this caution, however, it is interesting that recent population-based studies (Råstam et al. 1989) have found a similar ratio of 1:10 in an unselected general population.

The questions of why so few males develop eating disorders, and why those particular males, have not been satisfactorily answered. Andersen and DiDomenico (1992) evaluated the popular magazines most widely read by males and females ages 18–24 years and found essentially a "dose-response" relationship between reinforcement factors, such as number of magazine articles and advertisements promoting dieting, and the ratio of males to females with eating disorders, suggesting sociocultural reinforcements rather than intrinsic, gender-related biological or psychological differences to account for the 1:10 ratio. Groups in which males are exposed to relentless reinforcements for slimming or change in body shape have produced high rates of eating disorders.

Individuals at Risk

The clinical picture of the young, white female with avoidant personality features being predisposed to anorexia nervosa has not changed. Recent studies (Kishchuk et al. 1992), however, suggest that lower socioeconomic status, previously thought to be somewhat protective from anorexia nervosa, may in fact not be protective at all, and the lower rates in lower socioeconomic groups may simply reflect differential access to medical facilities. Studies have documented specific quantitative risk increases with certain populations requiring weight loss, such as ballet dancers (Frisch et al. 1980) and wrestlers (Steen et al. 1988).

Unresolved is the issue of whether individuals who are at risk can be prospectively identified with valid and reliable psychological instruments. The primary goal of medicine is prevention rather than treatment. Identification of patients with probable eating disorders in situ would represent a major advance. Cooper et al. (1989) developed a more specific and reliable questionnaire than the Eating Attitudes Test (Garner et al. 1982) or the Eating Disorders Inventory (Garner et al. 1983). Unresolved also is whether males differ in their risk factors quantitatively or qualitatively compared with females with similar demographic features. Males may, for example, have more obsessional features to their personality.

Severity of Illness

Unchanged for 15 years is the recognition that patients are often medically as well as psychologically very ill on admission for treatment of anorexia nervosa or bulimia nervosa and may die from their eating disorder. Since the inception of the treatment program at Johns Hopkins, although patients appear to have presented with progressively more severe illness, fewer have died than would be predicted by earlier studies.

Unresolved, however, is whether early admission for an adequate length of time to treat the disorder definitively leads to improved outcome compared with multiple short admissions. Many reimbursement policies are structured such that repetitive short admissions are inevitable. I propose as a necessary future study to compare and contrast these two different methods of treatment to evaluate subsequent severity of illness and degree of improvement on a long-term basis.

Prevailing Sociocultural Norms

In the last 50 years, society has continued its overvalued belief in the superlative qualities of thinness. The thin, tanned, bony picture of the model Twiggy in the 1960s, however, has given way to the more fit, muscular, tubular form favored by athletically fit young women now featured in popular magazines. According to anecdotal reports from our patients, this emphasis has led to patients' seeking breast reduction operations if the voguish, tubular appearance now valued has not been endowed by nature or earned by compulsive exercise, or if the formerly sought hourglass figure desired in the 1940s was conferred instead.

The appearance of the next abusive and abnormal demand on body size and shape remains to be seen. Society, both cross-sectionally throughout the world at present and longitudinally from a historical perspective, has often demanded abusive changes in body shape or size that, in retrospect, appear absurd. However, this critical perspective is lost when one is submerged in the culture in which these demands are the status quo.

Program Principles

The program at the Johns Hopkins Hospital has maintained a relatively enduring set of constant features in regard to its program principles since 1975 (Table 6–2). However, some aspects have changed, or emerged, and, as with the other areas of discussion, a number of issues remain unresolved.

Initial Priority in Treatment

A consensus emerged in the 1970s that the first priority of treatment was to change promptly the abnormal behavior of self-starvation. More psychoanalytically oriented therapists were previously persuaded, in contrast, that only after the attainment of insight and working through of psychodynamic issues could change in behavior be requested or encouraged. Although the program at Johns Hopkins has never endorsed exclusively behavioral principles, it has maintained through its history that prompt and thorough changing of abnormal behaviors should take priority before or along with psychological work. We have found that not only can abnormal behavior such as self-starvation be promptly and thoroughly changed, but the rate of weight restoration can be substan-

Table 6–2. Johns Hopkins Eating Disorders Program: program principles 1975–1990

	Constant features	Changed features	Unresolved issues
Initial priority in treatment	Change the abnormal behavior promptly and thoroughly	Rate of weight gain increased from 2.2 to 3 pounds/week	1. What is the upper limit to rate of weight gain? 2. How much medical testing is appropriate?
Comprehensive emphasis	Changing the abnormal behavior is never enough	1. Recognition of how many and varied are the comorbidities 2. Emergence of identity issues 3. Cognitive-behavioral and interpersonal approaches both effective 4. *Perspectives of Psychiatry* by McHugh and Slavney	1. Tension between behavioral and psychodynamic emphasis continues—what can treatment expect to accomplish? 2. How to determine ideal body weight—group norms versus individualized methods?
Attitude toward patients	Be kind to patients: 1. Psychologically—don't blame them or their families 2. Medically—normal food eaten normally	1. Active psychoeducational patient involvement in addition to passive reception of kindness 2. Discontinuance of hyperalimentation on most medical services	1. What to do with chronically ill, noncompliant patients? Are they ill or irresponsible? 2. Are prokinetic agents useful or should patients tolerate discomfort until natural resolution of gastrointestinal distress?
Treatment personnel	Multidisciplinary team required	Separate and overlapping responsibilities of team members defined	1. Who is qualified to diagnose and treat eating disorder patients? 2. Do adjunctive therapies play a meaningful role? 3. Should there be separate treatment groups for anorexia nervosa versus bulimia nervosa, adolescents versus adults?
Psycho-pharmacology	Use medications, but selectively	1. Medications often given concomitant with, rather than sequential to, change in behavior 2. Emergence of fluoxetine as a widely used antidepressant	1. Is any medication effective for central psychopathology of anorexia nervosa? 2. Are antidepressants "anti-binge" as well as antidepressant?

Role of families	Families are vitally involved	1. Progression of conceptualization of role of parents from causative to dyadic interaction to family systems theory 2. Multigenerational emphasis	1. What is the role of family in treatment: enforcers versus supporters? 2. Can failure to thrive result from familial eating disorder psychopathology? 3. Are parents of eating disorder patients abnormal in weight?
Etiology and mechanism	Unknown, probably multifactorial, leading to pragmatic, integrative treatments	"Critical cluster" concept, with hierarchy of mechanisms as a function of stage of illness	1. Value of reductionistic, biomedical paradigm versus appreciation of conditioned emotional responses and complex psychodynamic and behavioral mechanisms 2. Proof of critical cluster of factors in predisposing, precipitating, promulgating, and "prevailing" phases of illness
Duration of treatment	Because illness may be long term, treatment must be extended as long as needed	Emergence of day hospital and other step-up/step-down approaches to long-term treatment	1. What are criteria for rehospitalization? 2. Is "cure" possible or is pessimism justified? 3. What is optimum sequence of psychotherapeutic methods?
Brain function	The brain may be abnormal in structure and function	1. Brain changes are probably secondary, not primary 2. Documentation of brain shrinkage in anorexia nervosa and abnormal positron-emission tomography scan in bulimia nervosa	1. How long for brain to return to normal after weight restored, or interruption of binge-purge behavior? 2. How to separate eating disorder brain changes from nonspecific changes or from comorbid processes? 3. Is an animal model possible for eating disorders?
Research	Conduct research along with treating eating disorders; it is necessary, interesting, and keeps you from getting bored or "burned out"	1. Multiplication of research methods in eating disorders—a growth industry with every form of modern technology 2. Description of presence of counterregulation in bulimia nervosa eating behavior 3. True medical anorexia is present in anorexia nervosa	1. How can we conduct better interinstitutional research by standardizing research criteria for comparability of patients (diagnosis, severity, comorbidity), specificity of treatment, and comprehensiveness of outcome research? 2. How are the regulatory aspects of eating behavior altered in eating disorder patients? 3. What is perceptual distortion?

tially increased from our former rate of approximately 1 kg per week to 3 pounds or more per week.

It has not been empirically determined what the upper limit to the rate of weight gain from "normal food eaten normally" is, but our appreciation of some increase in subjective gastrointestinal complaints and in pedal edema suggests that 3 pounds may be close to the maximum. Unresolved, also, is the question of how much medical testing is appropriate for initial evaluation of patients with starvation. When the history of anorexia nervosa is clear, the patient's illness and response to treatment generally assumes a fairly predictable physiological course, suggesting that medical tests formerly thought to be necessary may now be prudently limited to lower costs. Tests such as X rays of the gastrointestinal tract are usually not necessary.

Comprehensive Emphasis

Although the principle of changing the abnormal behaviors promptly and thoroughly has continued, so has the conviction that changing abnormal behavior never, by itself, constitutes adequate or complete treatment. Recent studies have documented a multiplicity of comorbidities in patients with eating disorders. Studies using the Schedule for Affective Disorders and Schizophrenia, Lifetime Version (Endicott and Spitzer 1978), have found from two to four psychiatric comorbidities in patients with subgroups of eating disorders (Andersen et al. 1988). Fairburn et al. (1991) demonstrated that an interpersonal approach to psychotherapy of these patients may, in fact, be as effective as a cognitive-behavioral approach. *The Perspectives of Psychiatry* by McHugh and Slavney (1983) emphasized multimodal influences on disorders of human behavior, with the implication that treatment must be broadly based.

The tension continues, however, between a behavioral and a psychodynamic emphasis, even in an apparently uniform and consistent treatment program, especially when changes occur in the attending physicians and other staff. Other questions remain. What can treatment be expected to accomplish? Should the goal be the achievement of humans so free from any defects, quirks, whims, or abnormalities that they would be healthier than unselected members of the general population? Or, rather, should treatment be confined to eliminating clearly defined disorders or toward promoting human growth and development?

What constitutes adequate weight restoration also remains unclear. Various population-based norms, such as the Metropolitan Height and

Weight Tables (Metropolitan Life Insurance Co 1983), have themselves changed. For its first 10 years, the Johns Hopkins program simultaneously used the Metropolitan tables for adults, the nomograms of Frisch and McArthur (1974) for adolescents, and the Kemsley (1951) population-based norms for research analysis.

Attitude Toward Patients

A theme of kindness to patients, psychologically and medically, has been a stated goal of the treatment team at Johns Hopkins Hospital. This may seem to be a universally accepted theme that does not need reiteration. However, in our experience during the first several years of the program, we frequently received patients who had been told that they or their families were to blame for their disorders. Also, through the teaching of Professor Gerald Russell, and following the example of Gull (1874) more than a century ago, the medical nutritional emphasis has been on refeeding patients with normal food eaten in a normal manner. Documentation of the adverse consequences of hyperalimentation has supported this decision in retrospect.

The attitude toward patients has evolved, however, from being passively kind to patients, asking them to accept prudent and conservative treatment, to promoting an active, psychoeducational, collaborative relationship. The publication of teaching material regarding psychoeducation by Garner et al. (1985) has given specific information and techniques to help with active patient involvement.

Staff attitude, however, has remained mixed, and sometimes conflicted, toward chronically ill, noncompliant patients, with some staff undecided about whether these patients are ill or irresponsible. Even though "normal food eaten normally" has been a thematically constant program feature, the role of "prokinetic" agents to decrease gastric discomfort has not been resolved. We have demonstrated that gastrointestinal symptomatology improves with refeeding alone, without the addition of prokinetic agents (Waldholtz and Andersen 1990). Other studies, however, have suggested use of these agents routinely (Saleh and Lebwohl 1980).

Treatment Personnel

The view that a multidisciplinary team is essential to treatment has remained, but the separate and overlapping responsibilities of team members have been increasingly well defined (Hedblom et al. 1981). The issue of just who is qualified to diagnose and treat patients with eating disorders, however, is unresolved. Although this is not problematic within the Johns Hopkins program, we receive patients from many health professionals of various degrees of expertise and discharge patients to the same variety of therapists. Efforts to credential or license diagnostic or treatment facilities have not yet succeeded. What used to be an esoteric, academic disorder, diagnosed in university hospitals by specialized psychiatrists, has given way to diagnosis by family members, teachers, social workers, nurses, and pediatricians—a helpful advance, but not without potential problems.

It is not clear yet whether adjunctive therapies such as dance therapy and movement therapy play a meaningful role or simply make treatment more pleasant. It is also not agreed on yet whether there should be different treatment facilities for the different subtypes of eating disorders or for patients of different ages.

Psychopharmacology

The principle of using psychopharmacological agents in a selective manner, when necessary, has not changed. What has changed, however, has been the concomitant use of psychopharmacological agents rather than the delay of their use until the full response to nutritional rehabilitation can be observed. This is partly due to the pressure of third-party payers and decreased lengths of stay as well as to increased confidence in diagnosis of affective disorders in individuals and families.

Fluoxetine has emerged as a widely used antidepressant primarily for patients with bulimia nervosa but also to some extent as a possible means of altering the central psychopathology of anorexia nervosa. It is unresolved, however, whether any psychopharmacological agent can significantly or even slightly change the central psychopathological features of overvaluation of thinness and phobic avoidance of fatness. Whether antidepressants are directly effective in reducing the tendency to binge or whether their effect on bingeing is through their effect on associated depressive disorders is not settled. Some antidepressants, however, do appear to reduce bingeing even in nondepressed bulimic patients.

Role of Families

The principle of family involvement was outlined in detail by Lasègue (1873) more than a century ago, and his work remains a vital document for family treatment. The prior conceptualization of families as having a causative role in the onset of anorexia nervosa has yielded first to a dyadic concept of patient-parent interaction and more recently to a family systems theory. In addition, an appreciation of the multigenerational contributions to family structure and function has evolved and led to broader evaluation techniques.

Whether family members should be enforcers of treatment or supporters who simply encourage patients but leave the treatment to professionally trained staff has not been established. A darker side of family interaction has emerged with our finding that some cases of failure to thrive in children may result from maternal fear of fatness being translated into behavioral deprivation of children's food.

Etiology and Mechanism

We have continued to maintain, in the absence of more empirical data, the principle that eating disorders and other disorders of motivated behavior are of unknown origin, but are probably multifactorial, leading us to pragmatic and integrative treatments rather than to specific, rational methods based on understanding of fundamental pathogenic mechanisms. This diffuse multifactorial concept of origin has been conceptually refined somewhat, however, to involve a concept of a "critical cluster" of factors in the origin of eating disorders and a sequential cascade of possibly very different mechanisms that subserve the subsequent different stages of illness. Still unresolved is whether these disorders can be entirely subsumed into a paradigm of operantly conditioned emotional responses. Although a critical cluster concept of multiple factors for etiology and mechanism that differ in the sequential stages of predisposition, precipitation, promulgation, and amelioration makes sense, no definite proof has been demonstrated based on clear research methodology to make this more than an organizing concept.

Duration of Treatment

Although the need for extended treatment continues to be recognized, there has emerged a "step-up" and "step-down" approach to care by the development of several steps between weekly outpatient care and 24-hour inpatient care. The day hospital especially has emerged as a programmatically sophisticated treatment.

When to readmit patients is unresolved and is a decision perhaps determined more by access to adequate facilities and reimbursement policies than by rational psychiatric and medical criteria. How long patients should remain in treatment remains unresolved because the definition of "cure" remains vague. In practice, many therapists have an unduly pessimistic attitude toward patients with eating disorders, and there is no evidence that a majority of patients cannot be freed completely from symptoms. I have suggested a sequence of psychotherapeutic methods for patient care that appreciates the different strengths and needs of patients coming into treatment centers (Andersen 1989). This sequence begins with supportive and psychoeducational efforts and proceeds to cognitive-behavioral, psychodynamic, and existential stages of psychotherapy.

Brain Function

The hypothalamus has been, in many ways, the all-purpose source of explanation for unknown mechanisms of behavioral abnormality, remaining a "black hole" of understanding of these more complicated motivated behaviors. Research during the last 15 years has suggested that brain changes are definitely present in both anorexia nervosa and bulimia nervosa—structurally, functionally, and biochemically—but these changes are almost certainly consequences rather than primary causes. The brain diminishes in size as the body is severely starved and is not invulnerable as previously thought.

It is not clear, however, how long it takes for the brain to return to normal weight and function after body weight is restored or binge behavior is interrupted. It has been suggested that an animal model is not possible for eating disorders (Stricker and Andersen 1980), but certain aspects of the eating disorders may well be susceptible to induction, observation, and treatment in nonhuman species.

Research

A principle of conducting research along with treatment has continued at Johns Hopkins Hospital. In addition to the implied demands for research based on being a research institution and a university hospital, research efforts also keep staff from suffering from boredom or becoming "burned out," a vague but observable state of dissatisfaction. Research, however, has evolved from a more descriptive and passive observational approach into active testing of prospective, hypothesis-driven research proposals. Research on patients with bulimia nervosa has demonstrated, for example, that counterregulatory aspects of eating behavior may be central to perpetuating bulimia nervosa. Although the term *anorexia nervosa* was formerly considered by us to be flawed because of the absence of true medical anorexia, recent studies have demonstrated that true loss of appetite is present in anorexia nervosa in proportion to starvation (Rolls et al., in press).

Comparisons between patient groups in different institutions remain limited, however, because of the lack of standardized research criteria for defining patients in terms of severity and comorbidity and because of the difficulty in validating whether the stated thematic emphasis of a given program is, in fact, the one practiced. Many aspects of regulatory behavior of eating disorder patients remain unknown. The term *perceptual distortion* is used widely but its essential meaning as a useful and discrete phenomenon has been challenged.

Program Practices

Table 6–3 provides an overview of the program practices of the Johns Hopkins Eating Disorders program.

Nutrition

Unchanged at Johns Hopkins is the utilization of nutritional rehabilitation by progressively increasing energy (calorie) intakes, beginning with 1,200–1,500 calories per day, increasing to higher levels. What has changed has been the introduction of a specified and rapid stepwise progression to a maximum of 3,500–4,500 calories per day, increasing by 500-calorie increments every 4 days. Micronutrients such as zinc have been suggested as playing a role in the pathogenesis or maintenance of these disorders, but no conclusive evidence has emerged to confirm the role of micronutrients. Unresolved also is the issue of how fast feeding can take place, and especially how to decrease the length of stay without provoking increased gastrointestinal symptomatology or refeeding edema, either peripherally or centrally.

Nursing Supervision

Because of the patient's conflicted attitudes toward weight restoration and fears of ingestion of normal amounts of food, the principle of close

Table 6-3. Johns Hopkins Eating Disorders Program: program practices 1975–1990

	Constant features	Changed features	Unresolved issues
Nutrition	Begin with 1,200–1,500 calories/day, increasing slowly to 3,500 calories/day	1,500 calories/day, increasing rapidly to 3,500–4,500 calories/day	1. Role of micronutrients in treatment—trace minerals, vitamins? 2. Will more rapid refeeding increase gastrointestinal symptoms and refeeding edema?
Nursing supervision	Concept of 1:1 nursing supervision; moderate length of constant observation, decreasing in slow steps to maintenance phase	1. Increase from literal 1:1 to 1:5–10 patients supervised at meals 2. Strict level of constant observation, with rapid decrease only after attaining goal weight	Will video cameras and constant measurement of food intake and eating behavior be implemented?
Goal weight	3 standards: Metropolitan Life, Frisch and McArthur, Kemsley	1 standard: Metropolitan Life, with 2 ranges, one lower range for anorexia nervosa versus one higher range for overweight bulimia nervosa patients	Will we adopt 1990 Calloway, unified, gender-free, two-tier, age-related standard of optimal weight?
Exercise	Reasonable amount	Dependent on osteoporosis evaluation for bone mineral density	Is exercise useful as a method to attain optimal body shape and distribution during treatment?
Research	Observational and retrospective	Evolved concept: a. Every meal an experiment b. Every patient potentially a research subject	1. Are anorectic starved patients useful as models for Third-World malnutrition? 2. Comparability of osteoporosis in elderly and anorexia nervosa?
Recruitment practice	Passive recruitment	Active, noncompetitive, with coordinator and outreach program	Should we become more active, competitive, with marketing consultation?

one-to-one nursing supervision has continued to be strongly emphasized at Johns Hopkins Hospital. Beginning, however, with a very staff-
intensive, literal, one-to-one supervision of patients with eating
disorders; having a separate primary nurse for each patient; and choos-
ing a single nurse for supervising a small group of patients while eating
has proved to be comparably satisfactory. Instead of a variable and very
individualized approach to nursing supervision, a protocol has been established in which strict 14-hour (8 A.M. to 10 P.M.), continued, direct observation of patients has been instituted and is maintained until patients
are at their goal weight or, if suffering from bulimia nervosa ongoing,
for at least 2 weeks.

More sophisticated methodologies using video cameras and constant
measurement of food intake may well be important for future treatment
as well as research, but such a technologically sophisticated, practical, and
clinical program has not yet evolved. In hospitals that utilize state-of-the-
art, highly evolved, technological approaches to subtle aspects of surgical
instrumentation, it is surprising how relatively crude are the methods for
behavioral assessment and treatments.

Goal Weight

As noted previously, in the past there were three different standards for
ideal weight for different subgroups or ages of patients. Currently only
one standard, the Metropolitan Life, is used, with a lower normal-weight
range applied to patients emerging from anorexia nervosa and a higher
normal-weight range for those patients with bulimia nervosa who have
been overweight.

Just as these changes have been accepted, however, a new, much
broader normal-weight range has been suggested by C. W. Calloway (personal communication, April 1990), proposing a gender-free, two-tier, age-
related standard for optimal weight. Perhaps in the future there will be a
change from any weight goal to other more physiologically significant
indices, such as percentage of body fat or waist-to-hip ratios, but these
have not yet been widely adopted in the treatment of patients with eating
disorders. The enduring goal is to free patients from being committed to
an unhealthy weight range.

Exercise

The practice of giving to patients a reasonable but subjective and individualized amount of exercise during their nutritional rehabilitation

has yielded to preexercise evaluations of bone mineral density using dual photon spectrometry. The recognition of possibly significant amounts of osteoporosis in these patients with eating disorders has required evaluation of this potentially hidden but serious problem prior to significant exercise.

Exercise, however, plays an unresolved role in the attainment of optimal body shape and distribution during in-hospital treatment. A major complaint of patients during treatment is the relatively larger amount of fat that appears to deposit selectively on the abdomen during early stages of refeeding. Whether a more acceptable body shape can be achieved during refeeding that will prevent future provocation of renewed efforts for slimming after discharge remains unresolved. Exercise is often perceived as being too low in technology or budget to receive the extraordinary attention and expense of more technically sophisticated approaches in medicine, which themselves have not necessarily been very effective.

Research

The practice of continuing to emphasize research has led to the goal that "every meal is an experiment; every patient is potentially a research subject." Patients, even though seeming to be uniform from a distance, are sufficiently diverse such that each one can teach the clinician something new, and, for associated research studies, can provide valuable information about both eating disorders and the extremes of human physiology. Researchers would be threatened with jail or other punishments if they caused humans to choose the extreme physiological states into which anorectic and bulimic patients regularly put themselves. These patients, therefore, provide extraordinary opportunities for both formal hypothesis testing as well as descriptive and observational research.

Whether patients with anorexia nervosa would serve as models for Third-World malnourished individuals and whether the osteoporosis in anorexia nervosa is comparable to that found in elderly patients remain unresolved, however. Programs comparing the response of patients with anorexia to different nutritional programs would be of value in comparing changes in blood lipids, distribution of body fat, and perhaps coronary artery consequences from very different kinds of caloric intake.

Recruitment Practice

The combination of public alarm from the widespread awareness of anorexia nervosa plus presence of relatively few treatment facilities led to a temporary situation during the late 1970s and early 1980s of treatment sites having long waiting lists of patients. This state was accompanied by a passive recruitment policy that has since had to evolve toward an active, coordinated recruitment policy, often with an outreach component, as programs have proliferated, patients have become restricted in health care cost coverage, and much of the backlog of patients has been treated.

Whether university hospitals should become active, competitive, marketing groups remains unresolved. More and more facilities are competing for an apparently stable, slowly growing number of patients.

Psychiatric Financing

Few topics evoke more emotional responses than medical financing. Society at large and the government in particular have accelerating medical costs and shrinking health care financial resources. A variety of thoughtless and ruthless responses have been promoted to cut costs. The financing of medical care in the United States has remained quite variable; it is significantly different from city to city and according to socioeconomic status. Table 6–4 overviews psychiatric financing at the Johns Hopkins Eating Disorders Program.

Source of Financing

A majority of eating disorder patients at Johns Hopkins continue to have care financed by third-party payers. In the last 10 years, however, health maintenance organizations have widely appeared and have on the whole ravaged fiscal support for psychiatric care. There is little uniformity among health maintenance organizations, which have a single, overriding, shared concern for minimizing costs by a variety of ruthless mechanisms. They, on the whole, have used attractive, misleading information to recruit healthy individuals who will not utilize the medical care required for chronic or severe illness. There have been increases in deductibles, increases in copayments, and decreases in lifetime benefits (often to a ridiculous amount), with a generally chaotic structuring de-

Table 6–4. Johns Hopkins Eating Disorders Program: psychiatric financing 1975–1990

	Constant features	Changed features	Unresolved issues
Source of financing	1. Third-party payers 2. Occasional self-pay	1. Health maintenance organizations appear widely 2. No free hospital care 3. Decreased state coverage	Will we obtain parity of medical and psychiatric coverage?
Classification of disorder for reimbursement	Psychiatric *or* medical classification possible and defensible	Comorbid psychiatric conditions may be primary diagnosis at admission	Should we promote a sequential classification of initial medical status followed by psychiatric designation?
Adequacy of reimbursement	Moderately to fully adequate	Moderately adequate to completely inadequate	Will we see continued increase in copayments, deductibles, and decreased maximum lifetime benefits?
Length of stay	90–100 days required for classical anorexia	31 days overall: all subtypes of eating disorders	1. Continued decrease in length of stay? 2. Adequacy of multiple short-term hospitalizations versus definitive care?
Frequency of case evaluation for reimbursement	Some form of case evaluation may be performed	Prospective and ongoing evaluation, with occasional retrospective denial	Will we see the evolution of concomitant, on-site, continuous review, and possible treatment dictation?
Location of program and billing practice	1. Department of psychiatry 2. Separate professional fees, independent of hospital charges	1. Moved physically from a separate building, psychologically isolated from the main hospital, to a unit within the medical hospital, perceived as more integrated 2. Single professional fee	1. Would an intensive care unit for eating disorder patients on admission serve a clinical purpose and provide increased staff and billing? 2. Change to unbundled billing versus one comprehensive fee for hospital plus professional fees?

signed to discourage patients from obtaining adequate benefits. Hospitals themselves no longer provide free care, and state coverage has decreased.

Unresolved is whether legislative action will bring parity in medical and psychiatric coverage. There is no rational reason why psychiatric costs should be financed at a lower level of coverage than medical costs. It could be well argued that the personal contributions to disorders such as coronary disease and cancer are as great or substantially greater than that for anorexia nervosa or bulimia nervosa.

Classification of Eating Disorders for Reimbursement

At the beginning of our program at Johns Hopkins, patients with anorexia nervosa could be classified as psychiatric or medically ill according to where they were hospitalized, at times having comparable patients within the same hospital on different services. Because of the increased recognition of the comorbid psychiatric conditions in eating disorder patients, the primary diagnosis at admission may, in fact, not be the eating disorder. It is unresolved whether eating disorders should be classified sequentially as being initially a medical disorder and later a psychiatric disorder according to whether they meet separate criteria for medical and psychiatric classification.

Adequacy of Reimbursement

Inpatient treatment teams of 10–15 years ago did not utilize much time in planning the financial aspects of treatment of patients with eating disorders. As reimbursement decreased and as requirements for documentation increased, a clinician may now spend more time on obtaining reimbursement than on providing psychotherapy for these patients. A relentless, whittling away of adequate reimbursement continues.

Length of Stay

Table 6–5 shows the decrease in length of stay of patients in the Johns Hopkins program from a high of 126 days to a recent 30-day average. For minimum optimal treatment of classical anorexia nervosa, 90–100 days of treatment are still required. This need for long admissions for anorexia nervosa has to be compensated for by locating patients with short admissions due to other diagnoses, to financial limitations, or other pressures limiting length of stay, such as vocational commitments and family obligations, to obtain an acceptable overall average length of stay. The daunting perspective faces us that length of stay may continue to be ratcheted down to completely inadequate levels of 7–14 days for patients with eating disorders, as is now present in some states.

Frequency of Third-Party Case Evaluation

Some form of retrospective case evaluation was routinely performed on only a subset of patients at the beginning of our treatment program. Over the next 15 years, evaluations became prospective as well as retro-

Table 6–5.   Change in length of stay and ratio of diagnostic subtypes: 1975–1990

Year	Patients (N)	Average age (years)	Average length of stay (days)	Males (n)	No. discharges against medical advice	Diagnostic subtypes as %[a] (ANR:ANB: BNH×AN:BN)
1975	1	43	126	0	0	
1976	6	30	82	0	0	
1977	16	21	69	2	3	85:15:0:0
1978	22	23	71	1	3	
1979	25	23	100	1	0	
1980	25	21	122	4	1	
1981	29	23	93	2	2	
1982	31	24	84	4	1	
1983	36	24	76	5	0	38:23:21:18
1984	36	26	62	4	3	
1985	50	24	69	5	1	
1986	46	25	78	5	2	
1987	58	26	51	7	1	
1988	66	26	49	9	3	
1989	89	27	35	8	10	31:33:11:25
1990	84	26	30	10	6	
Average		25.8 ± 1.3	74.8 ± 1.8	4.2 ± 0.8 (10.8%)	2.3 ± 0.7 (5.8%)	

Note. ANR = anorexia nervosa, restricting subtype. ANB = anorexia nervosa, bulimic subtype. BNHxAN = bulimia nervosa with history of anorexia nervosa. BN = bulimia nervosa without a history of anorexia nervosa.
[a]Three sample years are analyzed.

spective, and ongoing evaluations were initiated. There is the realistic prospect of essentially daily review and associated dictation of treatment if the present trend continues. Individuals of modest or inadequate clinical credentials have now assumed the role of dictating treatment length and content to experienced clinicians. Where this practice will lead is not clear but it has consumed an enormous amount of staff time in justifying essential admissions.

Location of Program and Billing Practice

The program at Johns Hopkins has been located in the Department of Psychiatry. As the department has moved from a physically separate building, psychologically isolated from the main hospital, to a unit within the main hospital, its perception of being an integral part of the medical institution has increased. We have not yet developed a separately billed, physically discrete "intensive care unit" for seriously ill eating disorder purposes that would serve both clinical and administrative goals, including adequate reimbursement for the increased staff required for these seriously ill patients during the initial phase of treatment.

Billing for professional fees has remained separate from hospital charges. Professional fees have evolved from an "unbundled" approach (i.e., charging for each aspect of care separately) to a single comprehensive professional fee, a change in the opposite direction of the trend in other specialties toward unbundling.

Conclusion of Program Analysis

This overview of a 15-year experience demonstrates that even a seemingly homogeneous and continuous program is, in fact, constantly changing and evolving for three primary reasons. First, new scientific knowledge must be translated into practical program changes as soon as possible. Second, attending staff members often have differing views or principles and practices. Third, financial coverage has changed remarkably.

Recognizing these forces for change, there are still several overarching thematic consistencies that have been maintained despite the advent and incorporation of new knowledge, staff differences, and decreased insurance coverage. These include altering abnormal behavior promptly, treating the patient comprehensively, limiting invasive procedures, treating with the most natural and least damaging methods even if they appear low budget and low technology, not blaming patients or families, maintaining a multifactorial approach to etiology, remaining pragmatic where fundamental knowledge is lacking, conducting research along with treatment, teaching at every level of clinical interaction, emphasizing patient psychosocial growth and development as well as relief from illness, and, where possible, conducting treatment trials that are scientifically valid and reliable.

The body exists to nourish the brain. The aspects of the brain that are most unique to humans are those that seek meaning, identity, and relationship. Based on these two bold-faced statements, we are led to the belief that eating disorders are, in the end, integrative, adaptive, self-sustaining, biobehavioral responses to issues of meaning, identity, and intimacy. Any view of eating disorders that purports to understand their origin or treatment on the basis of conditioned reflexes, strictly behavioral paradigms, or neurochemical function remains inadequate in our view. The opposite, polar approach of emphasizing only the issues of identity, meaning, and relationship without changing the abnormal life-threatening behaviors, physical consequences, or abnormal thinking has been clearly outdated for some time. As oil, vinegar, and herbs remaining separate are unpalatable in their discrete states, so single-modal conceptualizations of eating disorders regarding origin or treatment remain unsatisfactory. Only when radically different understandings, perspectives, and methods, seemingly incompatible, are shaken together in the same crucible does successful treatment emerge for the eating disorders. The challenge of keeping horses racing in opposite directions (behavioral versus neurochemical versus psychodynamic) harnessed together to jointly pull the treatment along remains the model for the treatment of eating disorders. Joining the seemingly disparate methods of nutritional rehabilitation, behavioral relearning, psychopharmacology, and cognitive psychodynamic and existential psychotherapy, whether in tandem or in sequence, represents currently the optimal approach to treatment of eating disorders, based on the Johns Hopkins experience of 15 years. Reductionism in medical science has a strong but specious appeal because of its clear methods and results. Clarity may be at the expense of truth, and oversimplification may be misleading. The 19th century paradigm of the infectious disease single etiology approach to medical understanding is inadequate as a model for disorders of motivated behavior.

Short-Term Results and Follow-Up

The results of treatment outcome of our program must prove or disprove these points of belief and rhetoric. Short-term inpatient results and a partial study of long-term outcome for women have been published (Andersen 1985). A follow-up study on men (Andersen and Mickalide 1983) found a gender-unrelated comparable outcome. Long-term comprehensive follow-up is in progress. In the meantime, available program results are summarized here. In addition, some new information is provided describing in more detail three years: 1977, the second full year of operation; 1983, the middle of the study period; and 1989, the last year for which results are available.

Treatment Response

Over a 15-year period, 620 patients were admitted, with a steady progression in patient admissions. Along with steadily increasing admissions has been a shortening in length of stay from more than 120 days to 30 days in 1991, a fourfold decrease.

The average age of patients has remained surprisingly high, 25.8 ± 1.3 years, reflecting the state of chronic illness that many patients are in before seeking treatment in a tertiary care, specialized program. The percentage of admissions by males, 10.8%, coincides, as noted before, with recent prevalence estimates of the ratio of males to females having eating disorders in the general population. Discharges against medical advice have averaged 5.8%, but the substantial increase in 1989 to more than 10% for that year probably reflects patient response to a more rigorous protocol requiring more prolonged nursing supervision of patients.

The final column in Table 6–5 reflects the changing pattern of diagnostic subgroups of eating disorders. Not surprisingly, in 1977, no patients were admitted with a diagnosis of bulimia nervosa, although in retrospect a subgroup of the anorectic patients that had bulimic symptomatology was present. By 1983, 39% of the patients met criteria for bulimia nervosa, a figure that has stayed relatively constant. The presence of a diagnosis of anorexia nervosa in the majority of inpatients contrasts with the data in Table 6–6, which show that in outpatient consultations a majority of the patients have bulimic diagnoses, suggesting that more anorectic patients proportionately need inpatient care than those with bulimic diagnoses. The guideline has remained consistent that most anorectic patients who meet diagnostic criteria need to be treated in the hospital whereas the majority of bulimic patients may be treated as outpatients.

The average increase in weight in patients meeting criteria for anorexia nervosa has been 24 pounds, representing approximately a 20% increase in ideal body weight, with most patients leaving the hospital at 90%–95% of ideal weight. Patients prior to developing illness were on the average 8%–12% above 100% of "ideal body weight," suggesting that they may not be fully restored to their full level of functioning at less than about 10% above so-called ideal weight, and 15% above the weight where they would like to maintain themselves. Studies finding continuing biological abnormality in "long-term recovered" patients who are not truly restored to a full pre-illness healthy weight probably reflect continuing low-weight symptomatology rather than predisposing features. The discharge weight in the low to mid-90% of an ideal weight represents a compromise between full restoration and practical considerations of patient response and insurance coverage. The real goal is to have patients accept a truly healthy body weight without reference to a particular number of pounds on a scale.

Bingeing and purging behavior decreases substantially on treatment in an inpatient program, not surprising in view of the high degree of supervision. But in addition to this decrease in the overt behavior, the bulimic subscales scores on the Eating Disorders Inventory also show a fall into the normal range.

In addition to improvements in the critical areas of body weight and bingeing and purging behavior, patients on discharge from inpatient care show improvement in their general psychological functioning and in specific markers of eating disorders psychopathology. The General

Table 6–6. Comparison of percentage of inpatient versus outpatient consultations: diagnostic categories of eating disorders

	Inpatient (%)	Outpatient (%)
Anorexia nervosa, restricting subtype	31	33
Anorexia nervosa, bulimic subtype	33	11
Bulimia nervosa with history of anorexia nervosa	11	26
Bulimia nervosa without history of anorexia nervosa	25	30

Health Questionnaire (Goldberg and Hiller 1978) falls from the very symptomatic range of 16 on admission (4 or below is normal) to 3.5 at discharge. The Eating Attitudes Test scores (30 and below represent probable absence of an eating disorder) falls from a range of 40 to 70 to below 30. The drive for thinness and body image distortion subscales on the Eating Disorders Inventory fall from the markedly abnormal to the normal range as well. The Montgomery and Åsberg Depression Scale (Montgomery and Åsberg 1979) is used to follow depressive disorders during inpatient stay and documents decreased depressive symptomatology at the time of discharge.

Regarding another vital but more difficult-to-document area—family therapy—61% of treatment objectives were completely achieved in 48 families, and 22% of treatment objectives were partially achieved; 17% of objectives were not achieved during treatment.

Regarding a crude but essential criterion for treatment response, there were no deaths experienced during inpatient treatment. There were only three major medical complications in 620 patients. One patient experienced gastric dilatation, which responded to gastric evacuation and supportive intravenous care for several days followed by return to regular feedings. Two patients required treatment in the medical intensive care unit, one for idiopathic Addison's disease and one for autonomic instability from septicemia associated with changing a suprapubic catheter from triplegia, both unrelated to an eating disorder. A minority of anorectic patients experience pedal edema, which has always responded to conservative medical treatment. None have experienced significant adverse cardiac or pulmonary consequences to refeeding.

Follow-Up

Comprehensive analysis of follow-up is still in progress. Table 6–7 summarizes the outcome of approximately 80 patients. The preliminary study has the flaw of being conducted primarily by telephone, but the advantage of being performed by the same staff person known to patients and with corroboration from a parent or a physician where possible.

Regarding body weight, only 4% are above an ideal body weight; 41% continue to be thinner in weight than desirable. These are patients who on the average had 4 years or more of illness prior to admission.

Menstrual outcome is directly related to the degree to which the patient has sustained a healthy body weight. As average body weight decreases, menses become irregular or absent.

The data in Table 6–7 confirm the impression that where bulimic symptoms are present, they are perpetuated by lowered weight. The probability of bulimic symptoms continuing increases with continuing lowered body weight.

On follow-up of 6 months to 6 years, approximately 75% of patients have reasonable social adjustment characterized by meeting with friends; in 47% of the cases, a dating relationship or other close social contact also exists.

Table 6–8 summarizes the best, average, and worst outcomes on follow-up after inpatient treatment. Not surprisingly, patients who did the best in the long run were those who were younger at age of admission (but not prepubertal), were less chronically ill, had fewer previous hospitalizations, were less severely lowered in weight, and were more likely to have a restricting rather than a bulimic form of anorexia nervosa.

Follow-up of males with eating disorders (Andersen and Mickalide 1983) refutes the idea that males have a necessarily worse outcome than females. They lost less than 1% of the body weight at discharge, remaining close to 92%, and fared as well or better than females overall in follow-up. There is no reason to suggest that maleness per se is an adverse risk factor for long-term outcome in patients with eating disorders.

Table 6–7.   Outcome results obtained on follow-up of discharged patients

Category	n	% of total n	Average
Body weight (IBW)	80		
Above 115%	3	4	135[a]
85%–115%	44	55	96[a]
Less than 85%	33	41	75[a]
Menstrual outcome	70		
Regular menses	23	33	98[b]
Irregular menses	13	19	94[b]
No menses	34	49	78[b]
Bulimic practice (IBW)	24		
Above 115%	1	4	
85%–115%	10	42	
Less than 85%	13	54	
Social adjustment	62		
Loners, no same-sex friends or dating	17	27	
Same-sex friends but no dating	16	26	
Date and have nondating friends	29	47	

Note. IBW = ideal body weight (1983 Metropolitan Life data).
[a]Average % IBW. [b]Average weight at present IBW.

Table 6–8. Best, average, and worst outcome after inpatient treatment for anorexia nervosa

	Best outcome	Average outcome	Worst outcome
Number of patients	11	90	14
Age at admission (years)	18.1	22	25.4
Sex	11 F	85 F, 5 M	13 F, 1 M
Years of illness	2.3	4.7	4.7
Number of previous hospitalizations	0.8	1.5	3
% of ideal body weight on admission	77	72.6	63.6
% of food-restricting anorexia nervosa	73	59	36
Months of follow-up	41	33	43
% of ideal body weight at follow-up	106	88.8	68.3

In summary, following the principles and practices outlined in the first part of this chapter, eating disorder patients in the Johns Hopkins program are regularly restored to a healthy weight range without significant medical complications and with substantial decrease in general and specific psychopathology. At a modestly long follow-up period, patients have maintained substantial gains, but a substantial minority remain chronically lowered in weight or afflicted with amenorrhea or bulimic symptomatology. This study is short in duration compared with that of Theander (1985); on the positive side, however, it documents a known outcome mortality on follow-up of less than 2%. There is every indication that the outcome of milder cases treated early and comprehensively is highly satisfactory. Ideal follow-up studies require a comparison of patients with similar severity of illness treated consistently by different methods, with comprehensive follow-up over several decades. In the meantime there is reason to believe that treatment of eating disorders alters the natural outcome of the illness in a favorable way and that prudent, vigorous, long-term, comprehensive multidisciplinary treatment can substantially ameliorate the symptoms of these disorders and in some cases provide a full resolution of the illness.

References

American Psychiatric Association: Diagnostic and Statistical Manual of Mental Disorders, 3rd Edition. Washington, DC, American Psychiatric Association, 1980

American Psychiatric Association: Diagnostic and Statistical Manual of Mental Disorders, 3rd Edition, Revised. Washington, DC, American Psychiatric Association, 1987

Andersen AE: Practical Comprehensive Treatment of Anorexia Nervosa and Bulimia. Baltimore, MD, Johns Hopkins University Press, 1985

Andersen AE: Prescribing psychotherapy. Directions in Psychiatry—Lesson 17 9:3–7, 1989

Andersen AE: A proposed mechanism underlying eating disorders and other disorders of motivated behavior, in Males With Eating Disorders. Edited by Andersen AE. New York, Brunner/Mazel, 1990, pp 221–254

Andersen AE, DiDomenico L: Diet vs. shape content of popular male and female magazines: a dose-response relationship to the incidence of eating disorders? International Journal of Eating Disorders 11:283–287, 1992

Andersen AE, Mickalide AD: Anorexia nervosa in the male: an underdiagnosed disorder. Psychosomatics 24:1066–1076, 1983

Andersen AE, Mickalide AD: Anorexia nervosa and bulimia: their differential diagnoses in 24 males referred to the Eating and Weight Disorders Clinic. Bull Menninger Clin 49:227–235, 1985

Andersen A, Spencer W, Simpson S, et al: Co-morbidities of anorexia nervosa and bulimia nervosa by subgroup using the SADS-Lifetime. Abstract presented at the 2nd International Conference on Eating Disorders, New York, April 22–24, 1988

Cooper Z, Cooper PJ, Fairburn CG: The validity of the eating disorder examination and its subscales. Br J Psychiatry 154:807–812, 1989

Endicott J, Spitzer RL: A diagnostic interview: the Schedule for Affective Disorders and Schizophrenia. Arch Gen Psychiatry 35:837–844, 1978

Fairburn C, Jones R, Peveler R, et al: Three psychological treatments for bulimia nervosa: a comparative trial. Arch Gen Psychiatry 48:463–469, 1991

Feighner JP, Robins E, Guze SB, et al: Diagnostic criteria for use in psychiatric research. Arch Gen Psychiatry 26:57–63, 1972

Frisch RE, McArthur JW: Menstrual cycles: fatness as a determinant of minimum weight for height necessary for their maintenance or onset. Science 185:949–951, 1974

Frisch RE, Wyshak G, Vincent L: Delayed menarche and amenorrhea of ballet dancers. N Engl J Med 303:17–19, 1980

Garner DM, Olmsted MP, Bohr Y, et al: The Eating Attitudes Test: psychometric features and clinical correlates. Psychol Med 12:871–878, 1982

Garner DM, Olmsted PM, Polivy J: Development and validation of a multidimensional eating disorder inventory for anorexia nervosa and bulimia. International Journal of Eating Disorders 2:15–34, 1983

Garner DM, Rockert W, Olmsted MP, et al: Psychoeducational principles in the treatment of bulimia and anorexia nervosa, in Handbook of Psychotherapy for Anorexia Nervosa and Bulimia Nervosa. Edited by Garner DM, Garfinkel PE. New York, Guilford, 1985, pp 513–572

Goldberg DP, Hiller VF: A scaled version of the General Health Questionnaire. Psychol Med 8:1–7, 1978

Gull WW: Anorexia nervosa. Transactions of the Clinical Society of London 7:22–28, 1874

Hedblom JE, Hubbard F, Andersen A: Anorexia nervosa: a multidisciplinary treatment team for patient and family. Soc Work Health Care 7:67–86, 1981

Kemsley WFF: Body weight at different ages and heights. Annals of Eugenics 16:316–334, 1951

Kishchuk N, Gagnon G, Bélisle D, et al: Sociodemographic and psychological correlates of actual and desired weight insufficiency in the general population. International Journal of Eating Disorders 12:73–81, 1992

Lasègue C: On hysterical anorexia. Medical Times and Gazette 2:265–266, 367–369, 1873

Metropolitan Life Insurance Co: 1983 Metropolitan Height and Weight Tables for Men and Women, Vol 64, No 1, January–June 1983. New York, Metropolitan Life Insurance Co, 1983

McHugh PR, Slavney PR: The Perspectives of Psychiatry. Baltimore, MD, Johns Hopkins University Press, 1983

Montgomery SA, Åsberg M: A new depression scale designed to be sensitive to change. Br J Psychiatry 134:382–389, 1979

Morton R: Phthisiologica: Or a Treatise of Consumptions. London, Smith & Walford, 1694

Ortega DF, Waranch HR, Maldonado AJ, et al: A comparative analysis of self-report measures of bulimia. International Journal of Eating Disorders 6:301–311, 1987

Råstam M, Gillberg C, Garton M: Anorexia nervosa in a Swedish urban region: a population-based study. Br J Psychiatry 155:642–646, 1989

Rolls BJ, Andersen AE, Moran TH, et al: Food intake, hunger, and satiety after preloads in women with eating disorders. Am J Clin Nutr (in press)

Russell GFM: Bulimia nervosa: an ominous variant of anorexia nervosa. Psychol Med 9:429–448, 1979

Saleh JW, Lebwohl P: Metoclopramide-induced gastric emptying in patients with anorexia nervosa. Am J Gastroenterol 74:127–132, 1980

Steen SN, Oppliger RA, Brownell KD: Metabolic effects of repeated weight loss and regain in adolescent wrestlers. JAMA 260:47–50, 1988

Stricker EM, Andersen AE: The lateral hypothalamic syndrome of anorexia nervosa. Life Sci 26:1927–1934, 1980

Theander S: Outcome and prognosis in anorexia nervosa and bulimia: some results of previous investigations compared with those of a Swedish long-term study. J Psychiatr Res 19:493–508, 1985

Waldholtz BD, Andersen AE: Gastrointestinal symptoms in anorexia nervosa: a prospective study. Gastroenterology 98:1415–1419, 1990

Chapter 7

Critique of Follow-Up Studies

L. K. George Hsu, M.D.

O utcome studies for anorexia nervosa and bulimia nervosa are conducted primarily to provide empirical data on the course, outcome, and prognostic indicators of the disorders. However, apart from satisfying the intellectual curiosity of researchers, such data are useful for several purposes. First, they may provide clinicians who treat these sometimes chronic and occasionally fatal disorders with a proper perspective and focus. Second, they may allow clinicians and researchers to evaluate the effectiveness of particular treatment approaches. Third, they may help researchers in their efforts to classify the nosology of these disorders.

Common Flaws

Unfortunately, methodologically robust outcome studies for the eating disorders are rare. There are several flaws among recent studies that are most common.

High Rate of Failure to Trace

The high rate of failure to trace is probably the most common flaw in studies and can seriously bias the findings. Because the long-term crude mortality rate of anorexia nervosa is approximately 15%, a failure-to-trace rate of more than 15% would render the findings of a study un-interpretable.

Insufficient Outcome Information

Insufficient information occurs either in the form of inadequate out-come definition or missing data. Most studies classify outcome in terms of categories. Unfortunately, many fail to define what constitutes a good or poor outcome. Also, it is unlikely that the many aspects of a patient's functioning can be captured adequately in a single category. For exam-ple, an individual who has a normal body weight might become de-pressed and withdrawn. Therefore, in addition to stating whether the patient had a good or bad outcome, data on body weight, eating habits, menstrual function, and mental status should be provided in detail. Standardized instruments should be used for the assessment of out-come in terms of eating habits, mental status, and psychosocial func-tioning.

All deaths should be reported, and causes of death should be de-scribed. Subjective judgments of whether a death is related to the eating disorder should not interfere with the reporting of such data. Death due to bronchial carcinoma might seem unrelated to anorexia nervosa, but heavy smoking for the purpose of suppressing appetite is common among some anorectic patients. Therefore, the standardized mortality ratio should be calculated so that the mortality finding can be compared with that in the general population, or with the standardized mortality ratios of other studies.

Undefined Diagnostic Criteria

Although debate continues on the identity of the eating disorders, there are at least several well-accepted diagnostic criteria currently available so that an operational definition of anorexia nervosa or bulimia nervosa is possible. Fortunately, inadequately defined cases are now rare in the more recent studies.

Uneven or Inadequate Duration of Follow-Up

More than 20 years ago, Russell (1970) stated that the minimum dura-tion of follow-up for anorexia nervosa should be at least 4 years to allow the illness to run its full course. Several recent studies on anorexia nervosa have heeded this advice and confined their follow-up duration to at least 4 years from the time of discharge from the hospital (e.g., Morgan and Russell 1975), the time of initial assessment (e.g., Hsu et al. 1979), or the onset of illness (e.g., Hall et al. 1984). However, several long-term studies have indicated that even a duration of 4 years might not be long enough (Hsu et al. 1990; Ratnasuriya et al. 1989; Theander 1985). An apparently recovered woman in her mid- or late 20s (the mean age of patients at time of follow-up in most studies) may still be at risk of a relapse of her eating disorder. There is therefore little justification for retrospective studies with a follow-up duration of less than 4 years. Because the outcome pattern may change with time, studies in which there is great variability in the subjects' follow-up duration (e.g., Bassoe and Eskeland 1982) become difficult to interpret.

Use of Indirect Methods of Follow-Up

It is generally agreed that direct face-to-face interviews are more likely than telephone interviews or mailed questionnaires to yield valid and reliable information. Given the secretiveness of pathological eating and weight-control behaviors, direct interviews are probably essential for gathering follow-up data on patients with eating disorders.

Idiosyncratic Data Presentation

As already mentioned, a minimum outcome should be described in terms of body weight, eating habits, menstrual status for females, mental state, and psychosocial functioning. However, there is obviously no perfect format for the presentation of such data, and investigators may of course present them according to personal preferences. Nevertheless, to facilitate comparison across studies, it may be advisable to adopt uniform schemes for presenting data in the five areas outlined above. Many recent studies have adopted the Morgan and Russell (1975) outcome categories, and this has certainly facilitated data comparison. In addition, more studies are now using standardized instruments to measure eating habits, mental status, and psychosocial functioning. I have only one recommendation for describing mental state outcome: the psychiatric diagnoses (lifetime and current) of the patients should be described (including subthreshold cases), and patients should be divided into those who still have an eating disorder and those who have recovered. This may allow us to understand the course of the eating disorders and changes in psychopathology. The data may then benefit clinicians in their treatment planning and researchers in their attempt to classify the eating disorders.

Outcome of Anorexia Nervosa

For intermediate-term outcome (4–12 years after onset of illness), I discuss mainly the seven studies that have avoided most but by no means all of the aforementioned pitfalls (Bassoe and Eskeland 1982; Burns and Crisp 1984; Hall et al. 1984; Hsu et al. 1979; Morgan and Russell 1975; Morgan et al. 1983; Tolstrup et al. 1985) (Tables 7–1 and 7–2). Except for the study by Bassoe and Eskeland, all the other six studies used the Morgan and Russell outcome criteria (Morgan and Russell 1975) and thus allowed for direct comparison. For a review of the mortality findings, I also include three studies (Patton 1988; Steinhausen and Glanville 1983; Theander 1970) (Table 7–3) that provide good data on mortality but unfortunately not on outcome pattern.

For long-term outcome (at least 18 years after onset), I discuss the Swedish study by Theander (1985) and the Maudsley study by Russell and

Table 7–1.   Intermediate-term outcome: anorexia nervosa

Study	n			Followed		Duration[a]	Method
	Females	Males	Inpatients	n	%	(years)	
Morgan and Russell 1975	38	3	41	41	100	4–10 disc	Direct 79%
Hsu et al. 1979	105	0	49	102	97	4–8 eval	Direct 75%
Bassoe and Eskeland 1982	?	?	?	77	100	4 minimum eval	Indirect eval
Morgan et al. 1983	73	5	42	75	96	4–8 eval	Direct 88%
Burns and Crisp 1984	0	27	20	27	100	2–20 eval	Direct 85%
Hall et al. 1984	50	0	36	49	98	4–12 onset	Direct 86%
Tolstrup et al. 1985	140	11	?	142	94	4–22 eval	Direct 80%

[a]Duration of follow-up: disc = from time of discharge; eval = from time of initial evaluation; onset = from time at onset.

colleagues (Ratnasuriya et al. 1989). For long-term mortality, I also in-clude my own study (Hsu et al. 1990).

Intermediate-Term Outcome Studies

All the studies have explicit diagnostic criteria that included emaciation or weight loss, amenorrhea in females, and the mental characteristic of weight phobia. Thus, although different criteria were used—for exam-ple, Hall et al. (1984) used Feighner's criteria (Feighner et al. 1972), Morgan and Russell (1975) used Russell's diagnostic criteria (Russell 1970), and Hsu et al. (1979) used Crisp's criteria (Crisp 1980)—it is likely that most if not all of the patients in the 10 studies were suffering from bona fide anorexia nervosa. Except for the patients in Theander's study who had received no formal psychiatric treatment, all the patients in the other studies had at least some medical and psychiatric treat-ment, although a small number (perhaps less than 10%) had an evalua-tion only.

Given the methodological similarities, it is not surprising that the re-sults among these studies (Table 7–2) were quite similar. Overall, about 50% had a good outcome in terms of weight and menstrual function (in the case of males, weight and normal sexual functioning), about 5% had died, about 20% were still anorectic, and the remainder (about 25%) were in various stages of recovery.

It is perhaps significant to note that the one study that had the most favorable outcome (Bassoe and Eskeland 1982) also had more method-

Table 7–2.   Overall outcome pattern

	Good		Intermediate		Poor		Dead	
Study	n	%	n	%	n	%	n	%
Morgan and Russell 1975	16	39	11	27	12	29	2	5
Hsu et al. 1979	47	45	32	30	21	20	2	2
Bassoe and Eskeland 1982[a]	58	62	13	17	12	16	0	
Morgan et al. 1983	45	58	15	19	15	19	1	1
Burns and Crisp 1984	12	44	7	26	8	30	0	
Hall et al. 1984	18	36	18	36	13	26	1	2
Tolstrup et al. 1985	60	40	44	29	29	19	9	6
Mean (%)	46		26		23		2.3	

[a]Undefined criteria.

ological flaws, the main ones being the reliance on mailed questionnaires for gathering follow-up data and the failure to define normal body weight. To underscore further the importance of how methodological differences can affect the findings, I have included the findings from four short-term studies (Hawley 1985; Kohle and Mall 1983; Martin 1985; Nussbaum et al. 1985) (Table 7–4) and from six studies with a large proportion of untraced patients (Becker et al. 1981; Santonastaso et al. 1987; Steinhausen and Glanville 1983; Toner et al. 1986; Touyz and Beumont 1984; Vandereycken and Pierloot 1983) (Table 7–5). It is immediately apparent that the outcome pattern in these studies is more variable.

Mortality. The crude mortality at intermediate-term follow-up is usually less than 5% (Table 7–3). Three other studies have been included here. Theander (1970) published what was probably the first detailed outcome study on anorexia nervosa: 94 female patients admitted to different hospitals in Southern Sweden between 1931 and 1960 were followed after at least 8 years from time of admission. None of the patients had any formal psychiatric treatment for their disorder. Steinhausen and Glanville (1983) reported on 31 patients followed for 4–28 years after

Table 7–3. Intermediate-term mortality

Study	Total deaths		Suicide		Complications		Other	Standardized mortality rate[a]
	n	%	n	%	n	%		
Morgan and Russell 1975	2	5	1	3	1	3	0	?
Hsu et al. 1979	2	2	0		2	2	0	?
Bassoe and Eskeland 1982	0		0		0		0	0
Morgan et al. 1983	1	1	1	1	0		0	?
Burns and Crisp 1984	0		0		0		0	0
Hall et al. 1984	1	2	?		?		?	?
Tolstrup et al. 1985	9	6	6	4	3	2	0	?
Theander 1970	12	13	3	3	9	9	0	?
Steinhausen and Glanville 1983	0		0		0		0	0
Patton 1988	11	3	?		?		?	601

[a]The mortality rate of the cohort compared with the general population matched for sex and age over the period of follow-up.

onset, and, although 10 (32%) refused to participate in the follow-up, thus making the overall outcome pattern difficult to interpret, the authors were nevertheless able to ascertain that they are all alive. Patton (1988) reported on a 4- to 15-year follow-up of 332 anorectic patients seen at the Royal Free Hospital in London and found a crude mortality rate of 3.3%, which represented a standardized mortality ratio (mortality rate compared with the expected mortality rate in the general population matched for sex and age and duration of study) of 6.01. That is, anorectic women are six times more likely to die (from whatever causes) than

Table 7–4. Short-term anorexia nervosa studies

Study	Total N	Good n	Good %	Intermediate n	Intermediate %	Poor n	Poor %	Dead n	Dead %	Unknown n	Unknown %
Hawley 1985	21	9	43	6	29	3	14	0		3	14[a]
Kohle and Mall 1983	36	9	25	17	47	9	25	1	3	0	
Martin 1985[b]	22	19	86	?		3	14	0		0	
Nussbaum et al. 1985[b]	70	45	64	12	17	6	9	?		7	10

[a]All known to be alive. [b]Authors used different outcome classification.

Table 7–5. Anorexia nervosa studies with large numbers of untraced patients

Study	Total N	Good n	Good %	Intermediate n	Intermediate %	Poor n	Poor %	Dead n	Dead %	Unknown n	Unknown %
Becker et al. 1981[a]	38	14	37	7	18	6	16	5	13	6	16
Santonastaso et al. 1987	55	25	45	7	13	6	11	2	4	15	27
Steinhausen and Glanville 1983	31	6	19[b]	?		4	13[b]	0		10	32
Toner et al. 1986[a]	149	23	15	16	11	16	11	5	3	89	60
Touyz and Beumont 1984	49	18	37	9	18	4	8	2	4	16	33
Vandereycken and Pierloot 1983[c]	26	15	58[b]	?		?		?		About 50% overall	

[a]Different outcome category used by authors. [b]At least. [c]Taking only patients followed for at least 5 years.

women in the general population. Unfortunately, Patton did not report on the overall outcome pattern of his sample. In all these studies, the most common causes of death are suicide or complications of anorexia nervosa (Table 7–3).

Eating pattern.   This is an area of outcome where standardized instruments are needed for evaluation. Because none of the studies used such instruments and because each study used a somewhat different format for reporting eating behavior (actually a few made no mention of eating behavior), the meaning of the findings was obscure, and comparison between studies was impossible. A detailed review is unlikely to be rewarding, but it is apparent that abnormal behaviors such as bulimia, vomiting, and laxative abuse were common, not only among those who were still anorectic but also among those who had recovered in terms of weight and menstrual function. I believe that future studies will benefit by separating those who are anorectic and those who are not, and then describing the eating behavior in the two groups, including how many of them would qualify for bulimia nervosa or atypical eating disorder.

Mental status.   This is another area of outcome where standardized interview instruments are needed for evaluation. Data that focused on symptoms without defining severity and duration are unsatisfactory. The findings of the Toronto group (Toner et al. 1986) should point us to the importance of a detailed mental state evaluation in future studies: 60% of anorectic patients had a lifetime and 1-year prevalence of both mood and anxiety disorders.

Furthermore, the anorectic patients, restricting subtype, had a higher prevalence of obsessive-compulsive disorder than the anorectic patients, bulimic subtype (23% versus 10%); the bulimic anorectic patients had a higher prevalence of substance use disorder than the restricting anorectic patients (43% versus 0%). Unfortunately, it is unclear if the excess of these disorders occurred also among those who have already recovered from their eating disorder; that is, it is unclear whether these disorders occurred concurrently with an eating disorder. As already mentioned, a more uniform way of reporting mental state outcome by separating recovered from nonrecovered patients may clarify the course of this sometimes chronic disorder.

Psychosocial and psychosexual functioning.   Psychosocial and psychosexual functioning are also not reported in a standardized fashion. Most studies suggested that better psychosocial functioning (including sexual attitudes) occurred among those whose anorectic symptoms had improved. Several studies reported the percentage of patients married at follow-up (e.g., Burns and Crisp 1984, 30%; Hall et al. 1984, 40%) or of those who had borne children (e.g., Bassoe and Eskeland 1982, 29% of females), but without comparison groups such data were difficult to interpret. In the Danish study (Brinch et al. 1988), 50 of 140 women had borne children during the follow-up interval (mean, 12.5 years); none of the 11 males had fathered a child. The patients were older at age of first delivery of a child than the national average (26.1 years versus 24.1 years), and the number of children per women for the patients was 0.6, compared to the national average of 1.7 for women age 32. At the time of pregnancy, 36 of the 50 patients were considered to have recovered from their anorectic illness, and overall the mothers had a better outcome than those who were not mothers. In the offspring, perinatal complications were common; prematurity was twice the expected rate; and perinatal mortality was six times the expected rate. Unfortunately, the authors did not report on details such as whether there was a correlation between perinatal complications or mortality and the mother's clinical status. Clearly, more data are needed in this area. Work and school performance were almost always satisfactory at follow-up, even among patients who were still anorectic.

Prognostic indicators.   Prognostic indicators varied among the series; methodological differences (such as criteria for each prognostic item and statistical methods used) probably accounted for such discrepancies. Table 7–6 lists the four factors that have been found in five of the studies (Burns and Crisp 1984; Hsu et al. 1979; Morgan and Russell 1975; Mor-

Table 7–6.   Prognostic indicators

Study	Longer duration	Lower weight	Poor family relationships	Failed treatment
Morgan and Russell 1975	X	X	X	X
Hsu et al. 1979	X	X	X	X
Morgan et al. 1983	X		X	
Burns and Crisp 1984	X	X	X	X
Steinhausen and Glanville 1983		X		X

gan et al. 1983; Steinhausen and Glanville 1983) to predict a poor outcome: longer duration of illness, lower minimum weight, previous treatment that failed to bring about a lasting remission, and a premorbid
disturbed relationship with the family. The first three factors suggest the
presence of a severe, chronic, and treatment-resistant illness, and they
therefore make intuitive sense (i.e., chronicity begets chronicity). The
last factor (poor relationship with family) suggests either a family system
interaction disturbance or else a disturbed personality. Unfortunately,
the criteria for assessing quality of family relationships or premorbid personality were poorly defined, and, because the assessment was retrospective, subjective bias could not be reliably excluded.

Summary of findings at intermediate-term outcome.   The outcome at
a minimum of 4 years after onset of illness in properly diagnosed anorectic patients is quite uniform in terms of weight and menstrual functioning: about 75% improved to various degrees, 5% died, and the remainder
were unimproved. Therefore, any study reporting a significantly different
outcome pattern should be examined in terms of its adherence to the
methodological criteria described above.

Beyond the weight, menstrual, and mortality data, few generalizations
can be made. Available data suggest that those who have recovered from
their emaciation and amenorrhea are less likely to suffer from affective
or anxiety symptoms. Schizophrenic symptoms are not more frequent
than expected. Psychosocial functioning (except perhaps work or school
performance) and psychosexual functioning are better in those who have
recovered from their anorectic symptoms. Among the prognostic indicators, those that suggest the presence of a severe, chronic, and treatment-
resistant illness are more likely to predict a worse outcome.

Long-Term Outcome of Anorexia Nervosa

If there was any optimism over the intermediate-term outcome of anorexia nervosa, it was shattered when Theander (1985), in Lund, Sweden, published his long-term follow-up of the 94 patients that he
originally reported on in 1970: the crude mortality rate at a minimum of
24 years (mean of 33 years) after onset of illness was 20% (19 of 94)
(Table 7–7). Five patients (5%) had died as a result of suicide, 12 (13%)
of the complications of anorexia nervosa, and 2 (2%) of cancer. This
grim outlook is ameliorated somewhat by the finding that more patients
have recovered at the 24-year follow-up (71%) than at the 6-year follow-

up (52%). Unfortunately, Theander did not report the standardized mortality ratio of his cohort. A third finding of significance in Theander's study is that about half of the patients who died (10 of 94, 11%) had succumbed within 8 years of onset of illness (i.e., early deaths), whereas the remainder (9 of 94, 10%) died after 17 years (i.e., late deaths). Some investigators (i.e., Crisp 1980; Hsu 1990) suggested that the lower rate of early deaths in the more recent studies may be related to more effective treatment.

Russell at the Maudsley Hospital in London also completed a long-term follow-up (minimum of 18 years, mean of 20 years from time of admission to the Maudsley Hospital) of patients on whom he had reported earlier (Morgan and Russell 1975). The result (Ratnasuriya et al. 1989) indicated that of 41 patients, 12 (29%) recovered according to weight and menstrual function, 13 (32%) had an intermediate outcome, 8 (20%) had a poor outcome, and 7 (17%) had died. Of those who died, 3 (7%) died from suicide, 3 (7%) from complications of the illness, and 1 (2%) from an unrelated cause (murder) (Table 7–8). Thus, a similarly high long-term mortality rate is seen in the Maudsley cohort. However, the overall good outcome pattern reported by the Swedish study (Theander 1985) is not confirmed by the Maudsley study. If anything, the Maudsley group had a worse outcome at 20-year follow-up than at 5-year follow-up. This discrepancy could probably be explained by the fact that the Maudsley patients are younger: at 20-year follow-up their mean age was 40 years, whereas the Swedish cohort at 24-year follow-up had a mean age of 51 years; that is, the illness in the Maudsley cohort may still not

Table 7–7. Twenty-year mortality of anorexia nervosa

Study	Total N	0–12 years n	0–12 years %	12–24 years n	12–24 years %	Total deaths n	Total deaths %	Standardized mortality rate
Theander 1985	94	10	11	9	10	19	20	?
Ratnasuriya et al. 1989	41	2	5	5	12	7	17	?
Hsu and Callender, unpublished, 1989	63	3	5	5	8	8	13	471
Hsu and Crisp, unpublished, 1989	105	2	2	2	2	4	4	136

Table 7–8. Causes of death in long-term studies

Study	Total N	Anorexia nervosa		Suicide		Other		Total	
		n	%	n	%	n	%	n	%
St. George's	105	2	2	1	1	1	1[a]	4	4
Aberdeen	63	3	5	4	6	1	2[a]	8	13
Sweden	94	12	13	5	5	2	2	19	20
Maudsley	41	3	7	3	7	1	2[b]	7	17

[a]Cancer. [b]Murder.

have run its full course. Of significance is the lower early mortality (2 of 41, 5%) in the Maudsley series, which, as already mentioned, may be due to better treatment. However, the benefits of treatment do not seem to extend beyond 12 years because the late mortality rate (5 of 41, 12%) is actually higher in Maudsley than in Sweden. The high suicide rate is particularly disturbing.

I have conducted a preliminary long-term follow-up (minimum 17 years from onset) of the St. George's cohort (N = 105, all female) under Professor Crisp in St. George's Hospital in London, a cohort on which I have previously reported (Hsu et al. 1979). For comparison, I have also followed 63 female patients entered into the Aberdeen Case Register, in Scotland, between 1965 and 1973; they represent patients who were treated in catchment area medical or psychiatric facilities and not referred to a specialist clinic, as is the case for many of the other published series (Table 7–9). At the time of follow-up in 1989, 97 (92%) of the 105 St. George's patients were known to be alive, 4 (4%) had died (2 from complications of anorexia nervosa, 1 from suicide, 1 from cancer), and 4 were untraced although not recorded as dead at either the National Health Central Registry or the Birth and Death Registry. Of the 63 Aber-

Table 7–9. Clinical features of St. George's and Aberdeen cohorts

Cohort	Total N	Age at onset (years)	Duration of illness (years)	Age at follow-up (years)	Duration of follow-up (years)
St. George's	105	16.8 ± 3.8	3.7 ± 4.1	38.8 ± 6.7	21.8 ± 5.1
Aberdeen	63	19.1 ± 5.3	2.0 ± 2.4	40.9 ± 7.5	22.1 ± 4.9
t		3.27	3.0	1.8	1.1
P		<.01	<.01	NS	NS

Note. NS = not significant.

deen patients, 53 (84%) are alive, 8 (13%) have died, and 2 (3%) were untraced (again not recorded as dead). The expected mortality for the two cohorts, calculated from age- and sex-specific mortality of the respective populations (England and Wales and Scotland) in 1981, midpoint of the follow-up period, was 2.95 for the London cohort and 1.70 for the Aberdeen cohort. The standardized mortality ratio for the London cohort was therefore 136 (4:2.95, that is, anorectic women were 1.36 times more likely to die than women of the same age in England and Wales during the period 1973 to 1989), and 471 (8:1.70, that is, anorectic women were 4.71 times more likely to die than women of the same age in Scotland during the period 1973 to 1989) in Aberdeen. The data are summarized in Tables 7–7 and 7–8.

The point of interest is the difference in standardized mortality ratio and the difference in late mortality in the two cohorts. The relatively low early mortality of the Aberdeen series is consistent with the Maudsley finding, and the standardized mortality ratio of the Aberdeen cohort is similar to that of the Royal Free Hospital series (Patton 1988), which in fact had a shorter follow-up interval. Again, these findings lend support to the contention that better treatment may reduce early mortality. For the St. George's cohort, the low overall mortality rate and, in particular, the low late mortality rate are unexpected. Because patient selection factors are unlikely to have worked in its favor (being a specialist center, St. George's Hospital tends to treat more chronic and treatment-resistant cases), the low mortality at St. George's Hospital strengthens the case that competent and comprehensive treatment may reduce not only early mortality but also late mortality. Effective treatment may also have contributed to its lower suicide rate (Table 7–8): in the other three series (Aberdeen, Maudsley, and Sweden), the suicide rate ranged from 5% to 7%, whereas the St. George's cohort had only one suicide (jumped from a height). Again, it is possible that the illness might not have run its full course in either the Aberdeen (mean age 40.9 ± 7.5 years at follow-up) or St. George's (mean age 38.8 ± 6.7 years) patients in view of their relatively young age in comparison with Theander's patients.

Although my study is a pilot attempt to determine primarily the feasibility of a full-scale follow-up study of the two cohorts, I was able to interview 16 patients (9 from London and 7 from Aberdeen) in an attempt to test the feasibility of the interview instruments. Nine of the patients had recovered and had no eating disorder (anorexia nervosa, bulimia nervosa, or eating disorder not otherwise specified) for at least 12 months before the interview (normal weight; eating at least two regular meals a day; no bingeing, vomiting, or purging behavior; normal men-strual cycles); one had normal-weight bulimia nervosa; and two had eat-ing disorder not otherwise specified (both had episodic binge eating but do not meet severity criteria for bulimia nervosa). The findings are sum-marized in Table 7–10. Among the nine patients who had recovered from anorexia nervosa, three had major depressive episodes not related to any eating disturbance, one also had panic disorder, and a second a simple phobia (flying). In contrast, psychiatric disorders were much more prev-alent during the times of active anorexia nervosa or bulimia nervosa. Psychometric measures that significantly distinguished the recovered from nonrecovered patients are summarized in Table 7–11. It is obvious that those who had significant eating disturbances had higher depression and anxiety scores.

Clearly, it is still too early to come to a definite conclusion about the

Table 7–10. DSM-III-R diagnosis at follow-up ($N = 16$)

	Lifetime	Current
Eating disorders		
Anorexia nervosa, restricting subtype	16	2
Anorexia nervosa, bulimic subtype	5 (4)	2
Bulimia nervosa, normal weight	1 (1)	1
Eating disorder not otherwise specified	5	2[a]
Disorders not concurrent with anorexia nervosa or bulimia nervosa		
Bipolar	1	0
Major depression	3	0
Psychoactive substance	1	0
Panic disorder	1 (1)	1
Simple phobia	1	0
Obsessive-compulsive disorder	1 (1)	1
Disorders concurrent with anorexia nervosa or bulimia nervosa		
Bipolar	1	1
Major depression	6 (1)	2
Delusional disorder	1	0
Psychoactive substance	3	1
Panic disorder	3	2
Social phobia	2 (1)	0
Obsessive-compulsive disorder	1 (1)	0
Hypochondriasis	1	1

Note. Subthreshold in parentheses.
[a]Bulimia nervosa.

long-term outcome for anorexia nervosa. However, from the 300 patients in the four series, it is clear that, in time, about one of seven patients (14%) may die as a result of suicide or complications of the illness. It is gratifying to find some support that treatment seems to have at least prevented early deaths. The overall outcome pattern is still unclear and must await further study.

Outcome of Bulimia Nervosa

Because bulimia nervosa was not delineated from anorexia nervosa until the late 1970s, it is perhaps not surprising that outcome studies are fewer and of shorter follow-up duration than those for anorexia nervosa. For this chapter, I confine my review to bulimic patients with a normal weight.

Short-Term Outcome of Bulimia Nervosa

I have been able to find nine studies that have at least a 1-year follow-up from time of evaluation (Abraham et al. 1983; Fairburn 1981; Fairburn

Table 7–11.   Recovered versus nonrecovered (mean ± SD)

Psychometric measure	Recovered ($n = 9$)	Nonrecovered ($n = 7$)	t^a	P
Eating Disorders Inventory[b]	15.1 ± 10.6	45.4 ± 27.5	3.05	.026
Thinness	0.56 ± 0.88	7.0 ± 7.30	2.65	.019
Ineffectiveness	2.22 ± 2.05	9.0 ± 7.62	2.58	.022
Distrust	1.33 ± 1.12	4.43 ± 2.82	3.03	.009
Hamilton Rating Scale for Depression[c]	3.22 ± 5.07	18.0 ± 14.73	3.83	.013
Maudsley Obsessive Compulsive Inventory[d]	3.78 ± 3.49	9.71 ± 5.91	2.52	.025
Hopkins Symptom Checklist—90[e]	14.67 ± 10.98	31.0 ± 14.60	2.56	.023
Depression	4.22 ± 3.70	12.71 ± 6.24	3.40	.004
Anxiety	1.78 ± 2.17	4.43 ± 2.07	2.47	.027
Crown-Crisp Experimental Index[f]				
Obsessionality	5.89 ± 2.85	9.57 ± 2.30	2.78	.015
Depression	4.78 ± 2.05	8.43 ± 7.55	2.59	.021
Social Adjustment Scale[g]	1.78 ± 0.67	3.86 ± 1.35	4.07	.001
Social	1.56 ± 0.88	3.86 ± 0.90	5.13	.001

Note. All df = 14.
[a]Two-tailed. [b]Garner et al. 1983. [c]Hamilton 1967. [d]Hodgson and Rachman 1977.
[e]Derogatis et al. 1974. [f]Crown and Crisp 1979. [g]Weisman et al. 1971.

et al. 1986; Hsu and Holder 1986; Johnson et al. 1986; Lacey 1983; Russell et al. 1987; Wilson et al. 1986; Yager et al. 1987) (Table 7–12). Apart from the studies by Fairburn et al. and Lacey, which have remarkably good results, the other studies found that about 75% of patients who have been treated are not diagnosable for a bulimic disorder at follow-up, although some of these patients may still have occasional episodes.

All the studies are treatment studies (i.e., patients underwent treatment at the respective centers) except for the one by Yager et al., which recruited patients from the community at large. Perhaps it is for the lack of specific treatment that the patients in Yager et al.'s study fared worse, because all the available controlled, randomized studies indicate that some form of cognitive-behavioral treatment is superior to nonspecific or supportive therapy (Fairburn et al. 1986; Freeman et al. 1985; Kirkley et al. 1985; Lacey 1983; Lee and Rush 1986; Mitchell et al. 1990; Ordman and Kirschenbaum 1985; Russell et al. 1987; Wilson et al. 1986).

Similarly, most of the controlled medication trials suggest that antidepressants are superior to placebo in decreasing bulimic episodes, including tricyclic antidepressants (Agras et al. 1987; Barlow et al. 1988; Hughes et al. 1986; Mitchell et al. 1989; Pope et al. 1983), monoamine oxidase inhibitors (Kennedy et al. 1988; Walsh et al. 1988), bupropion (Horne et al. 1988), and trazodone (Pope et al. 1989). Thus it is clear from the available evidence that cognitive-behavioral therapy and antidepressants are effective in the short term for bulimia nervosa.

Intermediate-Term Outcome Studies

Four studies have a follow-up duration of more than 2 years (Brotman et al. 1988; Hsu and Sobkiewicz 1989; Mitchell et al. 1989; Swift et al. 1987) (Table 7–13). Overall, between 16% and 50% of patients are still diagnosable as having bulimia nervosa at follow-up, and between 9% and 37% are still having occasional episodes. Again, the three studies (Brotman et al. 1988; Hsu and Sobkiewicz 1989; Mitchell et al. 1989) that used specific treatment seemed to have a better outcome than the one that used nonspecific treatment (Swift et al. 1987). However, the duration of follow-up in these studies is still relatively brief (not longer than 5 years), and thus the long-term outcome of bulimia nervosa remains to be clarified. With regard to mental status, the data are incomplete. Swift et al. found major depression at follow-up to be uncommon. Brotman et al. did not report such data, and the findings of the two

Table 7-12. Short-term outcome of bulimia nervosa

Study	Total N	n followed	Index treatment	Duration (months)	Follow-up method	Bulimia nervosa[a] Nondiagnosable (%)	Diagnosable (%)	Outcome body weight	Further treatment
Abraham et al. 1983	51	43	OP, I	14–72	Interview	65 (?)	35 (?)	Normal	ND
Fairburn 1981	11	6	OP, I	12	ND	83	17	Normal	None
Fairburn et al. 1986	24	22	OP, I	12	Interview	100	—	Normal	None
Hsu and Holder 1986	56	48	OP, I	12–35	Telephone	75	25	Normal	ND
Johnson et al. 1986	12	6	OP, I	12	ND	83	17	ND	ND
Lacey 1983	30	28	OP, I, G	Up to 24	ND	100	—	Normal	11%
Russell et al. 1987	23	23	IP, OP, I, F	12	Interview	At least 21	ND	Mostly normal	ND
Wilson et al. 1986	17	11	OP, G	12	Interview	73	27	Normal	36%
Yager et al. 1987	?	392	ND	20	Postal questionnaire	43 (?)	57 (?)	ND	ND

Note. OP = outpatient. I = individual. ND = not described. G = group. IP = inpatient. F = family. ? = not clearly stated.
[a]Percentages are based on patients successfully traced for follow-up.

Table 7–13. Intermediate-term outcome of bulimia nervosa

Study	Total N	n followed	Index treatment	Duration (months)	Follow-up method	Bulimia nervosa[a] Nondiagnosable (%)	Diagnosable (%)	Outcome body weight	Further treatment
Brotman et al. 1988	12	12[b]	OP, I, G, M	24–60	ND	58 in remission	17 (25 marked improvement)	ND	ND
Hsu and Sobkiewicz 1989	45	35	OP, I	48–60	Mostly telephone	47	16 (plus 16% symptomatic but nondiagnosable)	Normal 2% underweight	30%
Mitchell et al. 1989	100	91	OP, G	24–60	Telephone	66	25 (plus 9% symptomatic but nondiagnosable)	Normal 1% underweight 7% overweight	ND
Swift et al. 1987	38	30	IP, OP (?)	24–60	Interview	13	50 (plus 37% symptomatic but nondiagnosable)	Normal	100%

Note. OP = outpatient. I = individual. G = group. M = medication. ND = not described. IP = inpatient. ? = not clearly defined.
[a]Percentages are based on patients successfully traced for follow-up. [b]Taking only patients followed for at least 2 years.

studies that predominantly used telephone follow-up could not be evaluated. Prognostic indicators were not examined in these studies.

Comment

The eating disorders, especially anorexia nervosa, appear to be chronic disorders in some patients. Clinicians must therefore be prepared to monitor carefully the progress of their patients and not be satisfied with short-term "breakthroughs." Investigators should perhaps turn their attention to continuation or maintenance treatments rather than acute treatments.

In anorectic patients, it is probable that major depression is more prevalent than expected even among those who no longer have an eating disorder. Although the nature of the link between an affective disorder and an eating disorder is still unclear, I suggest that mood disturbances in anorectic patients, whether they occur concurrently or independently of the eating disturbance, be treated vigorously. Hopefully, successful treatment of the depression may improve both the overall outcome of anorexia nervosa as well as reduce its suicide rate. In this connection, the preliminary finding that fluoxetine may be beneficial in anorexia nervosa is noteworthy (Gwirtsman et al. 1990).

Available findings indicate that anorexia nervosa may progress to bulimia nervosa in some patients, but the relationship of eating disorder not otherwise specified to either anorexia nervosa or bulimia nervosa is unclear. Eating disorder not otherwise specified as a diagnostic category is unsatisfactory because it encompasses patients with subthreshold restricting anorexia nervosa as well as subthreshold bulimia nervosa in normal-weight or overweight individuals. Some attempt should be made to separate eating disorder not otherwise specified into these components, and studies to determine the outcome of each would be worthwhile.

Finally, the fear of fatness seems to persist even in patients who have been recovered for some time from their eating disorder (Hsu et al. 1992). This finding is consistent with an "accretion" process in which certain abnormal eating behaviors become added onto the abnormal attitude of weight phobia in the development of an eating disorder, whereas during recovery such behaviors desist but the attitude remains. Elsewhere (Hsu 1990) I have suggested that simple abnormal eating occurring in the presence of certain risk factors (such as a mood disturbance) may become amplified and develop into an eating disorder.

Although this linear model may appear simplistic to some investigators and empirical data to support it are minimal, I still believe that an attempt should be made to determine if this accretion process in fact occurs during the progression of eating disturbances.

References

Abraham S, Myra M, Llewellyn-Jones D: A study of outcome. International Journal of Eating Disorders 2:175–180, 1983

Agras WS, Dorian B, Kirkley BG, et al: Imipramine in the treatment of bulimia: a double-blind controlled study. International Journal of Eating Disorders 6:29–38, 1987

Barlow J, Blouin J, Blouin A, et al: Treatment of bulimia with desipramine: a double-blind crossover study. Can J Psychiatry 33:129–133, 1988

Bassoe HH, Eskeland I: A prospective study of 133 patients with anorexia nervosa: treatment and outcome. Acta Psychiatr Scand 65:127–133, 1982

Becker H, Korner P, Stoffler A: Psychodynamics and therapeutic aspects of anorexia nervosa: a study of family dynamics and prognosis. Psychother Psychosom 36:8–16, 1981

Brinch M, Isager T, Tolstrup K: Anorexia nervosa and motherhood: reproductional pattern and mothering behavior of 50 women. Acta Psychiatr Scand 77:90–104, 1988

Brotman AW, Herzog DB, Hamburg P: Long-term course in 14 bulimic patients treated with psychotherapy. J Clin Psychiatry 49:157–160, 1988

Burns T, Crisp AH: Outcome of anorexia nervosa in males. Br J Psychiatry 145:319–325, 1984

Crisp AH: Anorexia Nervosa: Let Me Be. London, Plenum, 1980

Crown S, Crisp AH: Crown-Crisp Experimental Index. London, Hodder & Stoughton, 1979

Derogatis LR, Lipman RS, Rickels K, et al: The Hopkins Symptom Checklist (HSCL): a self-report symptom inventory. Behav Sci 19:1–15, 1974

Fairburn CG: A cognitive-behavioral approach to the management of bulimia. Psychol Med 11:707–711, 1981

Fairburn CG, Kirk J, O'Connor M, et al: A comparison of two psychological treatments for bulimia nervosa. Behav Res Ther 24:629–643, 1986

Feighner JP, Robins E, Guze SB, et al: Diagnostic criteria for use in psychiatric research. Arch Gen Psychiatry 26:57–63, 1972

Freeman C, Sinclair F, Turnbull J, et al: Psychotherapy for bulimia: a controlled study. J Psychiatr Res 19:473–478, 1985

Garner DM, Olmsted MP, Polivy J: Development and validation of a multidimensional eating disorder inventory for anorexia nervosa and bulimia. International Journal of Eating Disorders 2:15–34, 1983

Gwirtsman HE, Guze BH, Yager J, et al: Fluoxetine treatment of anorexia nervosa: an open clinical trial. J Clin Psychiatry 5:378–382, 1990

Hall A, Slim E, Hawker F, et al: Anorexia nervosa: long-term outcome in 50 female patients. Br J Psychiatry 145:407–413, 1984

Hamilton M: Development of a rating scale for primary depressive illness. British Journal of Social and Clinical Psychology 6:278–296, 1967

Hawley RM: The outcome of anorexia nervosa in younger subjects. Br J Psychiatry 146:657–660, 1985

Hodgson RJ, Rachman S: The Maudsley Obsessive Compulsive Inventory. Behav Res Ther 15:389–395, 1977

Horne RL, Ferguson JM, Pope HG, et al: Treatment of bulimia with bupropion: a multicenter controlled trial. J Clin Psychiatry 49:262–266, 1988

Hsu LKG: Eating Disorders. New York, Guilford, 1990a

Hsu LKG: The experiential aspects of bulimia nervosa: implications for cognitive behavioral therapy. Behav Modif 14:50–65, 1990b

Hsu LKG, Holder D: Bulimia nervosa: treatment and short term outcome. Psychol Med 16:65–70, 1986

Hsu LKG, Sobkiewicz TA: Bulimia nervosa: four to six year outcome. Psychol Med 19:1035–1038, 1989

Hsu LKG, Crisp AH, Harding B: Outcome of anorexia nervosa. Lancet 1:62–68, 1979

Hsu LKG, Chesler BE, Santhouse R: Bulimia nervosa in eleven sets of twins. International Journal of Eating Disorders 9:275–282, 1990

Hsu LKG, Crisp AH, Callender JS: Recovery in anorexia nervosa: the patient's perspective. International Journal of Eating Disorders 11:341–350, 1992

Hughes PL, Wells LA, Cunningham CJ, et al: Treatment of bulimia with desipramine: a double-blind, placebo-controlled study. Arch Gen Psychiatry 43:182–186, 1986

Johnson WG, Schlundt DG, Jarrell MP: Exposure with response prevention in bulimia nervosa. International Journal of Eating Disorders 5:35–45, 1986

Kennedy SH, Piran N, Warsh JJ, et al: A trial of isocarboxazid in the treatment of bulimia nervosa. J Clin Psychopharmacol 8:391–396, 1988

Kirkley BB, Schneider JA, Agras W, et al: Comparison of two group treatments for bulimia. J Consult Clin Psychol 53:43–48, 1985

Kohle K, Mall H: Follow-up study of 36 anorexia nervosa patients treated on an integrated internistic-psychosomatic ward. International Journal of Eating Disorders 2:215–219, 1983

Lacey JH: Bulimia nervosa, binge eating and psychogenetic vomiting: a controlled treatment study and long-term outcome. Br Med J 286:1609–1613, 1983

Lee N, Rush PAJ: Cognitive-behavioral group therapy for bulimia. International Journal of Eating Disorders 5:599–613, 1986

Martin FE: The treatment and outcome of anorexia nervosa in adolescents: a prospective study and five year follow-up. J Psychiatr Res 19:509–514, 1985

Mitchell JE, Pyle RL, Hatsukami D, et al: A 2 to 5 year follow-up study of patients treated for bulimia. International Journal of Eating Disorders 8:157–165, 1989

Mitchell JE, Pyle RL, Eckert ED, et al: A comparison study of antidepressants and structured intensive group psychotherapy in the treatment of bulimia nervosa. Arch Gen Psychiatry 47:149–160, 1990

Morgan HG, Russell GFM: Value of family background and clinical features as predictors of long-term outcome in anorexia nervosa: four year follow-up study of 41 patients. Psychol Med 5:355–371, 1975

Morgan HG, Purgold J, Welbourne J: Management and outcome in anorexia nervosa: a standardized prognosis study. Br J Psychiatry 143:282–287, 1983

Nussbaum M, Shenker IR, Baird D, et al: Follow-up investigation in patients with anorexia nervosa. J Pediatr 106:835–840, 1985

Ordman AM, Kirschenbaum DS: Cognitive-behavioral therapy for bulimia: an initial outcome study. J Consult Clin Psychol 53:305–313, 1985

Patton GC: Mortality in eating disorders. Psychol Med 18:947–952, 1988

Pope HG, Hudson JI, Jonas JM, et al: Bulimia treated with imipramine: a placebo controlled, double-blind study. Am J Psychiatry 140:554–558, 1983

Pope HG, Keck PE, McElroy SL, et al: A placebo-controlled study of trazodone in bulimia nervosa. J Clin Psychopharmacol 9:254–259, 1989

Ratnasuriya RH, Eisler I, Szmukler GI, et al: Outcome and prognostic factors after 20 years of anorexia nervosa. Ann N Y Acad Sci 575:567–568, 1989

Russell GFM: Anorexia nervosa: its identity as an illness and its treatment, in Modern Trends in Psychological Medicine, Vol 2. Edited by Price JH. London, Butterworth, 1970, pp 131–164

Russell GFM, Szmukler GI, Dare C, et al: An evaluation of family therapy in anorexia nervosa and bulimia nervosa. Arch Gen Psychiatry 44:1047–1056, 1987

Santonastaso P, Favaretto G, Canton G: Anorexia nervosa in Italy: clinical features and outcome in a long-term follow-up study. Psychopathology 20:8–17, 1987

Steinhausen HC, Glanville K: A long-term follow-up of adolescent anorexia nervosa. Acta Psychiatr Scand 68:1–10, 1983

Swift WJ, Ritholz M, Kalin NH, et al: A follow-up study of thirty hospitalized bulimics. Psychosom Med 49:45–55, 1987

Theander S: Anorexia nervosa: a psychiatric investigation of 94 female patients. Acta Psychiatr Scand Suppl 214:1–94, 1970

Theander S: Outcome and prognosis in anorexia nervosa and bulimia: some results of previous investigations, compared with those of a Swedish long-term study. J Psychiatr Res 19:493–508, 1985

Tolstrup K, Brinch M, Isager T, et al: Long-term outcome of 151 cases of anorexia nervosa: the Copenhagen anorexia nervosa follow-up study. Acta Psychiatr Scand 71:380–387, 1985

Toner BB, Garfinkel PE, Garner DM: Long-term follow-up of anorexia nervosa. Psychosom Med 48:520–529, 1986

Touyz SW, Beumont PJV: Anorexia nervosa: a follow-up investigation. Med J Aust 141:219–222, 1984

Vandereycken W, Pierloot R: Long-term outcome research in anorexia nervosa: the problem of patient selection and follow-up duration. International Journal of Eating Disorders 2:237–242, 1983

Walsh BT, Gladis M, Roose SP, et al: Phenelzine vs placebo in 50 patients with bulimia. Arch Gen Psychiatry 45:471–478, 1988

Weisman MM, Paykel ES, Siegel R, et al: The social role performance of depressed women. Am J Orthopsychiatry 41:390–410, 1971

Wilson GT, Rossiter E, Kleifield EL, et al: Cognitive behavioral treatment of bulimia nervosa. Behav Res Ther 24:277–288, 1986

Yager J, Landsverk J, Edelstein CK: A 20-month follow-up of 628 women with eating disorders, I: course and severity. Am J Psychiatry 144:1172–1177, 1987

Section IV

Neuroendocrinology, Neuropeptides, and Metabolism

Chapter 8

Neuroendocrine and Reproductive Function

Karl Martin Pirke, M.D.
Elizabeth Philipp, M.D.
Ulrich Schweiger, M.D.
Andrew Broocks, M.D.
Thomas Wilckens, M.D.

⸻

E ating disorders—anorexia nervosa and bulimia nervosa—are characterized by various abnormal behaviors. In these syndromes, we find self-imposed food restriction that is either permanent (anorexia nervosa) or intermittent (bulimia nervosa). Bingeing and vomiting are obligatory in bulimia nervosa but occur also in many anorectic patients. Hyperactivity is observed in many patients with anorexia nervosa (Kron et al. 1978) and occurs, far less frequently, in bulimia nervosa. It is therefore of great interest to study the consequences of the behaviors mentioned on brain neurotransmitter systems. This could provide insight into the nature of neuroendocrine and other physiological dysregulations seen in eating disorders. It could also throw some light on secondary changes of psychophysiological regulations (e.g., hunger and satiety). Because no methods are yet available to conduct such studies in patients, animal models for eating disorders are of great interest. Mrosowsky (1984) reviewed animal mod-

els in which self-imposed starvation occurred. No model accounts for all
the different behavioral abnormalities in eating disorders.

We present here an animal model that allows us to study the combined
effects of starvation and hyperactivity, which are characteristic of anorexia nervosa. Richter (1922) observed that hyperactivity can be induced in rats living in a running wheel when access to food is restricted
to 1 hour/day. The rats run more and more and reduce feeding even
during the hour of food availability. They die if the experiment is not
terminated in time (Epling and Pierce 1989).

We have studied this model intensively, especially with regard to neurotransmitter and neuroendocrine regulations (Broocks et al. 1990). We
modified the experimental conditions slightly. Instead of reducing the
time of feeding, we supplied only 50% of the ad lib intake in the beginning. After the hyperactivity developed, the amount of food was adjusted
in such a way that body weight was kept constant at 70% of the original
weight. High running activity at 18–20 km/day was maintained as long as
the experiment was continued. Both male and female rats show this phenomenon. However, hyperactivity developed faster and remained higher
in female rats. There was a remarkable difference between male and fe-

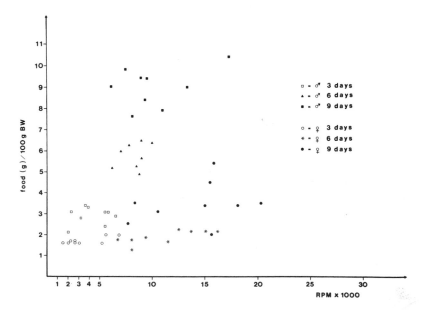

Figure 8–1.   Food intake versus running activity (rpm) in male and female rats
on Days 3, 6, and 9 of semistarvation-induced hyperactivity. BW =
body weight.

male animals with regard to food consumption during the first 9 days of the experiment. Figure 8–1 shows food intake per 100 g of body weight versus running activity at different points in time. In the beginning of the experiment, both sexes had similar food intake. After 6 days, and even more so after 9 days, the female rats needed much less food than male rats to run a certain distance. Because the energy cost of running is unlikely to be different between sexes, we can assume that the basal energy requirement is probably more effectively reduced in female rats than in male rats.

Basal energy metabolism is regulated in mammals to a great extent by thyroid hormones. Hypothyroidism is characterized by low basal energy metabolism. Table 8–1 shows triiodothyronine levels in the experimental groups. Starvation alone reduces triiodothyronine values in rats, as it does in dieting and starving humans (Pirke et al. 1989) and in anorectic and bulimic patients (Heufelder et al. 1985). Hyperactive semistarved rats show a further reduction in triiodothyronine values; this reduction, however, is not different between male and female rats.

Hypothalamic-Pituitary-Gonadal Axis

In both male and female rats, reproductive function is rapidly lost during the experiment described above. Female rats lose their menstrual cycle in the second week. Male semistarved running rats have decreased luteinizing hormone (LH) values (5.63 ± 0.5 versus 10.91 ± 0.4 ng/ml) and decreased testosterone values (0.58 ± 0.08 versus 2.95 ± 0.2 ng/ml)

Table 8–1. Triiodothyronine and corticosterone in semistarved and hyperactive rats on Day 10

Rat group	Body weight (g)	Triiodothyronine (ng/ml)	Corticosterone (ng/ml)
Semistarved running	185.9 ± 1.7	0.08 ± 0.03	313.6 ± 42.5
Semistarved sedentary	183.9 ± 2.4	0.30 ± 0.05	220.4 ± 24.4
Ad libitum running	290.0 ± 5.6	0.87 ± 0.05	66.4 ± 11.6
Ad libitum sedentary	306.0 ± 3.0	0.84 ± 0.03	80.9 ± 10.4

Note. See text for description of experiment.

when compared with ad lib fed controls. When semistarved running rats were compared with semistarved sedentary rats, no difference in LH and T values were found, indicating that semistarvation and not hyperactivity causes hypogonadism (Broocks et al. 1990). These data are in agreement with observations in female athletes (Schweiger et al. 1988), showing the importance of insufficient calorie intake for the development of menstrual disturbances. Several studies have been undertaken to reveal the mechanism underlying the hypogonadism seen in starved rats (Küderling et al. 1984; Pirke and Spyra 1981, 1982; Warnhoff et al. 1983). Neither endorphin nor prostaglandin mechanisms seem to be involved. None of the starvation-induced changes of the neurotransmitters seem to be responsible.

The following endocrine observation may, however, shed some light on the problem. Table 8–1 shows the 24-hour mean values of corticosterone in the different experimental groups. Starvation causes a significant increase of corticosterone. Semistarvation-induced hyperactivity causes an even higher glucocorticoid increase. The circadian rhythm parallels the running activity. It is well known that increased activity of the hypothalamic-pituitary-adrenal (HPA) axis can suppress the pituitary-gonadal axis. Corticotropin-releasing hormone can impair gonadotropin secretion at the hypothalamic level (Rivier and Vale 1984). Glucocorticoids can decrease gonadal hormone secretion (Doerr and Pirke 1976). The endocrine finding in the animal model closely parallels the situation in anorectic patients: a high activity of the HPA axis is associated with an impaired reproductive function. This relation is discussed later in this chapter.

Neurotransmitter Activity

Norepinephrine

We have previously demonstrated that total starvation and semistarvation reduce norepinephrine turnover in the hypothalamus (Pirke and Spyra 1981, 1982). Turnover was measured using different methods; the alpha-methyl paratyrosine method and the measurement of 3-methoxy-4-hydroxyphenylglycol (MHPG) both show a decreased norepinephrine turnover (Pirke and Spyra 1982; Schweiger et al. 1985). Figure 8–2 shows the circadian pattern of MHPG-sulfate in the medial basal hypothalamus. MHPG values in semistarved rats are significantly decreased when compared with controls fed ad lib *(shaded area)*. A clear circadian rhythm is observed, with a maximum at feeding time at noon. Semi-starved running rats show an even more pronounced circadian pattern, reaching a maximum at 4 P.M. Running significantly increases MHPG levels in semistarved rats and in controls fed ad lib (data not shown). The average 24-hour MHPG levels in the medial basal hypothalamus are significantly elevated in the semistarved running rats.

Similar observations were made for the dopaminergic system (Broocks et al. 1989). Semistarvation reduced dihydrophenylacetic acid (DOPAC) concentrations in the hypothalamus, and semistarvation-induced hyperactivity caused an increase in dopamine metabolites. Different observations were obtained in the serotonergic system (Broocks et al. 1989, 1990). Figure 8–3 shows that semistarvation alone increases hypothalamic concentrations of 5-hydroxyindoleacetic acid (5-HIAA). This

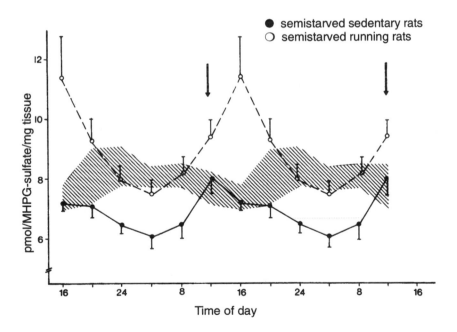

Figure 8–2. Mean ± SE levels of 3-methoxy-4-hydroxyphenylglycol (MHPG)–sulfate in the medial basal hypothalamus of semistarved sedentary rats and semistarved running rats plotted over a 2-day period. *Arrows* indicate the time of feeding. *Shaded area* represents mean ± SE in sedentary rats fed ad libitum. Data from Broocks et al. 1990.

finding is in agreement with the literature (Kantak et al. 1978). Semi-starvation-induced hyperactivity further increases 5-HIAA. Serotonin inhibits food intake in experimental animals and in humans. We might therefore speculate that the impairment of food intake during prolonged running described earlier may be mediated by the increased serotonergic activity.

We have tried to evaluate further the role of the serotonergic system in the development of semistarvation-induced hyperactivity (Wilckens et al., in press). Hyperactivity was suppressed by serotonin agonists that show a high affinity to the 5-HT$_{1c}$ receptor (TfMPP, mCPP, DOI, and quipazine). This seems to be a specific effect because the agonist effects can be prevented by antagonists sharing a high affinity for the 5-HT$_{1c}$ receptor (mianserin, metergoline, and mesulgerine). Figure 8–4 shows the dose-dependent depression of hyperactivity by mCPP *(top)* and the antagonizing effect of mianserin *(bottom)*. Ketanserin, cyanopindolol, and propranolol, which are mainly active at other serotonin receptors, do not antagonize the mCPP effect. These data clearly indicate that alterations

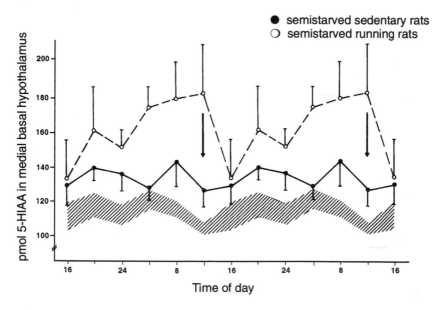

Figure 8–3. Mean ± SE levels of 5-hydroxyindoleacetic acid (5-HIAA) in the medial basal hypothalamus of semistarved sedentary rats and semistarved running rats. *Shaded area* represents mean values ± SE of the sedentary group fed ad libitum. Data from Broocks et al. 1990.

in the serotonergic system are not responsible for the development of semistarvation-induced hyperactivity: serotonin does not induce hyperactivity, but inhibits it.

Another candidate playing a role in the development of hyperactivity is the norepinephrine system. As indicated earlier, we observe greatly elevated norepinephrine values. If we inhibit the norepinephrine neurons

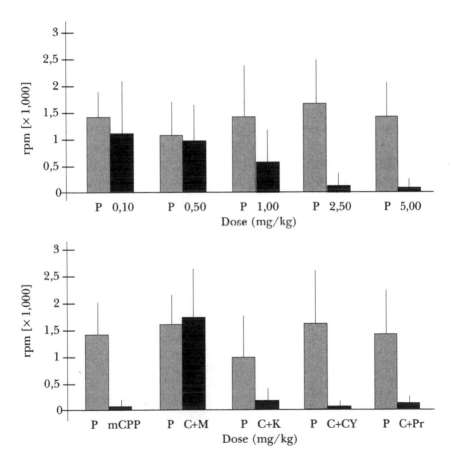

Figure 8–4. Effect of mCPP on running activity in semistarved hyperactive rats. In each group, 12 animals were studied. *Top:* Dose-response curve of the activity-suppressing effect of mCPP (C). P = day previous to testing. *Bottom:* Antagonistic effect of mianserin (M) but not of ketanserin (K), cyanopindolol (CY), and propranolol (Pr) on the suppressive effect of mCPP on running; P = day previous to treatment. Means ± SE are given. Data from Wilckens et al., in press.

by giving alpha$_2$ agonists (clonidine, guanfacine), the running activity is blocked. This is a specific alpha$_2$ effect because it can be antagonized by alpha$_2$ antagonists like yohimbine. Alpha$_1$ and beta agonists do not influence running behavior. The fact that norepinephrine antagonists do not influence running activity argues strongly against a causal role of norepinephrine in semistarvation-induced hyperactivity.

In summarizing these animal experiments, we can state that the mechanism causing hyperactivity in semistarved rats remains unclear. The data, however, do support the hypothesis that the stimulation of the serotonin turnover caused by hyperactivity may be responsible for the reduced food intake observed in this animal model.

Clinical Studies

Cholecystokinin and Gastrin

Cholecystokinin (CCK) is known to regulate satiety in experimental animals and in humans (Gibbs and Smith 1977). It is well established that CCK binds to A receptors at the vagus nerve. Thus, the message of satiety—generated by CCK release after fat- and protein-rich meals—is transported to the hypothalamus and stops feeding. A second, less-well-documented mechanism is the direct effect of smaller CCK molecules that may penetrate the blood-brain barrier like CCK-4. However, because the satiety effect of CCK can be abolished by cutting the vagus nerve, the direct effect of CCK at the brain seems to be less important. A third mechanism should also be considered: CCK activates the pylorus muscle, thus inhibiting gastric emptying. Satiety is also caused by distension of the stomach. A delayed gastric emptying has been observed in anorectic patients (Dubois et al. 1984). Thus, CCK may indirectly prolong the feeling of satiety. We have studied patients with anorexia nervosa, patients with bulimia nervosa, and age-matched healthy control subjects before and after a standardized fluid test meal rich in fat and protein. CCK-8-S was measured after extraction from plasma, separation by high-pressure liquid chromatography (HPLC), and radioimmunoassay of the CCK-8-S fraction. Figure 8–5 shows that basal CCK-8-S levels in plasma were similar in all groups. The increase after the test meal was significantly lower in patients with bulimia nervosa when compared with that of anorectic patients and control subjects. Gastrin levels, which became higher after the test meal, did not differ between groups. These results suggest that impaired feeling of satiety in bulimic patients was accompanied by a low CCK-8-S secretion.

Reproductive Function in Eating Disorders

It has long been established that amenorrhea—an obligatory symptom in anorexia nervosa—is caused by hypothalamic dysregulation (Boyar et al. 1974; Marshall and Kelch 1979; Pirke et al. 1979). Amenorrhea in anorexia has been mainly attributed to weight deficit (Frisch and Revelle 1970). It was therefore surprising that a high percentage of patients with bulimia nervosa who have normal body weight also suffer

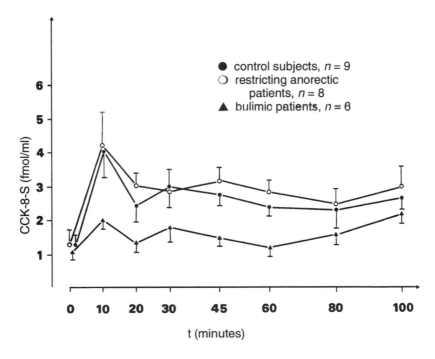

Figure 8–5. Cholecystokinin (CCK)–8-S response to a fat- and protein-rich test meal in eight restricting anorectic patients, six bulimic patients, and nine healthy sex- and age-matched control subjects. CCK-8-S was measured after extraction from plasma, separation by high-pressure liquid chromatography (HPLC), and radioimmunoassay of the CCK-8-S fraction. Means ± SE are given. Data from Philipp et al. 1991.

from menstrual cycle disturbances. In two endocrine studies in 30 patients with bulimia nervosa (Pirke et al. 1988, 1989), we studied gonadotropins (LH and follicle-stimulating hormone) and gonadal hormones (estradiol and progesterone) longitudinally throughout one menstrual cycle or over a period of 6 weeks, when no cycle was observed. All these patients were inpatients treated in a psychosomatic hospital. Half of the patients had anovulatory cycles, and 30% showed luteal phase defects characterized by low progesterone and a luteal phase shorter than 8 days. Only 20% had normal cycles.

Figure 8–6 gives an example of the three types of cycle observed. *Panel A* shows a normal cycle, during which estradiol is slowly increasing in the follicular phase. The values then decrease after ovulation and reach a second maximum during the luteal phase. Progesterone becomes elevated after the ovulation and stays high for 10 days during the luteal phase. In *Panels B* and *C*, two patients with luteal phase defects are seen. Estradiol values still increase properly during the follicular phase. However, during the luteal phase, estradiol and progesterone remain low. In *Panels D* and *E*, two anovulatory cycles are shown. The gonadal hormones remain low throughout the observation period. Two questions arise: 1) What causes the reproductive failure in many bulimic patients, and 2) What are the endocrine mechanisms involved?

A series of studies conducted recently in our laboratory have clearly demonstrated that not only weight deficit but also moderate weight loss can cause disturbances of the menstrual cycle in normal-weight young women (Pirke et al. 1985a, 1986, 1989; Schweiger et al. 1987). In these studies, moderate dieting caused weight loss of 1 kg/week throughout one menstrual cycle. None of the subjects had less than 90% of their ideal body weight at the end of the study. When control cycles were compared with diet cycles, two-thirds of the subjects developed either anovulatory cycles or luteal phase defects.

In summarizing these studies we found:

1. The greater the weight loss, the more likely are menstrual cycle disturbances.
2. Younger women are more susceptible than older women to the effects of dieting.
3. Vegetarian diets are more damaging than mixed diets.
4. Menstrual disturbances caused by dieting are at least partly caused by impairment of the episodic gonadotropin secretion.

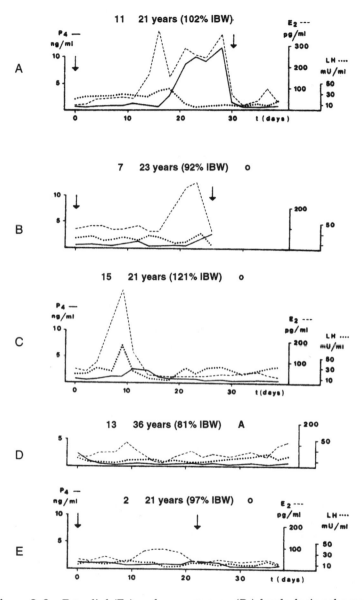

Figure 8–6. Estradiol (E2) and progesterone (P4) levels during the menstrual cycle in patients with bulimia nervosa. *Panel A:* Normal pattern in a bulimic patient. *Panels B* and *C:* Patients with luteal phase disturbances. *Panels D* and *E:* Bulimic patients with anovulatory cycles. IBW = ideal body weight. LH = luteinizing hormone. O = oligomenorrhea. A = amenorrhea. *Arrows* indicate beginning and end of menstrual cycle. Data from Pirke et al. 1987, 1988.

Bulimic patients show intermittent periods of dieting to keep their weight low. This was established in a systematic analysis of eating behavior using food diaries (Woell et al. 1989). The intermittent dieting in bulimia nervosa was also convincingly demonstrated by metabolic and endocrine signs of insufficient food intake: bulimic patients had low plasma glucose, low insulin, elevated free fatty acids, high beta-hydroxybutyric acid and acetoacetate, and low triiodothyronine and norepinephrine (Pirke et al. 1985b). From these observations, we can safely conclude that intermittent dieting contributes to the development of menstrual cycle disturbances in bulimic patients. This does not, however, exclude the possibility that stressful life events or the inability to cope with these events could contribute to the development of infertility.

What endocrine mechanisms are involved in the development of menstrual cycle disturbances in bulimia nervosa? In a recent study of bulimic patients (and 20 healthy control subjects), we evaluated the episodic LH secretion by sampling blood every 15 minutes over a 12-hour period (Schweiger et al. 1992). Figure 8–7 illustrates the findings. In *Panel A,* seven control subjects are shown. In *Panels B* and *C,* the LH secretion pattern of bulimic patients is shown. As can be seen, some bulimic patients with anovulatory cycles have no episodes of LH secretion, whereas others have rather normal LH patterns.

Interpretation of these data is difficult. We could assume that bulimic patients have intermittent periods of regular LH secretion alternating with periods without LH secretion episodes. This pattern might be insufficient for adequate gonadal stimulation. This assumption would explain why we see regular LH patterns in some but not in other bulimic patients with anovulatory cycles. A second explanation would assume that there are different causes for anovulatory cycles in bulimic patients. Some patients have a hypothalamic form of hypogonadism (with disturbed LH secretion), whereas in other cases other mechanisms might be important. Mechanisms acting on the hypothalamic, pituitary, or gonadal level should be considered. The question arises whether hyperprolactinemia could cause menstrual disturbances in bulimia nervosa. Studies in patients with adenoma of the pituitary gland showed a suppression of gonadotropin and gonadal hormone secretion. We demonstrated earlier that bulimic patients show decreased, not increased, prolactin secretion (Pirke and Tuschl 1988). It is therefore unlikely that prolactin plays a role in the development of infertility in bulimia.

Insulin has been shown to be gonadotropic. Patients with bulimia nervosa indeed have reduced plasma insulin levels (Schreiber et al.

1992). However, bulimic patients with infertility did not have different insulin values than bulimic patients with normal menstrual cycles (Schweiger et al. 1992). This observation does not support a role for hypoinsulinemia in infertile bulimic patients.

Norepinephrine is a tropic hormone at the ovary (Ojeda and Lara 1989). It is well known that norepinephrine concentrations are decreased in the plasma of bulimic patients (Heufelder et al. 1985). We compared the orthostatic norepinephrine increase of plasma norepinephrine in bulimic patients with and without hypogonadism. We found no significant differences. We can therefore exclude the possibility that alterations

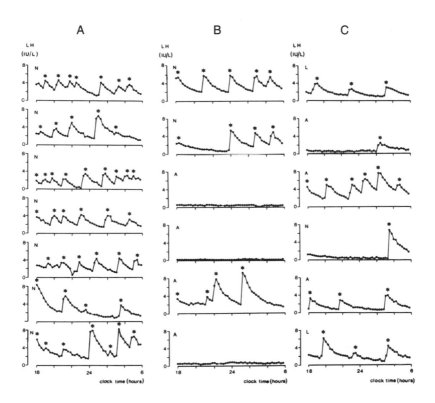

Figure 8–7.   *Panel A:* Episodic luteinizing hormone (LH) secretion in healthy normal control subjects on Days 4–6 of the menstrual cycle. *Panels B* and *C:* Episodic LH secretion in bulimic patients with normal cycles (N), with luteal phase defects (L), and with anovulatory cycles (A). Episodic LH secretions are marked by *asterisks.* Data from Schweiger et al. 1992.

of the sympathetic nervous system cause infertility in bulimia nervosa.

Hyperactivity of the HPA axis may impair the hypothalamic-pituitary-gonadal axis at different levels. Corticotropin-releasing hormone can inhibit gonadotropin-releasing hormone release from the median eminence of the hypothalamus (Rivier and Vale 1984). Glucocorticoids can inhibit gonadal hormone secretion by directly acting at the gonadal level (Doerr and Pirke 1976). We have studied cortisol secretion in bulimic patients and in healthy age- and sex-matched control subjects by measuring plasma levels at half-hour intervals between midnight and 6 A.M. As can be seen in Figure 8–8, patients with anovulatory cycles have significantly

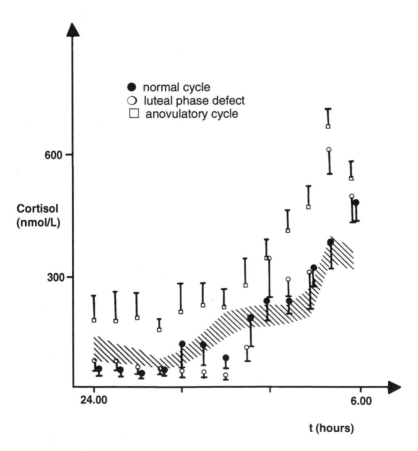

Figure 8–8. Plasma cortisol levels measured between midnight and 6:00 A.M. in bulimic patients with normal cycles, with luteal phase defects, or with anovulatory cycles and in healthy age- and sex-matched control subjects. *Shaded area* shows mean ± SE.

higher cortisol levels at all points in time. These data suggest that hypercortisolism may be involved in the impairment of the reproductive function in bulimia nervosa.

References

Boyar RM, Katz J, Finkelstein JW, et al: Anorexia nervosa: immaturity of the 24-hour luteinizing hormone secretory pattern. N Engl J Med 291:861–865, 1974

Broocks A, Liu J, Pirke KM: Influence of hyperactivity on the metabolism of central monoaminergic neurotransmitters and reproductive function in the semi-starved rat, in The Menstrual Cycle and Its Disorders. Edited by Pirke KM, Wuttke W, Schweiger U. Heidelberg, Springer-Verlag, 1989, pp 88–96

Broocks A, Liu J, Pirke KM: Semistarvation induced hyperactivity compensates for decreased norepinephrine turnover in the mediobasal hypothalamus of the rat. J Neural Transm 79:113–124, 1990

Doerr P, Pirke KM: Cortisol induced suppression of plasma testosterone in normal adult males. J Clin Endocrinol Metab 43:622–629, 1976

Dubois A, Gross HA, Ebert MH: Gastric function in primary anorexia nervosa, in The Psychobiology of Anorexia Nervosa. Edited by Pirke KM, Ploog D. Heidelberg, Springer, 1984, pp 87–92

Epling WF, Pierce WD: Excessive activity and anorexia in rats, in The Menstrual Cycle and Its Disorders. Edited by Pirke KM, Wuttke W, Schweiger U. Heidelberg, Springer, 1989, pp 79–87

Frisch RE, Revelle R: Height and weight at menarche and a hypothesis of critical body weight and adolescent events. Science 169:397–398, 1970

Gibbs J, Smith GP: The influence of CCK on satiety. Am J Clin Nutr 30:758–761, 1977

Heufelder A, Warnhoff M, Pirke KM: Alpha-adrenergic receptors and adenylate cyclase in patients with anorexia nervosa and bulimia. J Clin Endocrinol Metab 61:1053–1060, 1985

Kantak KM, Wayner MJ, Stein JM: Effects of various periods of food deprivation on serotonin turnover in the lateral hypothalamus. Pharmacol Biochem Behav 9:529–534, 1978

Kron L, Katz JL, Gorzynski G, et al: Hyperactivity in anorexia nervosa: a fundamental clinical feature. Compr Psychiatry 19:433–440, 1978

Küderling I, Dorsch G, Warnhoff M, et al: The actions of prostaglandin E-2, naloxone and testosterone on starvation induced suppression of LH. Neuroendocrinology 39:530–537, 1984

Marshall JC, Kelch RP: Low dose pulsatile gonadotropin releasing hormone in anorexia nervosa: a model of human pubertal development. J Clin Endocrinol Metab 49:712–718, 1979

Mrosowsky N: Animal models: anorexia yes, nervosa no, in Psychobiology of Anorexia Nervosa. Edited by Pirke KM, Ploog D. Heidelberg, Springer, 1984, pp 22–34

Ojeda SR, Lara HE: Role of sympathetic nervous system in the regulation of ovarian function, in The Menstrual Cycle and Its Disorders. Edited by Pirke KM, Wuttle W, Schweiger U. Heidelberg, Springer, 1989, pp 33–41

Philipp E, Pirke KM, Kellner MB, et al: Disturbed cholecystokinin secretion in patients with eating disorders. Life Sci 48:2443–2448, 1991

Pirke KM, Spyra B: Influence of starvation on testosterone-LH feedback. Acta Endocrinol (Copenh) 96:413–421, 1981

Pirke KM, Spyra B: Catecholamine turnover in the brain and the regulation of LH and corticosterone in starved male rats. Acta Endocrinol (Copenh) 100:168–176, 1982

Pirke KM, Tuschl RJ: Prolactin concentrations during menstrual cycles disturbed by weight reducing diets or exercise. Infertility 11:185–192, 1988

Pirke KM, Fichter MM, Lund R, et al: Twenty-four hour sleep-wake pattern of plasma LH in patients with anorexia nervosa. Acta Endocrinol (Copenh) 92:193–204, 1979

Pirke KM, Schweiger U, Lemmel W, et al: The influence of dieting on the menstrual cycle of healthy young women. Journal of Clinical Endocrinology 60:1174–1179, 1985a

Pirke KM, Pahl J, Schweiger U, et al: Metabolic and endocrine indices of starvation in bulimia: a comparison with anorexia nervosa. Psychiatry Res 15:33–39, 1985b

Pirke KM, Schweiger U, Laessle R, et al: Dieting influences the menstrual cycle vegetarian versus nonvegetarian diet. Fertil Steril 46:1063–1067, 1986

Pirke KM, Fichter MM, Chlond C, et al: Disturbances of the menstrual cycle in bulimia nervosa. Clin Endocrinol (Oxf) 27:245–251, 1987

Pirke KM, Dogs M, Fichter MM, et al: Gonadotropins, estradiol and progesterone during the menstrual cycle in bulimia nervosa. Clin Endocrinol 29:265–270, 1988

Pirke KM, Schweiger U, Strowitzki T, et al: Dieting causes menstrual irregularities in normal weight young women through impairment of episodic luteinizing hormone secretion. Fertil Steril 51:263–268, 1989

Richter CP: A behavioristic study on the activity of the rat. Comp Psychol Monogr 1:1–55, 1922

Rivier C, Vale W: Influence of corticotropin releasing factor on reproductive function in the rat. Endocrinology 114:914–921, 1984

Schweiger U, Warnhoff M, Pirke KM: Norepinephrine turnover in the hypothalamus of adult male rats: alteration of circadian patterns by semistarvation. J Neurochem 45:706–709, 1985

Schweiger U, Laessle R, Pflister H, et al: Diet induced menstrual irregularities: effects of age and weight loss. Fertil Steril 48:746–751, 1987

Schweiger U, Laessle RG, Schweiger M, et al: Caloric intake, stress and menstrual function in athletes. Fertil Steril 49:447–450, 1988

Schweiger U, Pirke KM, Laessle RG, et al: Gonadotropin secretion in bulimia nervosa. J Clin Endocrinol Metab 74:7722–7727, 1992

Warnhoff M, Dorsch G, Pirke KM: Effect of starvation on gonadotropin secretion and on in vitro release of LHRH from the isolated median eminence of the rat. Acta Endocrinol (Copenh) 103:293–301, 1983

Wilckens T, Schweiger U, Pirke KM: The role of 5-HT receptors in the regulation of starvation induced hyperactivity in the rat. Psychopharmacology (in press)

Woell C, Fichter MM, Pirke KM, et al: Eating behavior of patients with bulimia nervosa. International Journal of Eating Disorders 8:557–568, 1989

Chapter 9

Neuropeptide Abnormalities

Walter H. Kaye, M.D.

⸻⸻►◄⸻⸻

A ccording to DSM-III-R (American Psychiatric Association 1987), anorexia nervosa and bulimia nervosa are disorders of unknown etiology that are characterized by alterations of appetitive behavior and distortions of body image. Patients with eating disorders frequently develop dysphoric mood (Hudson et al. 1983) and various forms of hypothalamic-pituitary dysfunction. Little is known about the pathophysiology of these disorders. Several lines of evidence raise the possibility that disturbances of one or more brain neuropeptide systems may contribute to the symptom complex. Data in animals and humans suggest that brain neuropeptide systems modulate homeostatic functions such as feeding, water balance, and neuroendocrine activity as well as mood and cognition.

Although anorexia nervosa and bulimia nervosa are categorized as eating disorders, pathological eating behavior has tended to be viewed as derivative and not the primary pathophysiology. In the past decade, a better understanding of the modulation of feeding behavior has generated a body of knowledge that allows us to test the hypothesis of whether patients with eating disorders have a defect in some system that modulates feeding behavior (Leibowitz 1984; Morley and Blundell 1988). In this chapter, I focus on many of the neuropeptides known to be disturbed in patients with eating disorders. In addition, I address the question of whether neuropeptide disturbances are state or trait related.

Neuropeptide Function in the Central Nervous System

Neuropeptides are substances composed of chains of several to more than 40 amino acids. Their actions in the brain were initially related to hypothalamic and pituitary modulation of neuroendocrine function. More recently, research has shown that these peptides are located outside of the hypothalamus and produce many extra-endocrine effects. Bissette and Nemeroff (1988) noted that neuropeptides regulate such basic homeostatic behaviors as food and water conservation, sexual behavior, maternal behavior, sleep, and body temperature. In addition, neuropeptides modulate pain and autonomic function.

A variety of neuropeptides have now fulfilled many of the criteria for neurotransmitter status. Neuropeptides and biogenic amines coexist in many neurons. In fact, there are several examples of amines and peptides being stored in the same nerve-ending vesicles (Hokfelt et al. 1984).

Many of these peptides have been demonstrated to be phylogenetically ancient (Widerlov 1988). For example, peptides related to insulin and adrenocorticotropic hormone (ACTH) have been found in unicellular organisms (LeRoith et al. 1980), suggesting that neuropeptides have played a role as biochemical messengers for several billion years. Of particular interest to our field of psychiatry is that most neuropeptides have been found in both the brain and the gut. In fact, most peptides were first discovered in the gut and later in the brain (Widerlov 1988). Although little is known about this gut-brain peptide link, it is possible that such relationships developed during evolution as a means of communicating messages about metabolic needs to organisms. Limited data suggest that patients with eating disorders have disturbances of certain neuropeptide systems. A better understanding of neuropeptide activity holds a promise for a better understanding of the pathophysiology of patients with eating disorders.

Subgroups of Patients With Eating Disorders

A considerable literature (Beaumont et al. 1976; Casper et al. 1980; Garfinkel et al. 1980; Garner et al. 1985; Halmi and Falk 1982; Strober et al. 1982) suggests that certain factors distinguish subgroups of patients with eating disorders. These factors include the amount of weight lost, type of pathological eating behavior, and certain psychopathological characteristics (Herzog and Copeland 1985). Little is known about whether this psychopathology is related to disturbances of brain neuropeptides or whether differences in biological abnormalities differentiate these subgroups.

The terminology used to differentiate these subgroups has been in flux. The best-known eating disorder is anorexia nervosa, whose most distinguishing characteristic is severe emaciation. Two types of consummatory behavior are seen in anorexia nervosa. Restrictor or fasting anorexic patients, who tend to fit the DSM-III-R criteria for anorexia nervosa, lose weight by pure dieting. Bulimic anorexic patients, who qualify for a DSM-III-R diagnosis of both anorexia nervosa and bulimia nervosa, also lose weight but have a periodic disinhibition of restraint and engage in bingeing and purging. Compared with restricting anorectic patients, bulimic anorectic patients have been characterized as displaying significantly more evidence of premorbid behavioral instability, a higher incidence of premorbid and familial obesity, a greater susceptibility to depression, and a higher incidence of behaviors suggestive of impulse disorder (Beaumont et al. 1976; Casper et al. 1980; Garfinkel et al. 1980; Strober et al. 1982). In this chapter, I include both subtypes of patients with anorexia nervosa together.

The third eating disorder is normal-weight bulimia, or bulimia nervosa by DSM-III-R criteria. This disorder is at least 10 times more prevalent than anorexia nervosa (Halmi et al. 1981; Pope et al. 1984; Stangler and Printz 1980). These patients periodically binge and purge, usually by vomiting, but never become emaciated. That is, they maintain a body weight above 85% of average body weight (Garner et al. 1985). Normal-weight bulimic people resemble bulimic anorectic people in terms of impulsivity and a predisposition to obesity (Garner et al. 1985). In this chapter, this group will be described as normal-weight bulimic.

Methodological Issues

State- Versus Trait-Related Disturbances

Teasing apart cause-and-effect relationships in patients with eating disorders is a major methodological dilemma. It is impractical to study eating disorder patients prospectively. However, studies of subjects with eating disorders can be done when subjects are at a stable and normal weight and dietary intake. At such time they are more likely to be free of confounding nutritional influences. If a neuropeptide disturbance is found, then it is more likely to be trait related. Such studies can be done in anorexia nervosa by studying anorectic patients at various stages in their illness—while underweight and at intervals after weight restoration. Similarly, normal-weight bulimic patients can be studied during pathological eating behavior and after being abstinent from bingeing and purging behavior for some length of time.

Methods Used to Assess Neuropeptide Activity

Few methods are available to assess central nervous system (CNS) neuropeptide activity in humans. One commonly used method is to measure concentrations of neuropeptides in cerebrospinal fluid (CSF) or blood. In regard to CSF, studies of concentrations of neuropeptides and neuromodulators invariably raise the question of the physiological relevance of such measurements. For example, concentrations of CSF neuromodulatory substances might not reflect changes in neurotransmission, but might reflect alterations in metabolism or clearance of these substances from CSF. Alternatively, findings are difficult to interpret because of the multiplicity of CNS neuromodulatory pathways and the fact that there is no methodology presently available that can identify the specific pathways that contribute to altered CSF neuromodulator levels. It should be noted, however, that the ability to determine CSF neuromodulatory levels has been very useful in studies of human CNS disease. Somatostatin has been shown to be low in postmortem brain studies of Alzheimer's disease (Davies and Terry 1981; Rossor et al. 1980). Other studies show that CSF somatostatin levels are reduced in patients with Alzheimer's disease (Oram et al. 1981). Despite the limitations inherent in CSF studies, little alternative technology exists at present to study these brain neuromodulators directly in humans in vivo.

Neuropeptide Abnormalities in Anorexia Nervosa

Corticotropin-Releasing Hormone

The possibility of corticotropin-releasing hormone (CRH) hypersecretion in anorexia nervosa is of considerable interest because it is well recognized that underweight anorectic patients have pronounced hypercortisolism (Casper et al. 1979; Walsh et al. 1978). There has been considerable controversy concerning the pathophysiology of hyper-cortisolism in anorexia nervosa. Some studies (Gold et al. 1986; Hotta et al. 1986) have supported the probability that hypercortisolism in an-orexia nervosa is due to hypersecretion of endogenous CRH. Increased CNS CRH activity is of theoretical interest in anorexia because adminis-tration of CRH injected intracerebroventricularly to experimental ani-mals produces many of the physiological and behavioral changes classically associated with anorexia nervosa, including hypothalamic hypogonadism (Rivier and Vale 1984), decreased sexual activity (Sirinathsinghji et al. 1983), decreased feeding behavior (Britton et al. 1982), and hyperactivity (Sutton et al. 1982). Moreover, CRH hyper-secretion has been linked to the symptom complex of depression (Gold et al. 1984; Nemeroff et al. 1984).

Several studies (Hotta et al. 1986; Kaye et al. 1987a) reported elevated CSF CRH levels in underweight anorectic patients (Figure 9–1). We found a normalization of elevated CSF CRH levels after weight gain. Moreover, normalization of CSF CRH in anorexia nervosa was associated with relative normalization of pituitary-adrenal function.

The hypersecretion of CRH in underweight anorectic patients may represent a response to weight loss per se. Hypercortisolism occurs in individuals with protein-calorie malnutrition (Smith et al. 1975), and weight loss in healthy (Berger et al. 1983) or obese (Edelstein et al. 1983) individuals is accompanied by pituitary-adrenal resistance to dexametha-sone. We cannot rule out the possibility that hypersecretion of CRH may precede weight loss in some anorectic patients, particularly those with an affective disorder (i.e., because we found a positive correlation between CSF CRH and depression in the weight-corrected state, but not in under-weight patients). The profound inanition in underweight patients may produce a complex of confounding biochemical, psychological, and cog-nitive changes that may obscure an underlying relationship between CSF CRH and depression.

Opioid Peptides

A question has been raised as to whether altered endogenous opioid activity might contribute to disturbed feeding behavior in anorexia nervosa (Donohoe 1984; Marrazzi and Luby 1986; Moore et al. 1981; Szmukler and Tantam 1984). Such speculation has been fueled by con-siderable data, derived primarily from animal experimentation (Morley et al. 1983), which suggest that opioid agonists increase and opioid antagonists decrease food intake. It should be noted that assessment of brain opioid activity is problematic. First, there are multiple neuropeptides in the CNS that have opioid activity. We are not able to measure most of these peptides in vivo in humans. Second, there is a multiplicity of opioid receptors in the brain. Third, there are limitations placed on clinical research by the relative nonspecificity of pharmacologic probes.

CNS beta-endorphin is one opioid system that can be assessed by measuring levels of immunoreactive beta-endorphin in CSF. Our group (Kaye et al. 1987b) reported that underweight anorectic patients had significantly reduced CSF beta-endorphin concentrations compared with

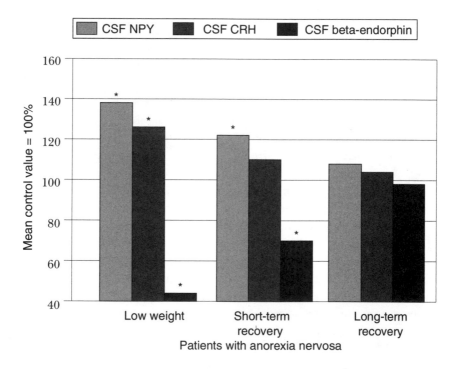

Figure 9–1. Cerebrospinal fluid (CSF) concentrations of neuropeptide Y (NPY), corticotropin-releasing hormone (CRH), and beta-endorphin in patients with anorexia nervosa at three stages of treatment. Values for each neuropeptide are expressed as a percentage of the values found in matched healthy volunteer women, which are set at 100% for each neuropeptide. *Asterisks* indicate a significant difference (*P* < .05) between anorectic patients and control subjects.

healthy volunteers. CSF beta-endorphin levels remained significantly below normal after short-term weight restoration. Long-term weight-restored anorectic patients had normal CSF beta-endorphin concentrations. In contrast, a radioreceptor assay, which measures overall opioid activity, showed that underweight anorectic patients had an increase of CSF opioid activity (Kaye et al. 1982). Finally, CSF dynorphin levels have been reported to be normal in all stages of anorexia nervosa (Lesem et al. 1991). Other opioid peptides cannot be reliably measured in CSF.

Plasma opioids have also been studied in anorectic patients. Brambilla et al. (1985) reported that anorectic patients had increased levels of plasma beta-endorphin and that beta-endorphin levels did not correlate with weight loss; rather, they corresponded with depressive symptomatology. It is important to emphasize that plasma beta-endorphin and CNS beta-endorphin reflect two different, and possibly unrelated, endogenous opioid systems.

Beta-endorphin has been shown to stimulate feeding behavior in rats when injected intraventricularly or into the medial hypothalamus (Leibowitz and Hor 1982; Tseng and Cheng 1980). Assuming that beta-endorphin activity contributes to feeding behavior in humans and that reduced CSF concentrations reflect decreased activity of this system, then it is possible that reduced beta-endorphin activity contributes to food refusal in acutely ill anorectic patients. It should be noted that values of beta-endorphin in CSF (Kaye et al. 1987b) were found to be less than 1% of the values for total opioid activity measured by the radioreceptor assay (Kaye et al. 1982). Other investigators have reported a discrepancy between measurements of beta-endorphin and total opioid activity (Nybert et al. 1983; Recant et al. 1983). Thus, elevated concentrations of one or more of the other endogenous opioid peptides may account for the radioreceptor assay results. Such a possibility remains to be explored.

Brain opioid pathways contribute to the modulation of reproductive function. Opioids suppress pulsatile gonadotropin secretion in rats and sexually mature humans (Grossman 1983; Pfeiffer and Herz 1984). The relationship of opioid activity and reproductive activity has been studied in anorexia nervosa by the use of an infusion of naloxone, an exogenous opiate antagonist (Ropert et al. 1981). Naloxone has been administered to a small number of underweight anorectic patients in three studies. Baranowska et al. (1984) gave a 4-mg naloxone bolus followed by 2.8 mg/hour for 4 hours. They found that 11 of 24 underweight anorectic patients had an increase in luteinizing hormone (LH) secretion after naloxone, and these patients had a history of amenorrhea preceding weight loss. In contrast, the other 13 patients, who had no increase in LH after naloxone, had the onset of amenorrhea after weight loss began. Two other groups (Baraban et al. 1986; Giusti et al. 1988) gave naloxone to 10 underweight anorectic patients and found no increase in LH secretion. Although the study by Baranowska et al. did not measure maturational state, the likelihood that underweight anorectic patients have immature LH patterns suggests that factors other than maturational state may be related to opioid activity in anorexia nervosa. Reduced levels of beta-endorphin argue against the possibility that beta-endorphin inhibits gonadotropin secretion in anorectic patients but raises the possibility that a disturbance of some other endogenous opioid peptide is responsible.

It is also possible that a disturbance of opioid function could contribute to hypercortisolism in anorexia nervosa. Opioids, probably acting through hypothalamic mechanisms (Grossman 1983; Pfeiffer and Herz 1984), inhibit ACTH and cortisol release in humans.

Neuropeptide Y

Neuropeptide Y (NPY), a fairly recently discovered 36-amino-acid peptide (Allen et al. 1983), is of considerable theoretical interest in anorexia nervosa. NPY is among the most potent endogenous stimulants of feeding behavior within the CNS. NPY stimulates feeding behavior in satiated rodents when injected intracerebroventricularly or into the paraventricular nucleus of the hypothalamus (Morley et al. 1987; Stanley and Leibowitz 1984) and is selective for carbohydrate-rich foods (Stanley et al. 1985). NPY is among the most abundant peptides in the CNS (Allen et al. 1983) and is found in the hypothalamus, which provides anatomical support for its site of action on feeding behavior.

Intracerebroventricular administration of NPY to experimental animals produces many of the physiological and behavioral changes classically associated with anorexia nervosa. NPY administration has gonadal steroid–dependent effects on LH secretion (Kalra et al. 1986), suppresses sexual activity (Clark et al. 1985), increases CRH in the hypothalamus (Haas and George 1987), and produces hypotension (Fuxe et al. 1983).

We (Kaye et al. 1990) found that underweight anorectic patients had significantly elevated concentrations of CSF NPY compared with healthy volunteers (Figure 9–1). CSF NPY levels remained significantly elevated after short-term weight restoration. Although CSF NPY levels normalized in the group of long-term weight-restored anorectic patients, those long-term weight-restored anorectic patients who continued to have amenorrhea or oligomenorrhea had significantly elevated CSF NPY concentrations compared with healthy control subjects.

The explanation for elevated levels of CSF NPY in underweight anorectic patients is unclear. Animal studies offer limited support to the possibility that such elevations may represent a homeostatic mechanism to stimulate feeding (Sahu et al. 1988). However, elevated CSF NPY levels appear to be an ineffective stimulant of feeding in underweight anorectic patients because they are notoriously resistant to weight restoration. It is important to note, however, that anorectic patients typically display an obsessive and paradoxical interest in dietary intake and food preparation. We cannot discount the possibility that increased NPY activity could contribute to these cognitions. Alternatively, chronic elevation of NPY could be associated with a down-regulation of the NPY receptors that modulate feeding, more consistent with the food refusal and avoidance of sweet foods typically found in ill anorectic patients.

Anorectic patients invariably have amenorrhea that is thought to be related to a defect at, or above, the hypothalamus (Boyar et al. 1977). The neuropeptide disturbance(s) responsible have not been identified. NPY is intimately involved in the release of luteinizing hormone–releasing hormone (LHRH) into the hypophyseal portal circulation and directly affects pituitary LH response to LHRH (Crowley and Kalra 1987; Kalra et al. 1986). Thus increased NPY secretion, in a reduced gonadal steroid environment, may contribute to inhibition of LHRH or LH release in anorexia nervosa. Weight gain is thought to be important for the reversal of hypothalamic amenorrhea in anorexia nervosa (Jeuniewic et al. 1978), but normal menstrual cycles may not return for months or years after normalization of body weight (Falk and Halmi 1982). These data raise a question about whether persistent elevations of CSF NPY after weight gain contribute to persistent menstrual pathophysiology.

Vasopressin and Oxytocin

Vasopressin and oxytocin are structurally related neuropeptides that are transported from the hypothalamus to the posterior pituitary for release into systemic circulation. In the periphery, vasopressin controls free-water clearance of the kidney (Martin and Reichlin 1987), whereas oxytocin promotes uterine contraction during parturition and milk secretion during the postpartum period (Forsling 1986). In addition, both are distributed in the brain and function as long-acting neuromodulators and to exert complex behavioral effects. Oxytocin administration to rats disrupts memory consolidation and retrieval (Bohus et al. 1978), whereas vasopressin administration enhances memory function (De Weid 1965). Importantly, effects of oxytocin appear to be reciprocal to the effects of vasopressin. For example, oxytocin antagonizes vasopressin's promotion of consolidation of learning acquired during aversive conditioning (Bohus et al. 1978; De Weid 1965). In addition, studies in humans show that oxytocin modulates activation of the hypothalamic-pituitary-adrenal axis by antagonizing vasopressin-induced ACTH release from the anterior pituitary (Legros et al. 1982).

Underweight patients with anorexia nervosa have abnormally high levels of centrally directed vasopressin in association with a profound defect in the osmoregulation of plasma vasopressin (Gold et al. 1983). Demitrack et al. (1990) found that underweight restricting anorectic patients had reduced CSF oxytocin levels. Such abnormalities tend to normalize after weight restoration.

Demitrack et al. (1990) hypothesized that a low level of centrally directed oxytocin could act in concert with a high level of CSF vasopressin in underweight anorectic patients so as to enhance the retention of cognitive distortions of the aversive consequences of eating (i.e., to impair the extinction of aversively conditioned learning). Thus such changes in these neuropeptides may exacerbate the tendency for restricting anorectic patients to have perseverative preoccupation with the adverse consequences of food intake.

State-Related Neuropeptide Alterations

That these neuropeptide disturbances are corrected by weight restoration implies that such disturbances are secondary to malnutrition and weight loss and are not the cause. However, it is important to note that although such neuropeptide disturbances are not a permanent or pathognomonic feature of anorexia nervosa, they are strongly entrenched and are not easily corrected by improved nutrition.

The etiology of anorexia nervosa is unknown. It has been postulated that intrinsic biological alterations, dieting, psychosocial influences, and stresses are among the contributing factors to the onset of this illness. Whatever the cause, once weight loss and malnutrition occur, anorectic patients appear to enter a downward spiral, with malnutrition sustaining and perpetuating the desire for more weight loss and dieting.

Starvation-induced alterations of neuropeptide activity probably contribute to neuroendocrine dysfunctions in anorexia nervosa. It is most likely that CRH alterations contribute to hypercortisolism, and it is possible that NPY alterations contribute to amenorrhea. Alterations of neuropeptide activity (Table 9–1) could contribute to several other characteristic psychophysiological disturbances in acutely ill anorectic patients. Such neuropeptide disturbances could contribute to the vicious cycle that has been hypothesized to occur in anorexia nervosa; that is, the consequences of malnutrition perpetuate pathological behavior. For example, starvation-induced increases of CRH activity and reduced beta-endorphin activity could reduce appetite. However, the same reasoning would suggest that elevated NPY activity would stimulate feeding. Further studies are needed to determine the effects of these neuropeptides on feeding behavior in anorexia nervosa.

Normal-Weight Bulimia Nervosa

Neuropeptide disturbances have been found in patients with normal-weight bulimia nervosa in several systems known to contribute to the

Table 9–1. Hypothetical relationships between symptoms in underweight anorectic patients and neuropeptide effects

Symptoms	Underweight anorectic patients	Increased NPY	Increased CRH	Decreased beta-endorphin	Increased vasopressin	Decreased oxytocin
Feeding	↓	↑	↓	↓		
Motor activity	↑		↑			
Blood pressure	↓	↓				
Sexual interest	↓	↓	↓			
Hypothalamic-pituitary-gonadal axis	↓	↓	↓	↑		
Hypothalamic-pituitary-adrenal axis	↑	↑	↑	↑	↑	↑
Depression	↑		↑	↑		
Cognitive distortions	↑				↑	↑

Note. NPY = neuropeptide Y. CRH = corticotropin-releasing hormone.

modulation of feeding behavior. Studies of pathophysiology have only been done in patients with normal-weight bulimia nervosa who were actively bingeing and purging or who were abstinent from bingeing and purging for short periods of time (up to 4 weeks). We argue that even a month of abstinence is not long enough for neurobiological systems to recover fully. Thus it is not known whether neuropeptide alterations are state or trait related. In terms of state-related factors, Pirke et al. (1985) demonstrated that many women with normal-weight bulimia nervosa show signs of starvation. This study is important because it indicates that these women, despite being of normal weight, are often malnourished. Thus malnutrition could contribute to neuropeptide disturbances in normal-weight bulimic women. In addition, neuropeptide disturbances could be related to bingeing, purging, a state of withdrawal, stress, fluid or electrolyte abnormalities, or the presence of an affective disorder. Alternatively, neuropeptide disturbances could predate the onset of symptoms and contribute to the pathogenesis of this disorder.

Peptide YY

Peptide YY (PYY) is a neuropeptide related to NPY. As noted earlier in this chapter, these peptides are of considerable theoretical interest. It has been claimed (Morley et al. 1985; Stanley et al. 1986) that administration of NPY and PYY stimulates feeding to a greater extent than any other neurochemically specific manipulations examined to date. Both peptides stimulate feeding behavior in satiated rodents when injected intracerebroventricularly (Morley et al. 1985, 1987) or injected into the paraventricular nucleus of the hypothalamus (Stanley and Leibowitz 1984; Stanley et al. 1985). Moreover, both peptides are selective for carbohydrate-rich foods.

    There is a difference between these peptides in their behavioral potency. Paraventricular nucleus PYY injections are approximately three times as potent as NPY injections in stimulating feeding. Both of these peptides are found in the hypothalamus, a finding that provides anatomical support for their site of action on feeding behavior. NPY is one of the most abundant peptides in the CNS (Allen et al. 1983). PYY is contained in the CNS in much lower concentrations (Broome et al. 1985; Ekman et al. 1986). Both peptides, when injected into rat brains, are capable of overriding mechanisms of satiety and body-weight control. For example, Morley et al. (1985) injected PYY intracerebroventricularly into rats for

48 hours and found it caused massive food ingestion to which tolerance did not develop. This powerful effect on feeding behavior in animals has prompted Morley et al. to postulate that increased activity of PYY may contribute to bulimia nervosa.

In fact, several studies (Kaye et al. 1990; M. Lesem, personal communication, June 1989) have found that CSF PYY values were normal when bulimic patients were studied near in time to chronic bingeing and vomiting. However, after 30 days of abstinence from bingeing and vomiting, normal-weight bulimic patients had CSF PYY values that were significantly greater than healthy volunteer women and patients with anorexia

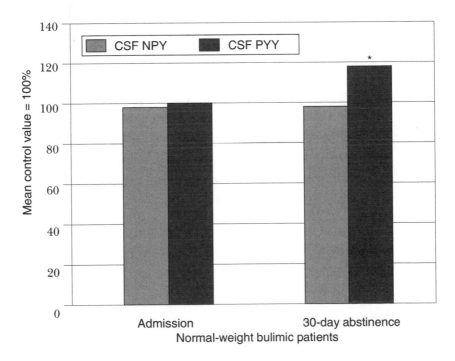

Figure 9–2. Cerebrospinal fluid (CSF) neuropeptide Y (NPY) and peptide YY (PYY) concentrations in patients with normal-weight bulimia nervosa studied on admission to the hospital and after 30 days in the hospital, when they were abstinent from bingeing and purging. Values for each neuropeptide are expressed as a percentage of the values found in matched healthy volunteer women, which are set at 100% for each neuropeptide. The *asterisk* indicates a significant difference (*P* < .05) between bulimic patients and control subjects.

nervosa (Figure 9–2). In contrast, CSF NPY levels were normal in both states.

It is not known why CSF PYY is elevated in bulimic patients abstinent from bingeing and vomiting. One possibility is that chronic bingeing or vomiting behavior, or other state-related factors, can reset the modulation of CNS PYY so that an abrupt cessation of bingeing or vomiting results in an overshoot of CNS PYY secretion. If this is so, then CSF PYY may normalize over a longer period. An alternative provocative interpretation is that bingeing and vomiting may normalize an intrinsic disturbance of CNS PYY release.

Whatever the cause of the high CSF PYY during abstinence from bingeing and vomiting, this disturbance is potentially important. Normal-weight bulimia nervosa is a disorder with a high rate of recidivism despite treatment (Garner et al. 1987; Pope and Hudson 1986). Abnormally elevated CNS PYY activity in the abstinent state may contribute to a persistent drive in feeding behavior, particularly a desire for sweet foods, and the resumption of bingeing behavior.

Cholecystokinin

Geracioti and Liddle (1988) measured blood levels of cholecystokinin (CCK) and subjective satiety in 14 women with bulimia nervosa and 10 healthy women volunteers before and after a mixed-liquid meal. The total integrated plasma CCK response to eating was significantly impaired in bulimic women as was postprandial satiety. Fasting CCK levels were similar in both populations. It has been demonstrated that exogenously administered CCK reduces food intake in animals and humans (Baile et al. 1986; Kissileff et al. 1981; Smith and Gibbs 1985; Stacher 1985). CCK-mediated transmission of satiety appears to occur by way of vagal afferents because vagotomy abolishes the effect of CCK on eating (Baile et al. 1986; Kissileff et al. 1981; Stacher 1985). The authors concluded that patients with bulimia nervosa do not have normal satiety and have impaired secretion of CCK in response to a meal.

Geracioti and Liddle (1988) studied five bulimic patients after a trial of antidepressants. They found that these patients had a significantly increased postprandial CCK response and that there was an increase in the satiety response to eating. Although it is possible that both of these abnormalities may be improved by treatment with tricyclic antidepressants, no data are available to determine if abstinence from bingeing and purging had any effect on CCK response.

Opioids

There has been considerable interest in opioid activity in patients with normal-weight bulimia nervosa. As noted above, opioid agonists increase and opioid antagonists decrease food intake in animals and humans (see review, Morley et al. 1983). Moreover, opioid administration seems preferentially to affect fat and protein consumption in animals and humans (Bhakthavatsalam and Leibowitz 1986; Drewnowski et al. 1989). Patients with normal-weight bulimia nervosa have stereotypic patterns of food consumption, such as bingeing on sweet, high-fat foods, that could reflect alterations in endogenous opioid activity (Drewnowski et al. 1989). In addition, brain opioid pathways contribute to the modulation of reproductive function. Reproductive abnormalities, either oligomenorrhea or amenorrhea, occur in more than 50% of normal-weight bulimic patients (Gwirstman et al. 1983; Pirke et al. 1987; Pyle et al. 1981). The pathogenesis of menstrual disturbances in bulimia nervosa is poorly understood. Disturbances of opioid activity is one possible contributing factor.

There is evidence of opioid disturbances in patients with bulimia nervosa. CSF beta-endorphin levels were reduced in two studies (Brewerton et al. 1992; W. Kaye, unpublished data, June 1985), whereas CSF dynorphin levels were normal (Brewerton et al. 1992; Lesem et al. 1991) (Figure 9–3). Plasma beta-endorphins have been reported to be increased in one study (Fullerton et al. 1986) and decreased in another study (Waller et al. 1986). Several studies have focused on determining whether opioid abnormalities were related to disturbances of feeding or menstrual function in bulimic patients. Several initial studies found that brief trials of opioid antagonists decreased bingeing (Jonas and Gold 1987; Mitchell et al. 1986). However, this was not confirmed by a more recent study (Mitchell et al. 1989). A 3-hour infusion of an opioid antagonist did not change LH secretion in four bulimic subjects (Baraban et al. 1986).

It appears likely that there is a disturbance of beta-endorphin in bulimia nervosa. Whether this disturbance or alterations of any other opioid systems contribute to pathological feeding in normal-weight bulimic patients remains an open question.

Summary

Theoretically, bingeing behavior is consistent with reduced peripheral CCK release, increased brain PYY activity, or faulty opioid modulation.

It may be that neuropeptide disturbances in ill normal-weight bulimic patients are a consequence of extremes of dietary intake, such as are found in anorexia nervosa. Even if this is the case, normal-weight bulimic patients may enter a vicious cycle in which pathological feeding sustains and provokes pathological behavior. Normal-weight bulimia nervosa is a tenacious illness with a high rate of relapse. Thus, persistent disturbances of neuropeptide function after abstinence from bingeing and purging could contribute to the high rate of recidivism. Alternatively, we cannot rule out the possibility that bulimic patients have a trait-related disturbance of neuropeptide activity that contributes to their appetitive dysregulation. The possibility that some trait disturbance may predate the onset of pathological eating behavior in bulimic patients is supported by observations that some bulimic patients may

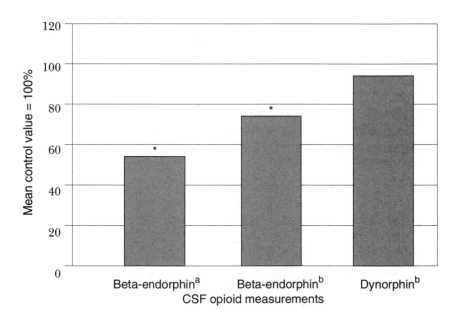

Figure 9–3. Cerebrospinal fluid (CSF) beta-endorphin and dynorphin concentrations in patients with normal-weight bulimia nervosa. Values for each neuropeptide are expressed as a percentage of the values found in matched healthy volunteer women, which are set at 100% for each neuropeptide. *Asterisks* indicate a significant difference ($P < .05$) between bulimic patients and control subjects. *Sources.* [a]W. H. Kaye, H. E. Gwirtsman, and W. H. Berrettini (unpublished data, June 1985). [b]Brewerton et al. (1992).

adopt binge-vomit cycles to counter a predisposition to developing obesity (Pyle et al. 1981) and that pathological eating begins as a weight-control technique (Chiodo and Latimer 1983).

Conclusions

With reference to eating disorders, our understanding of CNS pathophysiology has lagged behind the advances made in understanding many other psychiatric disorders. In part, this may be due to limited knowledge of the mechanisms that modulate appetite and relevant physiological functions. The past decade has seen a rapid increase in preclinical and clinical knowledge about the regulation of appetite. Such knowledge has the potential for offering new insights into understanding the neurobiology of eating disorders.

It has been theorized that a vicious cycle develops in anorexia nervosa in the sense that consequences of malnutrition perpetuate pathological behavior. In fact, starvation-induced alterations of CRH, beta-endorphin, NPY, vasopressin, and oxytocin activity probably contribute to neuroendocrine disturbances and may play a role in behavioral and appetitive abnormalities. The correction of these neuropeptide disturbances by weight restoration implies that such disturbances are secondary to malnutrition or weight loss and are not the cause.

Less is known about normal-weight bulimia nervosa. Data from several centers show that normal-weight bulimic patients have alterations of CCK, PYY, and opioid systems. It is not clear whether these alterations are trait or state related. Still, they are part of this disorder's neurobiological syndrome and imply that bulimia nervosa is not simply a variant of affective disorders. Finally, these data raise a question about whether antidepressants are therapeutic because they correct one or more of these neuropeptide disturbances.

References

Allen YS, Adrian TE, Allen JM: Neuropeptide Y distribution in the rat brain. Science 221:877–879, 1983

American Psychiatric Association: Diagnostic and Statistical Manual of Mental Disorders, 3rd Edition. Washington, DC, American Psychiatric Association, 1987

Baile CA, McLaughlin CL, Della-Fera MA: Role of cholecystokinin and opioid peptides in control of food intake. Physiol Rev 66:172–234, 1986

Baraban JM, Walsh BT, Gladis M, et al: Effect of naloxone on luteinizing hormone secretion in eating disorders: a pilot study. International Journal of Eating Disorders 5:149–155, 1986

Baranowska B, Rozbicka G, Jeske W, et al: The role of endogenous opiates in the mechanism of inhibited luteinizing hormone (LH) secretion in women with anorexia nervosa: the effect of naloxone on LH, follicle-stimulating hormone, prolactin, and beta-endorphine secretion. J Clin Endocrinol Metab 59:412–416, 1984

Beaumont PJV, George GCW, Smart DE: "Dieters" and "vomiters" in anorexia nervosa. Psychol Med 6:617–622, 1976

Berger M, Pirke K, Doerr P, et al: Influence of weight loss on the dexamethasone suppression test. Arch Gen Psychiatry 40:585–586, 1983

Bhakthavatsalam P, Leibowitz SF: Morphine-elicited feeding: diurnal rhythm, circulating corticosterone and macronutrient selection. Pharmacol Biochem Behav 24:911–917, 1986

Bissette G, Nemeroff CB: The role of neuropeptides in the pathogenesis and treatment of schizophrenia, in Neuropeptides in Psychiatric and Neurological Disorders. Edited by Nemeroff CB. Baltimore, MD, Johns Hopkins University Press, 1988, pp 49–75

Bohus B, Kovacs GL, De Weid D: Oxytocin, vasopressin and memory: opposite effects on consolidation and retrial processes. Brain Res 157:414–417, 1978

Boyar RM, Hellman LD, Roffwarg HP, et al: Cortisol secretion and metabolism in anorexia nervosa. N Engl J Med 296:190–193, 1977

Brambilla F, Cavagnini F, Invitti C, et al: Neuroendocrine and psychopathological measures in anorexia nervosa: resemblances to primary affective disorders. Psychiatry Res 16:165–176, 1985

Brewerton TD, Lydiard RB, Laraina MT, et al: CSF and β-endorphin and dynorphin in bulimia nervosa. Am J Psychiatry 149:1086–1090, 1992

Britton DR, Koob GR, Rivier J, et al: Intraventricular corticotropin-releasing factor enhances behavioral effects of novelty. Life Sci 31:363–367, 1982

Broome M, Hokfelt T, Terenius L: Peptide YY (PYY)-immunoreactivity neurons in the lower brain stem and spinal cord of rat. Acta Physiol Scand 125:349–352, 1985

Casper RC, Chatterton RT, Davis JM: Alterations in serum cortisol and its binding characteristics in anorexia nervosa. J Clin Endocrinol Metab 49:406–411, 1979

Casper RC, Eckert ED, Halmi KA, et al: Bulimia: its incidence and clinical importance in patients with anorexia nervosa. Arch Gen Psychiatry 37:1030–1035, 1980

Chiodo J, Latimer PR: Vomiting as a learned weight-control technique in bulimia. J Behav Ther Exp Psychiatry 14:131–135, 1983

Clark JT, Kalra PS, Kalra SP: Neuropeptide Y stimulates feeding but inhibits sexual behavior in rats. Endocrinology 117:2435–2442, 1985

Crowley WR, Kalra SP: Neuropeptide Y stimulates the release of luteinizing hormone-releasing hormone from medial basal hypothalamus in vitro: modulation by ovarian hormones. Neuroendocrinology 46:97–103, 1987

Davies P, Terry RD: Cortical somatostatin-like immunoreactivity in cases of Alzheimer's disease and senile dementia of the Alzheimer type. Neurobiol Aging 2:9–14, 1981

Demitrack MA, Lesem MD, Listwak SJ, et al: CSF oxytocin in anorexia nervosa and bulimia nervosa: clinical and pathophysiologic considerations. Am J Psychiatry 147:882–886, 1990

De Weid D: The influences of the posterior and intermediate lobe of the pituitary and pituitary peptides on the maintenance of a conditioned avoidance response in rats. International Journal of Neuropharmacology 4:157–167, 1965

Donohoe TP: Stress-induced anorexia: implications for anorexia nervosa. Life Sci 34:203–218, 1984

Drewnowski A, Gosnell B, Krahn D, et al: Opioids affect taste preferences for sugar and fat (New Research #396). San Francisco, CA, American Psychiatric Association Conference, May 1989

Edelstein CK, Roy-Byrne P, Fawy FI, et al: Effects of weight loss on the dexamethasone suppression test. Am J Psychiatry 140:338–341, 1983

Ekman R, Wahlestedt C, Bottcher G, et al: Peptide YY-like immunoreactivity in the central nervous system of the rat. Regul Pept 16:157–168, 1986

Falk CR, Halmi KA: Amenorrhea in anorexia nervosa: examination of the critical body weight hypothesis. Biol Psychiatry 17:799–806, 1982

Forsling ML: Regulation of oxytocin release, in Current Topics in Neuroendocrinology, Vol 6. Edited by Pfaff D, Ganen D. New York, Springer-Verlag, 1986, pp 19–53

Fullerton DT, Swift WJ, Getto CJ, et al: Plasma immunoreactive beta-endorphin in bulimics. Psychol Med 16:59–63, 1986

Fuxe K, Agnati LF, Harfstrand A: Central administration of neuropeptide Y induces hypotension, bradypnea and EEG synchronization in the rat. Acta Physiol Scand 118:189–192, 1983

Garfinkel PE, Moldofsky H, Garner DM: The heterogeneity of anorexia nervosa. Arch Gen Psychiatry 37:1036–1040, 1980

Garner DM, Garfinkel PE, O'Shaughnessy M: The validity of the distinction between bulimia with and without anorexia nervosa. Am J Psychiatry 142:581–587, 1985

Garner DM, Fairburn C, Davis R: Cognitive-behavioral treatment of bulimia nervosa: a critical appraisal. Behav Modif 4:398–431, 1987

Geracioti TD, Liddle RA: Impaired cholecystokinin secretion in bulimia nervosa. N Engl J Med 319:683–688, 1988

Giusti M, Torre R, Traverso L, et al: Endogenous opioid blockade and gonado-tropin secretion: role of pulsatile luteinizing hormone-releasing hormone administration in anorexia nervosa and weight loss amenorrhea. Fertil Steril 49:797–801, 1988

Gold PW, Kaye W, Robertson GL, et al: Abnormalities in plasma and cerebrospinal-fluid arginine vasopressin in patients with anorexia nervosa. N Engl J Med 308:1117–1123, 1983

Gold PW, Chrousos G, Kellner C, et al: Psychiatric implications of basic and clinical studies with corticotropin-releasing factor. Am J Psychiatry 141:619–627, 1984

Gold PW, Gwirtsman H, Avgerinos PC, et al: Abnormal hypothalamic-pituitary-adrenal function in anorexia nervosa: pathophysiologic mechanisms in underweight and weight-corrected patients. N Engl J Med 314:1335–1342, 1986

Grossman A: Brain opiates and neuroendocrine function. Clinics in Endocrinology Metabolism 12:725–746, 1983

Gwirstman HE, Roy-Byrne P, Yager J, et al: Neuroendocrine abnormalities in bulimia. Am J Psychiatry 140:559–563, 1983

Haas DA, George SR: Neuropeptide Y administration acutely increases hypothalamic corticotropin-releasing factor immunoreactivity: lack of effect in other rat brain regions. Life Sci 41:2725–2731, 1987

Halmi KA, Falk JR: Anorexia nervosa: a study of outcome discrimination in exclusive dieters and bulimics. Journal of the American Academy of Child Psychiatry 21:369–375, 1982

Halmi KA, Falk JR, Schwartz E: Binge-eating and vomiting: a survey of a college population. Psychol Med 11:697–706, 1981

Herzog DB, Copeland PM: Eating disorders. N Engl J Med 313:295–303, 1985

Hokfelt T, Hohansson O, Goldstein M: Chemical anatomy of the brain. Science 225:1326–1334, 1984

Hotta M, Shibasaki T, Masuda A, et al: The responses of plasma adrenocorticotropin and cortisol to corticotropin-releasing hormone (CRH) and cerebrospinal fluid immunoreactive CRH in anorexia nervosa patients. J Clin Endocrinol Metab 62:319–324, 1986

Hudson JI, Pope HG, Jonas JM, et al: Phenomenologic relationship of eating disorders to major affective disorder. Psychiatry Res 9:345–354, 1983

Jeuniewic N, Brown GM, Garfinkel PE, et al: Hypothalamic function as related to body weight and body fat in anorexia nervosa. Psychol Med 40:187–198, 1978

Jonas JM, Gold MS: Treatment of antidepressant-resistant bulimia with naltrexone. Int J Psychiatry Med 24:195–199, 1987

Kalra SP, Allen LG, Clark JT, et al: Neuropeptide Y—an integrator of reproductive and appetitive functions, in Neural and Endocrine Peptides and Receptors. Edited by Moody TW. New York, Plenum, 1986, pp 353–366

Kaye WH, Pickar D, Naber D, et al: Cerebrospinal fluid opioid activity in anorexia nervosa. Am J Psychiatry 139:643–645, 1982

Kaye WH, Gwirtsman HE, George DT, et al: Elevated cerebrospinal fluid levels of immunoreactive corticotropin-releasing hormone in anorexia nervosa: relation to state of nutrition, adrenal function, and intensity of depression. J Clin Endocrinol Metab 64:203–208, 1987a

Kaye WH, Berrettini WH, Gwirtsman HE, et al: Reduced cerebrospinal fluid levels of immunoreactive pro-opiomelancortin related peptides (including β-endorphin) in anorexia nervosa. Life Sci 41:2147–2155, 1987b

Kaye WH, Berrettini W, Gwirtsman H, et al: Altered cerebrospinal fluid neuropeptide Y and peptide YY immunoreactivity in anorexia and bulimia nervosa. Arch Gen Psychiatry 47:548–556, 1990

Kissileff HR, Pi-Sunyer FX, Thornton J, et al: C-terminal octapeptide of cholecystokinin decreased food intake in man. Am J Clin Nutr 34:154–160, 1981

Legros JJ, Chiodera P, Demy-Ponsart E: Inhibitory influence of exogenous oxytocin on adrenocorticotropin secretion in normal human subjects. J Clin Endocrinol Metab 55:1035–1039, 1982

Leibowitz SF: Noradrenergic function in the medial hypothalamus: potential relation to anorexia nervosa and bulimia, in The Psychobiology of Anorexia Nervosa. Edited by Pirke KM, Ploog D. Berlin, Springer-Verlag, 1984, pp 35–45

Leibowitz SF, Hor L: Endorphinergic and alpha-noradrenergic systems in the para-ventricular nucleus: effects on eating behavior. Peptides 3:421–428, 1982

LeRoith D, Shiloach J, Roth J, et al: Evolutionary origins of vertebrate hormones: substances similar to mammalian insulins are native to unicellular eukaryotes (Tetrahymena/Neurospora). Proc Natl Acad Sci USA 77:6184–6188, 1980

Lesem MD, Berrettini WH, Kaye WH, et al: Measurement of CSF dynorphin A 1-8 immunoreactivity in anorexia nervosa and normal weight bulimia. Biol Psychiatry 29:224–252, 1991

Marrazzi MA, Luby ED: An auto-addiction opioid model of chronic anorexia nervosa. International Journal of Eating Disorders 5:191–208, 1986

Martin JB, Reichlin S: Clinical Neuroendocrinology, 2nd Edition. Philadelphia, PA, FA Davis, 1987

Mitchell JE, Laine DE, Morley JE, et al: Naloxone but not CCK-8 may attenuate binge-eating behavior in patients with the bulimia syndrome. Biol Psychiatry 21:1399–1406, 1986

Mitchell JE, Christenson G, Jennings J, et al: A placebo-controlled, double-blind crossover study of naltrexone hydrochloride in outpatients with normal weight bulimia. J Clin Psychopharmacol 9:94–97, 1989

Moore R, Mills IH, Forster A: Naloxone in the treatment of anorexia nervosa: effect on weight. J R Soc Med 74:129–131, 1981

Morley JE, Blundell JE: The neurobiological basis of eating disorders: some formulations. Biol Psychiatry 23:53–78, 1988

Morley JE, Levine AS, Yim GK, et al: Opioid modulation of appetite. Neurosci Biobehav Rev 7:281–305, 1983

Morley JE, Levine AS, Grace M, et al: Peptide YY (PYY), a potent orexigenic agent. Brain Res 341:200–203, 1985

Morley JE, Levine AS, Gosnell BA, et al: Effect of neuropeptide Y on ingestive behaviors in the rat. Am J Physiol 252:R599–R609, 1987

Nemeroff CB, Widerkiv E, Bisetts G, et al: Elevated concentrations of CSF corticotropin-releasing factor-like immunoreactivity in depressed patients. Science 226:1342–1344, 1984

Nybert F, Wahlstrom A, Sjolund B, et al: Characterization of electrophoretically separable endorphins in human CSF. Brain Res 259:267, 1983

Oram JJ, Edwardson J, Millard PH: Investigation of CSF neuropeptides in idiopathic senile dementia. Gerontology 27:216–223, 1981

Pfeiffer A, Herz A: Endocrine actions of opioids. Horm Metab Res 16:386–397, 1984

Pirke KM, Pahl J, Schweiger U, et al: Metabolic and endocrine indices of starvation in bulimia: a comparison with anorexia nervosa. Psychiatry Res 15:33–39, 1985

Pirke KM, Fichter MM, Chlond C, et al: Disturbances of the menstrual cycle in bulimia nervosa. Clin Endocrinol (Oxf) 27:245–251, 1987

Pope HG, Hudson JI: Antidepressant drug therapy for bulimia: current status. J Clin Psychiatry 47:339–345, 1986

Pope HG, Hudson JI, Yurgelun-Todd D: Anorexia nervosa and bulimia among 300 suburban women shoppers. Am J Psychiatry 141:292–294, 1984

Pyle RL, Mitchell JE, Eckert ED: Bulimia: a report of 34 cases. J Clin Psychiatry 42:60–64, 1981

Recant L, Voyles N, Wade A, et al: Studies on the role of opiate peptides in two forms of genetic obesity: ob/ob mouse fa/fa rat. Horm Metab Res 15:589–593, 1983

Rivier C, Vale W: Influence of corticotropin-releasing factor on reproductive functions in the rat. Endocrinology 114:914–921, 1984

Ropert JF, Quigley ME, Yen SS: Endogenous opiates modulate pulsatile luteinizing hormone release in humans. J Clin Endocrinol Metab 52:583–585, 1981

Rossor MN, Emson PC, Mountjoy CQ, et al: Reduced amounts of immunoreactive somatostatin in the temporal cortex in senile dementia of the Alzheimer type. Neurosci Lett 20:373–377, 1980

Sahu A, Kalra PS, Kalra SP: Food deprivation and ingestion induces reciprocal changes in neuropeptide Y concentrations in the paraventricular nucleus. Peptides 9:83–86, 1988

Sirinathsinghji DJ, Rees LH, Rivier J, et al: Corticotropin-releasing factor is a potent inhibitor of sexual receptivity in the female rat. Nature 305:232–235, 1983

Smith GP, Gibbs J: The satiety effect of cholecystokinin: recent progress and current problems. Ann N Y Acad Sci 448:417–423, 1985

Smith GP, Bledsoe T, Chhetri MK: Cortisol metabolism and the pituitary-adrenal axis in adults with protein-calorie malnutrition. J Clin Endocrinol Metab 40:43–52, 1975

Stacher G: Satiety effects of cholecystokinin and ceruletide in lean and obese man. Ann N Y Acad Sci 448:431–436, 1985

Stangler RS, Printz AM: DSM-III psychiatric diagnosis in a university population. Am J Psychiatry 137:937–940, 1980

Stanley BC, Leibowitz SF: Neuropeptide Y: stimulation of feeding and drinking by injection into the paraventricular nucleus. Life Sci 35:2635–2642, 1984

Stanley BC, Daniel DR, Chin AS, et al: Paraventricular nucleus injections of peptide YY and neuropeptide Y preferentially enhance carbohydrate ingestion. Peptides 6:1205–1211, 1985

Stanley BC, Kyrkouli SE, Lampert S, et al: Neuropeptide Y chronically injected into the hypothalamus: a powerful neurochemical inducer of hyperphagia and obesity. Peptides 7:1189–1192, 1986

Strober M, Salkin B, Burroughs J, et al: Validity of the bulimia-restricter criteria in anorexia nervosa. J Nerv Ment Dis 170:345–351, 1982

Sutton RE, Koob GF, LeMoul M: Corticotropin-releasing factor produces behavioral activation in rats. Nature 297:331–333, 1982

Szmukler GI, Tantam D: Anorexia nervosa: starvation dependence. Br J Med Psychol 57:303–310, 1984

Tseng L, Cheng DS: Acute and chronic administration of β-endorphin and naloxone on food and water intake in rats. Federation Proceedings 39:606, 1980

Waller DA, Kiser RS, Hardy BW, et al: Eating behavior and plasma beta-endorphin in bulimia. Am J Clin Nutr 44:20–23, 1986

Walsh BT, Stewart JW, Levin J, et al: Adrenal activity in anorexia nervosa. Psychosom Med 40:499–506, 1978

Widerlov E: The future of neuropeptides in psychiatry and neurology, in Neuropeptides in Psychiatric and Neurological Disorders. Edited by Nemeroff CB. Baltimore, MD, Johns Hopkins University Press, 1988, pp 281–306

Chapter 10

Starvation-Related Endocrine Changes

Manfred M. Fichter, M.D.

B iological adaptation to times of famine was of great impor- tance for the evolution of the human race. There are numerous references in historical accounts to times of famine as a result of floods, severe droughts, the devastation of war, and earthquakes. Humankind would not have evolved and survived without the efficient biological mechanism of adaptation to famine and starvation. It is interesting to note that many religions prescribe rites of fasting at certain times of the year. Fasting is thought to purify the soul from sins and guilt and to purify the body. Fasting as a treatment has been advocated by Hippocrates, Celsius, and Sydenham for the cure of illnesses.

Fasting may also be used to put pressure on others; this dynamic is present in some families with a member with anorexia nervosa and in the use of fasting as a political weapon. The scientific exploration of the ef- fects of malnutrition and of deliberate fasting began fairly recently, at the end of the last century, with an experiment by the physician Tanner on himself (see Keys et al. 1950). About two decades later, Benedict (1915) conducted the Carnegie Nutrition Laboratory fasting experiment on healthy males and under conditions of semistarvation. The most exten- sive and widely cited fasting experiment—the Minnesota experiment— was conducted by Keys et al. (1950). A group of male "semi-volunteers" (conscientious objectors to military service) participated in this semi-starvation experiment over a period of 168 days. This study was the first to note mental changes during semistarvation in detail. The following disturbances were most common during semistarvation: tiredness, hunger, loss of appetite, sensitivity to noise, irritability, apathy, loss of concentration, loss of libido, loss of vigilance, emotional instability, depression, and decreased motor activity.

Sophisticated neuroendocrine assessments were not possible at the time the Minnesota experiment (Keys et al. 1950) was conducted. The first well-controlled study on neuroendocrine functioning in healthy subjects under conditions of complete food abstinence using modern radioimmunoassay techniques for determining plasma hormone levels was the Munich University starvation experiment (MUSE). The main hypothesis of this study was that reduced calorie intake (total food abstinence) in healthy subjects results in multiple endocrine changes. These changes can be seen as an adaptation of the human body to starvation (Fichter 1985; Fichter and Pirke 1986a, 1986b, 1990b; Fichter et al. 1986). Five healthy female paid volunteers were assessed over the four phases of the experiment: 1) a baseline phase, during which body weight was maintained at ideal (original) body weight; 2) a phase of fasting for 3 weeks under conditions of total food abstinence, resulting in a mean weight loss of 8.0 kg (15%) of ideal body weight; 3) a phase of restoration of body weight to the original level; and 4) a final baseline phase with maintenance of ideal body weight. Plasma concentrations of cortisol, luteinizing hormone (LH), follicle-stimulating hormone (FSH), growth hormone, thyroid-stimulating hormone (TSH), and prolactin were measured over 24 hours in 30-minute intervals before weight loss, after weight loss, and after weight restoration. At multiple times during the study, dexamethasone suppression tests (DSTs), thyrotropin-releasing hormone (TRH) tests, and clonidine tests were performed (for methodology and technical details, see Fichter and Pirke 1986a, 1986b).

The MUSE constitutes a fundamental analysis of neuroendocrine and neurotransmitter changes during starvation. Its results may help us to single out the causes of neuroendocrine and neurotransmitter dysfunctions in anorexia nervosa and bulimia nervosa. Reduced calorie intake or loss of body weight on the one hand and primary dysfunctions in the brain on the other could possibly result in neuroendocrine and neurotransmitter dysfunctions in eating disorders. It appears important to account for the variance of the effects of each of these possible causes. In studies of patients with eating disorders, these possible causes for endocrine changes could be confounded. Possible causes for neuroendocrine changes may also be confounded in studies of malnourished persons in Third-World countries, who show reduced calorie intake, protein deficiency, and vitamin deficiencies. This was the reason for designing the MUSE as an "experimentum crucis" to analyze the effects of total food abstinence with supplementation of minerals and vitamins in healthy subjects.

In this study, our major hypothesis—that reduced calorie intake causes multiple neuroendocrine changes—was confirmed. Reduced food intake in healthy subjects resulted in 1) hyperactivity of the hypothalamic-pituitary-adrenal (HPA) axis and insufficient cortisol suppression in the DST; 2) a diminished TSH response to stimulation with TRH; 3) regression in the 24-hour secretion pattern of gonadotropic hormones (LH, FSH); 4) increased basal growth hormone secretion after weight loss; and 5) a blunted growth hormone response to stimulation with the alpha$_2$-adrenergic receptor agonist clonidine after subsequent weight gain. Because very similar neuroendocrine disturbances in experimental starvation have been found in anorexia nervosa and to a lesser extent in bulimia nervosa, these results point to the importance of reduced calorie intake as a cause for neuroendocrine and neurotransmitter changes.

The results of the MUSE were confirmed and extended in studies by Schweiger et al. (1986) and Mullen et al. (1987) using a semistarvation paradigm and not the total food abstinence paradigm used in the MUSE. Mullen et al. studied 14 healthy female subjects, who received a low-calorie diet (1,000–1,200 kcal/day). As in the MUSE, insufficient cortisol suppression in response to dexamethasone was seen, and shortened rapid-eye-movement (REM) latencies in the sleep electroencephalogram were observed under conditions of reduced calorie intake. Both reduced REM latency (Kupfer 1984) and insufficient suppression in the DST (Carroll 1982) have been claimed to be "biological markers" for depression. These results and ours in the MUSE shed doubt on this notion and demonstrate that disturbances in the HPA axis in anorexia nervosa and bulimia nervosa are a result of (temporarily) reduced calorie intake.

In the study by Schweiger et al. (1986), two groups of 18 healthy normal-weight young women were studied under conditions of semistarvation (1,000 kcal/day). One group received a mixed diet (relatively high-protein, high-fat, and low-carbohydrate content), and another group received a largely vegetarian diet (low-protein, low-fat, and high-carbohydrate content). In accordance with the hypothesis of Wurtman et al. (1981), results of this study indicated reduced central serotonin metabolism as a consequence of a reduced tryptophan/large neutral amino acid quotient in women consuming few carbohydrates. Results of the clonidine test in the MUSE indicate reduced central metabolism of yet another neurotransmitter—norepinephrine—as a result of reduced calorie intake.

Gorozhanin and Lobkov (1990) exposed healthy volunteers to prolonged starvation (14 days), which resulted in an increase in plasma and urinary epinephrine, adrenocorticotropic hormone (ACTH), beta-endorphin, plasma cortisol, somatotropin, glucagon, cyclic adenosine monophosphate, and acetylcholine. Starvation resulted in a decrease in plasma norepinephrine, triiodothyronine (T_3), thyroxine (T_4), prolactin, insulin, C-peptide, FSH, LH, testosterone, histamine, prostaglandins A and E_2, and the pH level.

Jung et al. (1985) studied six healthy men before and after 36-hour periods of starvation. As expected, starvation resulted in a reduction of serum T_3 and a blunted TSH response to TRH. The LH response to gonadotropin-releasing hormone (GnRH) was significantly increased during starvation; the FSH response to GnRH was unaffected. Basal serum prolactin was not reduced after 36 hours of starvation. Prolactin responses to TRH and to the dopamine receptor blocker metoclopramide were unchanged during starvation, indicating that dopamine influence is of limited importance for neuroendocrine regulations during starvation.

In a number of studies, the effects of protein-calorie malnutrition in humans have been assessed. Cooke et al. (1964), Alleyne and Young (1967), and Smith et al. (1975) described increases in plasma cortisol concentrations, changes in 24-hour plasma cortisol pattern, prolonged half-life of plasma cortisol (indicating a slower cortisol catabolism), and insufficient suppression of cortisol secretion after application of dexamethasone in undernourished people in Third-World countries and in patients suffering from malnutrition due to various other organic diseases. Schelp et al. (1976, 1977, 1978) showed decreased levels for albumin, prealbumin, transferrin, proteinase inhibitors, inter-alpha-trypsin inhibitor, and alpha$_2$-macroglobulin in patients with protein-energy malnutrition with infection. The results provide evidence for the hypothesis that proteinase inhibitors limit the syntheses of albumin, prealbumin, and transferrin in protein-energy malnutrition with infection. There is a problem, however, in generalizing findings in protein-calorie malnutrition to anorexia nervosa and bulimia nervosa because—different from protein-calorie malnutrition—patients with anorexia nervosa and bulimia nervosa usually eat a high-protein, low-carbohydrate, and low-fat diet.

Animal Research on Starvation

LH and gonadal hormone secretion have been found to be depressed in starved rats (Campbell et al. 1977; Howland and Skinner 1973; Pirke and Spyra 1981; Pirke et al. 1984; Root and Russ 1972; Srebnik 1970). Pirke and Spyra (1982) showed suppressed LH plasma concentrations in male Wistar rats after only 2 days of food deprivation and a significant increase in plasma corticosterone after 5 days of starvation. Pirke and Spyra (1982) also showed a reduced catecholamine turnover (norepinephrine, dopamine) in the basal hypothalamus, the preoptic area, and the median eminence. Injection of the catecholamine precursor L-dopa and the alpha$_2$-agonist clonidine prevented the increase in plasma corticosterone. The decrease in plasma LH following food deprivation was not influenced by catecholamine precursors (L-dopa) or norepinephrine agonists (clonidine). Thus, it appears likely that a decreased activity of noradrenergic neurons may be responsible for the corticosterone increase during food deprivation. It is assumed that food deprivation mainly influences hypothalamic control because the pituitary gland can be stimulated by synthetic luteinizing hormone–releasing hormone (LHRH) in starved rats (Campbell et al. 1977; Pirke and Spyra 1981; Root and Russ 1972). Küderling et al. (1984) showed that in the terminal region of the hypothalamic LHRH system, the release of LHRH and the reaction of prostaglandin E$_2$ were not altered by starvation. The starvation-induced LHRH suppression was shown not to be due to a dysfunction at the pituitary level. The activity of the pituitary-gonadal axis appears to be impaired as a result of hypothalamic dysfunction in animals.

Broocks et al. (1989, 1990a, 1990b) analyzed the effects of semistarvation and running-wheel hyperactivity in male Wistar rats. Semistarvation over a 10-day period with continuous access to a running wheel resulted in a weight loss of 30% in the rats. Semistarved rats increased their activity up to 20 km/day; controls fed ad lib ran 2.3 km/day. Corticosterone was synergistically increased by semistarvation and activity; the reduction in T$_3$ as a result of semistarvation was significantly larger in rats with access to the running wheel. Although LH and testosterone were significantly decreased by semistarvation, hyperactivity did not result in an additional suppression of LH and testosterone. The hypothalamic norepinephrine turnover—as estimated by the concentration of its major metabolite, 3-methoxy-4-hydroxyphenylglycol (MHPG)—was significantly decreased in semistarved rats, and hyperactivity counteracted this effect. The same was found for the dopamine turnover, estimated by the concentrations of its major metabolite, dihydrophenylacetic acid (DOPAC), which was also decreased during semistarvation; this decrease was counteracted by hyperactivity. The circadian pattern of the running activity paralleled the pattern of the norepinephrine turnover. Semistarvation as well as hyperactivity resulted in a decrease in the norepinephrine precursor tyrosine, indicating that tyrosine availability does not appear to be the limiting factor for norepinephrine turnover in this paradigm (see Broocks et al. 1990b; Pirke et al., Chapter 8, this volume). Philip and Pirke (1987) and Schweiger et al. (1984) showed that tyrosine hydroxylase activity in the brain contributes to decreased norepinephrine turnover in starved rats.

Schumann and Haen (1988) assessed circadian plasma iron and plasma transferrin variations in rabbits during free access to food and during starvation. Starvation resulted in changes in circadian rhythm for plasma iron (decreased amplitude) but not for transferrin.

Mrosovsky (1984) investigated various animal models for insight into the understanding of anorexia nervosa. Animal research can increase our understanding of neuroendocrine and neurotransmitter changes when these issues cannot, for practical or ethical reasons, be studied in humans. However, the results of animal studies are of limited generalizability to humans with anorexia nervosa or bulimia nervosa.

In the following paragraphs, major endocrine changes are reported for anorexia nervosa and bulimia nervosa. These results are compared with findings in healthy starving subjects from the MUSE; details on the methodology of this study have been described elsewhere (Fichter and Pirke 1986a, 1986b). If not stated otherwise, our own data on anorexia nervosa are based on a study described by Fichter et al. (1982). Details on the methodology concerning our own studies with bulimia nervosa have been described elsewhere (Fichter and Pirke 1989; Fichter et al. 1990). Table 10–1 shows results from various studies concerning endocrine changes in starvation and in anorexia nervosa and bulimia nervosa.

Hypothalamic-Pituitary-Thyroid Axis

For anorexia nervosa, Casper and Frohman (1982), Norris et al. (1985), and Kiyohara et al. (1987) reported a blunted and delayed TSH response after injection of TRH. Tamai et al. (1986) reported significantly lowered serum T_4, free T_4, T_3, free T_3, TSH, binding proteins (thyroxine-binding globulin), and a delayed (in 66%) or blunted (in 24%) TSH response to TRH in patients with anorexia nervosa. After weight gain, the patients showed a significant increase in T_3, free T_3, T_4, TSH, and binding proteins (thyroxine-binding globulin).

In bulimia nervosa, we also found a blunted 30-minute TSH response to TRH. To analyze the effects of reduced calorie intake, we split the bulimic group at the median with respect to variables indicating reduced calorie intake (low calorie intake, high beta-hydroxybutyric acid plasma levels, and low T_3 plasma levels). Based on these calculations, we found a significantly decreased 30-minute TSH response for bulimic patients with a low percentage of carbohydrate intake as compared with healthy controls ($t = -28$, 23 df, $P = .004$) and compared with bulimic patients with high carbohydrate intake ($t = -1.9$, 19 df, one-tailed, $P = .035$) and a trend for a blunted TSH response to TRH for other variables indicating low calorie intake (Fichter et al. 1990). Norris et al. (1985) found a trend for a blunted TSH response to TRH in bulimic patients as compared with controls. Kiyohara et al. (1987) reported subnormal TSH responses to TRH in more than half of their normal-weight bulimic patients.

In the MUSE, healthy subjects showed a significantly reduced TSH response to TRH during the fasting phase as compared with the preceding baseline phase. The TSH response in healthy women normalized when body weight was restored. A blunted TSH response to TRH has been claimed to be a "biological marker" for depression (Loosen et al. 1980), and this issue has been extensively studied. Results on the TRH test in patients with anorexia nervosa and bulimia nervosa as well as in healthy starving subjects indicate the importance of reduced calorie intake for hypothalamic-pituitary-thyroid axis function. On the basis of these findings, blunted TSH responses to TRH in depression can be seen as a result of reduced appetite and consequent reduced calorie intake and weight loss, which are frequent symptoms in depression. Figure 10–1 shows our results concerning the TRH test for patients with bulimia nervosa and for healthy subjects during baseline and during starvation.

Reduced T_3 levels probably result in reduction in energy expenditure and conservation of protein during starvation. Thus changes in thyroid hormone metabolism during starvation are of an adaptive nature. Treatment with L-thyroxine to restore serum thyroid concentrations therefore does not appear appropriate in anorexia nervosa or conditions of starvation (Tibaldi and Surks 1985). Komaki et al. (1986) assessed 21 non-obese

Table 10–1. Endocrine changes in anorexia nervosa, in bulimia nervosa, and in starvation

Findings	Anorexia nervosa literature — Study	Own obs[a]	Bulimia nervosa literature — Study	Own obs[a]	Starvation literature — Study	Own obs[a]
Thyroid gland						
T$_4$ normal	Miyai et al. 1975; Moshang et al. 1975	NI	NI	NI	Palmblad et al. 1977	Yes
T$_3$ decreased	Miyai et al. 1975; Moshang et al. 1975	NI	NI	Yes	Palmblad et al. 1977	Yes
Decreased basal metabolism	Warren and van de Wiele 1973	NI	NI	NI	Brozek et al. 1946	NI
TSH normal to slightly decreased	Vigersky et al. 1976a	NI		NI	Palmblad et al. 1977	Yes
TSH response to TRF reduced	Vigersky et al. 1976b	Yes	NI	Yes	NI	Yes
Adrenal gland						
Increased plasma cortisol	Vigersky et al. 1976a; Walsh et al. 1978; Warren and van de Wiele 1973; Boyar et al. 1977	Yes	No; Walsh et al. 1987	No	Alleyne and Young 1967; Palmblad et al. 1977; Smith et al. 1975	Yes
Pathological 24-hour plasma cortisol secretory pattern		Yes				
Insufficient suppression of dexamethasone test	Walsh et al. 1978; Boyar et al. 1977; Walsh et al. 1978	Yes	Walsh et al. 1987; Walsh et al. 1987	Yes	Alleyne and Young 1967; Smith et al. 1975	Yes
Retarded cortisol catabolism		Yes		No	Alleyne and Young 1967; Smith et al. 1975	Yes
Increased cortisol production rate	Boyar et al. 1977; Walsh et al. 1978	Yes	No; Walsh et al. 1987	No	Smith et al. 1975	Yes

Finding	Reference				Reference	
Growth hormone						
Increased	Vigersky 1976a	NI	NI	(Yes)	Kling 1978[b]	Yes
Reduced growth hormone release after stimulation with clonidine	NI	NI	NI	Yes	NI	Yes
Prolactin						
Decreased nocturnal prolactin secretion	Brown et al. 1979	NI	NI	(Yes)	NI	Yes
Reduced prolactin response to TRF	Brambilla et al. 1981 Waldhauser et al. 1984	NI	NI	Yes	NI	NI
Gonadotropins						
Decreased plasma gonadotropin (LH/FSH)	Boyar et al. 1974	Yes	NI	Yes	Pirke and Spyra 1981[c]	Yes
Reduced response to LHRH	Halmi and Sherman 1975	NI	NI	NI	Pirke and Spyra 1981[c]	NI
Reduced response to clomiphene	Marshal and Fraspo 1971	NI	NI	NI	NI	NI
Regression of the 24-hour plasma LH secretory pattern	Boyar et al. 1974	Yes	NI	Yes	NI	Yes

Note. FSH = follicle-stimulating hormone. LH = luteinizing hormone. LHRH = luteinizing hormone–releasing hormone. NI = not investigated. No = finding not confirmed. Yes = finding confirmed. (Yes) = finding mainly confirmed. T_4 = thyroxine. T_3 = triiodothyronine. TSH = thyroid-stimulating hormone. TRF = thyrotropin-releasing hormone. [a]Own observation in patients with anorexia nervosa, patients with bulimia nervosa, or fasting test subjects. [b]Observations in subjects with increased body weight. [c]Animal experiments.

euthyroid patients with psychosomatic diseases following a 5-day fast, reporting decreased free T_4, T_3, and TSH plasma levels and increases in reverse T_3. Serum angiotensin-converting enzyme as an index of thyroid hormone action decreased significantly as a result of fasting, showing a further decrease during 5 days of refeeding (Komaki et al. 1988). Decreases in angiotensin-converting enzyme activity (not mediated by T_3) as a result of fasting were also reported by Butkus et al. (1987).

Growth Hormone, Growth Hormone Response to Clonidine, and Alpha$_2$-Adrenergic Functioning

Clonidine is an alpha$_2$-adrenergic receptor agonist that induces a temporary increase in growth hormone secretion in healthy subjects. Sev-

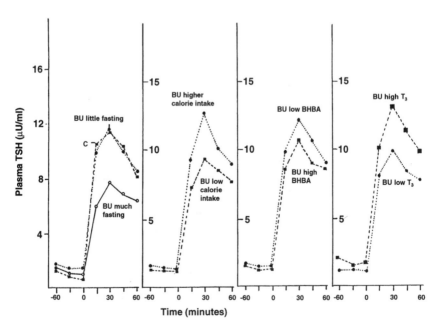

Figure 10–1.   Plasma thyroid-stimulating hormone (TSH) response to thyrotropin-releasing hormone (TRH) in patients with bulimia nervosa (BU) and in healthy control subjects (C). TSH response to TRH is lowered in bulimic patients with signs for reduced food intake—fasting, low kilocalories, high beta-hydroxybutyric acid (BHBA), low triiodothyronine (T_3).

eral studies have reported a blunted growth hormone response to clonidine in depression (Ansseau et al. 1988; Charney et al. 1982; Checkley et al. 1981). A blunted growth hormone response to clonidine has also been claimed to be a biological marker for depression; our data question this notion.

Because of its hypotensive side effects, a clonidine challenge test has so far not been performed with patients with anorexia nervosa. Cabranes et al. (1988) reported increased basal plasma growth hormone levels in both pubertal and postpubertal patients with anorexia nervosa; somato-medin-C concentrations were lower in pubertal but not in postpubertal anorectic patients. In a study of patients with bulimia nervosa, we found a significantly lower (blunted) growth hormone response in bulimic patients (excluding patients with basal growth hormone levels above 5 ng/ml) as compared with controls ($P < .05$). Because of the sensitivity of the clonidine test to the menstrual cycle, we also subdivided the patient group and the control group according to the phase of the menstrual cycle at the time of study. Blunting of the growth hormone response to clonidine was present only in bulimic patients during the luteal phase, whereas bulimic patients and control subjects did not differ in their response during the follicular phase (Fichter and Pirke 1990a, 1990b). Heufelder et al. (1985) reported increased capacity and decreased affinity of platelet $alpha_2$-receptors and an increased prostaglandin E_1 stimulatory and epinephrine inhibitory effects on cyclic adenosine monophosphate production in anorexia nervosa and bulimia nervosa, which largely normalized with weight gain.

In the MUSE, with healthy subjects under conditions of starvation, we found elevated basal growth hormone levels over 24 hours at the end of the fasting phase. Growth hormone responses were normal during baseline and after fasting but blunted after weight gain (paired t test, 2 df, $P < .05$). A blunted growth hormone response to clonidine presumably reflects a reduction in postsynaptic $alpha_2$-adrenergic receptor sensitivity. According to our results and further evidence presented by Pirke (1990), there is reduced sympathetic nervous system activity in patients with anorexia nervosa, in healthy starving subjects (with a time delay), and, to a lesser extent, in bulimic patients. Our results concerning bulimic patients are presented in Figure 10–2.

In humans, episodic release of growth hormone is infrequent and erratic; unlike release in the rat, release of growth hormone in humans apparently has no discernible ultradian periodicities. Ho et al. (1988) showed that 5 days of fasting led to an enhancement of circadian and

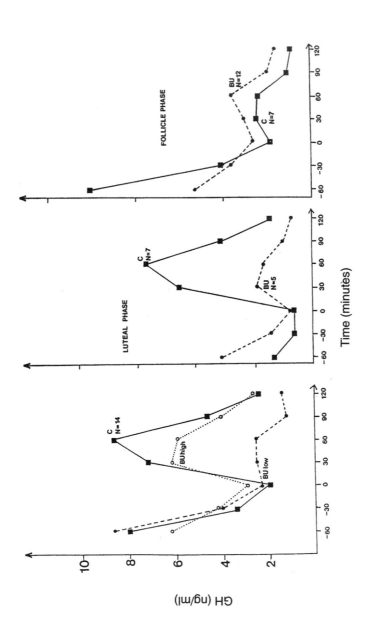

Figure 10–2. Response of growth hormone (GH) to the alpha₂-adrenergic receptor agonist clonidine in patients with bulimia nervosa (BU) and in healthy control subjects (C). High = high calorie intake, ≥1,880 kcal/day, $n = 6$; low = low calorie intake, <1,880 kcal/day, $n = 7$.

ultradian cycles of growth hormone release in humans. These changes in growth hormone release probably play a role in substrate homeostasis during starvation. Using epinephrine infusions in 11 normal-weight healthy subjects, Mansell et al. (1990) presented evidence for an enhancement of the chronotropic, lipolytic, and thermogenic effects of infused epinephrine by prior starvation despite lower plasma epinephrine levels.

Hypothalamic-Pituitary-Gonadal Axis

The hypothalamic-pituitary-gonadal axis has been studied extensively. The attainment and maintenance of ovulatory cycles requires a minimum degree of body fat (≥22% of total body weight). Fasting and weight loss result in alterations of body composition, with a reduction in fatty tissue; this is associated with impaired gonadotropin secretion, insufficient ovarian stimulation, and oligomenorrhea or amenorrhea. If women with suboptimal nutritional status do become pregnant, there is an increased risk for maternal and fetal morbidity and mortality as well as for future developmental problems in the child. The cessation of reproductive function in anorexia nervosa and other states of malnutrition represents an adaptive phenomenon. Treatment should therefore focus primarily on improving the nutritional state rather than on the induction of ovulation. However, with the recognition of an increased risk for osteoporosis in patients with anorexia nervosa with low plasma levels of estrogen, this issue has again become controversial because estrogen substitution reduces the risk for developing osteoporosis.

In our study (Fichter et al. 1982), 14 of 16 patients with anorexia nervosa had an infantile plasma LH secretion pattern on admission to inpatient therapy. All 16 patients developed a pubertal or adult secretion pattern either after 10% weight gain or by the time of discharge. The increase in average 24-hour LH plasma values per week was significantly higher in younger patients with anorexia nervosa as compared with older patients with anorexia nervosa, and longer duration of illness was associated with a slower duration of the LH pattern (Pirke et al. 1979). Devlin et al. (1989) confirmed our previous finding of fewer LH secretory spikes and lower mean 24-hour LH levels in both anorectic and bulimic patients; they also reported blunted LH responses to stimulation with GnRH in anorexia nervosa and elevated LH responses to GnRH in bulimia nervosa. The authors concluded that hypothalamic-pituitary-gonadal "axis abnormalities in eating disordered patients cannot entirely be attributed to emaciation and that factors other than subnormal weight contribute to disturbed hypothalamic-pituitary function in these patients" (p. 11). However, our results with patients with anorexia nervosa and bulimia nervosa and with healthy fasting subjects make it likely that not primarily body weight but a temporary reduction of calorie intake contributes to the observed changes in hypothalamic-pituitary-gonadal axis function. Treasure (1988) showed that estradiol levels increased when follicles became dominant (>1 cm in diameter) and that there was a linear relationship between uterine growth and plasma estradiol in patients with anorexia nervosa. She suggested pelvic ultrasonography as a simple method to determine hypothalamic-pituitary-ovarian axis function in anorexia nervosa.

In a sample of 24 patients with bulimia nervosa according to DSM-III (American Psychiatric Association 1980) criteria, we found significantly lowered LH and FSH average plasma levels at night, as compared with levels in healthy female control subjects (Fichter et al. 1990; Pirke et al. 1987). Gonadotropin plasma levels were significantly lower in bulimic patients with lower body weight, reduced calorie intake, or a higher number of "fasting days" with calorie intake below 1,000 kcal, as compared with levels in control subjects and with bulimic patients with nonreduced food intake. In a second study of 15 patients with bulimia nervosa according to DSM-III criteria and 9 healthy control subjects, the average nocturnal LH plasma concentration over 6 hours and the average LH peak amplitude were significantly lower in bulimic patients with anovulatory cycles as compared with those in healthy controls and bulimic patients with ovulatory cycles (Pirke et al. 1988). In this study, we also controlled for the phase of the menstrual cycle. In these 15 patients and an additional 15 bulimic patients, we studied the secretion of gonadotropins and gonadal hormones over the whole period of the menstrual cycle. Only 3 of the 30 bulimic patients (10%) showed a normal pattern of LH, estradiol, and progesterone secretion. Forty percent of the bulimic patients showed a luteal phase defect, and 50% showed continuously low estradiol and progesterone plasma levels, indicating the lack of a dominant follicle (Fichter and Pirke 1989). Figure 10–3 shows examples for a normal cycle, a luteal phase defect, and a defect in follicle as well as luteal phase of the menstrual cycle.

Our finding that 50% of the bulimic females studied showed anovulatory cycles with flat LH estradiol and progesterone secretion throughout the menstrual cycle is important when considering issues related to re-

productive functions and fertility as well as the development of osteoporosis. Estrogens are important for the calcification of bones. Patients with
anorexia nervosa or bulimia nervosa whose estrogen levels are low over
longer periods of time have an increased risk for developing osteoporosis. With the increase of eating disorders in the past decades and the
latency for developing osteoporosis, this is a "ticking time bomb" for the
future.

In the MUSE, a remarkable finding was that three of five healthy fe-

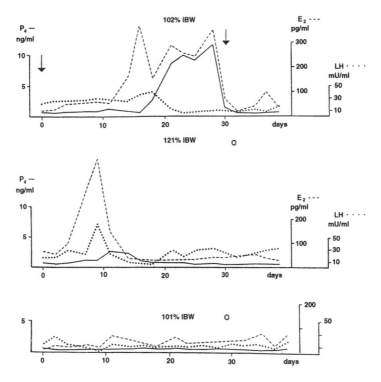

Figure 10–3. Plasma levels of estradiol (E₂) *(dashed lines)*, progesterone (P₄)
(solid lines), and luteinizing hormone (LH) *(dotted lines)* in
patients with bulimia nervosa over a complete menstrual cycle.
Top: Example of a bulimic patient with a normal menstrual
cycle. *Middle:* Example of a bulimic patient with a luteal phase
defect and normal follicular development. *Bottom:* Example of a
bulimic patient with a disturbance in follicular development.
IBW = ideal body weight according to Metropolitan Life
Insurance (1959) tables. O = oligomenorrhea (compare Fichter
and Pirke 1989).

male subjects showed total regression to an infantile plasma LH secretory pattern after 21 days of fasting. The remaining two subjects showed an adult plasma secretory pattern after fasting. The infantilization of the LH secretory pattern in starving healthy subjects occurred after only a minor weight loss (about 8 kg) when compared with the weight loss observed in anorexia nervosa, and it occurred within a relatively short period (14–23 days).

These findings in humans are in accordance with animal data. In orchidectomized rhesus monkeys, Dubey et al. (1986) showed that reduced food intake resulted in a complete cessation of gonadotropin secretion within 19 days. This inhibition of gonadotropin secretion was fully restored to previous gonadotropin (LH, FSH) plasma levels by intermittent intravenous infusions of GnRH. With normalization of body weight, gonadotropin plasma levels started to rise after about 1 week, returning to baseline levels. Cameron (1989) also showed that reduced food intake in monkeys resulted in a complete inhibition of LH secretion within 21 days; when the monkeys were then fed with a normal-calorie but protein-deficient diet, LH secretion quickly normalized. Thus, protein deficiency is apparently not a major cause of the LH regression of the LH secretory pattern.

Bergendahl et al. (1989) reported that pituitary GnRH receptors decreased by 50% in adult male rats after a 4- to 6-day period of food deprivation. Starvation also resulted in a significant decrease in serum and pituitary levels of LH, FSH, and prolactin; a decrease in testicular and serum levels of testosterone; and a decrease in testicular LH receptors and prolactin receptors. FSH receptors were not affected. Badger et al. (1985) found that a 4-day period of starvation in male rats resulted in decreases in serum LH and testosterone concentrations and testicular testosterone content, whereas urine output of LH and FSH were not affected, indicating that reduced calorie intake inhibits LHRH secretion.

Hypothalamic-Pituitary-Adrenal Axis

In patients with anorexia nervosa, the 24-hour plasma cortisol level was significantly elevated on admission to inpatient therapy (Doerr et al. 1980; Fichter et al. 1982). On admission, all but one of the anorectic patients showed insufficient cortisol suppression following application of dexamethasone. Hypercortisolism and insufficient cortisol suppression in the DST in anorexia nervosa normalized with minimal weight increase of only 10% of ideal body weight. In a longitudinal study with anorexia nervosa patients, Estour et al. (1990) confirmed earlier findings of insufficient cortisol suppression in response to intravenous dexamethasone and reported that reinvestigating the patients after refeeding and weight gain resulted in normal cortisol suppression in the DST in five patients. Insufficient cortisol suppression was found in four of nine patients, and the authors concluded that cortisol escape in the DST "is not related to the degree of starvation" (p. 45). However, body weight may not necessarily correlate with nutritional intake in the preceding days. According to our results, nutritional intake (and not body weight) is critical for insufficient cortisol suppression in response to dexamethasone. Kaye et al. (1989) reported starvation-related disturbances of peptides such as corticotropin-releasing hormone, beta-endorphin, and neuropeptide Y measured in the cerebrospinal fluid of patients with anorexia nervosa. They concluded that changes in the activity of neuropeptides induced by starvation may contribute to neuroendocrine and behavioral alterations in anorexia nervosa such as hypercortisolism, amenorrhea, and other symptoms, such as physical hyperactivity, depression, and abnormal feeding behavior.

Results concerning the HPA axis in bulimia nervosa are conflicting. In a sample of 24 patients with bulimia nervosa according to DSM-III criteria, we found no increased nocturnal plasma cortisol levels from 1 A.M. to 6:30 A.M. in bulimic patients as compared with healthy female control subjects (Fichter et al. 1990). The same result was found by Walsh et al. (1987). Kennedy et al. (1989) did find elevated basal cortisol levels in patients with bulimia nervosa. Gwirtsman et al. (1989) reported normal ACTH and cortisol levels in bulimic patients on hospital admission. However, after patients abstained from binge-purge episodes, the cerebrospinal fluid ACTH levels showed a significant decrease. In our study we found some evidence for insufficient cortisol suppression following ingestion of dexamethasone in bulimic patients as compared with healthy female control subjects; this difference did not, however, quite reach statistical significance using two-tailed t testing ($t = 2.0$, 36 df, $P = .058$). A trend for insufficient cortisol suppression was seen especially in bulimic patients with a high degree of calorie restriction and in bulimic patients with high beta-hydroxybutyric acid plasma levels—indicating reduced food intake in the preceding days. A higher degree of depression in bulimic patients was not associated with insufficient cortisol suppression in the DST.

In the MUSE, there was clear evidence for elevated 24-hour cortisol levels and increased plasma cortisol half-life in healthy subjects at the end of the fasting phase. Restoration of body weight resulted—as in patients with anorexia nervosa—in a normalization of the plasma cortisol level and half-life. The DST sufficiently suppressed cortisol in all 11 tests performed in the five subjects during the initial baseline phase. Of 14 DSTs, 7 (50%) showed insufficient suppression of cortisol during the fasting phase. All 11 DSTs, which were performed during the weight-gain phase, were sufficiently suppressed. Of 18 of the cortisol probes at 4 P.M. and at 9 P.M., 17 (94.4%) were normally suppressed in the final baseline phase. Dexamethasone plasma levels were significantly lower during fasting, indicating reduced absorption and transport of dexamethasone from the gastrointestinal tract to the circulating blood. Figure 10–4 shows the results of the DST for our healthy subjects before and during starvation and in patients with bulimia nervosa.

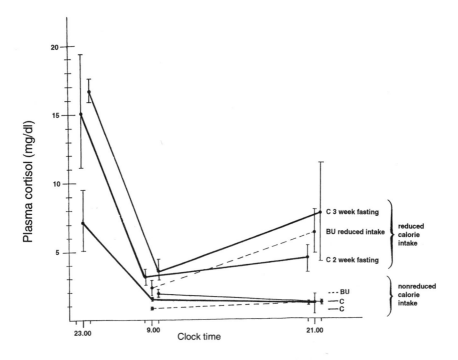

Figure 10–4. Dexamethasone suppression tests in patients with bulimia nervosa (BU; *dashed lines*) and in healthy control subjects (C; *solid lines*) with reduced or nonreduced calorie intake showing plasma cortisol levels before and after ingestion of dexamethasone (mean ± SE).

Other Changes Induced by Starvation

Evidence for depression-like symptoms were reported by Keys et al. (1950) and were found in the MUSE. There have also been some reports on "crash diet depression"—depressive symptoms resulting from harsh dieting (Robinson and Winnek 1973). Issues concerning dieting and depression have been reviewed by Smoller et al. (1987). There is some evidence that dieting involving foods with low-carbohydrate content (Schweiger et al. 1986) can induce depressive symptoms. Depressive symptoms in patients with eating disorders may therefore be partially a result of reduced calorie intake in general or specifically a result of reduced carbohydrate intake. More research is needed on the effects of food composition on mood, neurotransmitters, and hormones.

Tanaka et al. (1989) studied a large number of autopsies and reported that starvation or protein-calorie malnutrition caused decreases in the weight of different organs such as the liver (8% decrease) and kidney, heart, spleen, and adrenal gland (15%–20% decrease). However, the brain and thyroid gland showed almost the same weight as in control subjects, and the pituitary gland showed an 18% increase in weight. Cranial computer tomographic studies (Krieg et al. 1988, 1989) reported pseudoatrophy of the brain in anorexia nervosa and in some cases of normal-weight bulimia nervosa. These findings in anorexia nervosa normalized with refeeding. Pseudoatrophy of the brain in normal-weight bulimic patients can be the result of repeated dieting (temporary reduction of calorie intake) and the body weight fluctuating around ideal body weight. The finding in anorexia nervosa and bulimia nervosa that ventricular size is inversely correlated with plasma levels of T_3, which can be seen as an indicator of starvation, supports this assumption.

Scheithauer et al. (1988) studied patients who died of complications of anorexia nervosa, crash dieting, or inanition resulting from organic disease, and victims of fatal accidents (control subjects). The pituitary gland of patients with anorexia nervosa and organically ill patients with inanition showed relative hypogranulation of adrenocorticotropic cells and growth hormone cells. These changes were probably the result of chronic starvation because they were not present after the crash diet or in control subjects. Other studies also showed that mental alertness, assessed by total reaction time and moving time to a visual signal, was reduced in healthy subjects after 12 or 72 hours of fasting, respectively

(Fourest-Fontecave et al. 1987); mental alertness was also reduced in anorexia nervosa. An open question is to what extent the reduction in mental alertness is a result of hypoglycemia, neuroendocrine changes, or neurotransmitter changes during starvation. Diet, nutrition, and starvation may also be of importance for the bioavailability, binding, hepatic metabolism, and renal clearance of applied medication (Anderson 1988). Starvation can impair neuronal maturation; if it occurs during a critical phase of brain development, it may have lasting effects on behavior and intellectual performance (Zeisel 1986).

The role of neurotransmitters in eating disorders has been reviewed by Pirke (1990) and Leibowitz (1990). The synthesis of neurotransmitters in the brain may be affected by dietary intake of tryptophan and glucose (for synthesis of serotonin), tyrosine (for synthesis of dopamine and norepinephrine), and choline (for synthesis of acetylcholine). The paraventricular and ventromedial nuclei in the medial hypothalamus mediate the action of serotonin, which interacts antagonistically with norepinephrine and its alpha$_2$-noradrenergic receptors. During food intake, serotonin induces satiety for carbohydrates and may switch the macronutrient preference toward protein. In anorexia nervosa, plasma tryptophan, urinary 5-hydroxyindoleacetic acid (5-HIAA), platelet serotonin binding, and basal cerebrospinal fluid 5-HIAA are decreased and normalize with weight restoration. In bulimia nervosa, prolactin responses to serotonin agonists are blunted, indicating reduced postsynaptic responsiveness in the hypothalamic-pituitary serotonergic pathways.

"Yo-yo dieting" is widely practiced, especially by females in Western countries. Brownell et al. (1986) reported in rats significant increases in food efficiency (weight gain per kilocalorie of food intake) in the second food restriction phase and refeeding period compared with the first food restriction phase. In the second cycle of weight loss and gain, weight loss occurred at half the rate and weight gain at two times the rate as compared with the first cycle of weight loss and gain. Weight-cycled animals had a fourfold increase in food efficiency compared with control rats at the end of the experiment. Despite its relevance, this issue has so far received little attention in studies with humans. Bennett et al. (1989) found a lower resting metabolic rate in patients with severe bulimic symptoms as compared with healthy control subjects and patients with less severe bulimic symptoms. If dieting in the long range has the effect of increasing the food efficiency, this would in the long run be contrary to the hopes and expectations of dieters, who want to achieve or maintain a lower body weight. More research is needed to substantiate these findings for humans and to pinpoint the specific mechanisms for a possible increase in food efficiency following starvation, fasting, or dieting.

Conclusion

There are multiple neuroendocrine and neurotransmitter changes in anorexia nervosa, many of which are, to a lesser extent, also present in bulimia nervosa. A likely hypothesis to explain these changes is the nutritional hypothesis, which assumes that a temporary reduction of calorie intake (possibly accompanied by weight loss) causes substantial changes in neurotransmitters and various hormone axes. This hypothesis is substantiated by the finding that most of these changes in anorectic patients normalize with weight restoration and by findings in healthy subjects and animals under conditions of restricted food intake followed by refeeding. Neuroendocrine and neurotransmitter changes in anorexia nervosa and bulimia nervosa appear to be largely adaptations to a temporary state of starvation.

References

Alleyne GAO, Young VH: Adrenocortical function with severe protein-calorie malnutrition. Clin Sci 33:189–195, 1967

American Psychiatric Association: Diagnostic and Statistical Manual of Mental Disorders, 3rd Edition. Washington, DC, American Psychiatric Association, 1980

Anderson KE: Influences of diet and nutrition on clinical pharmacokinetics. Clin Pharmacokinet 6:325–346, 1988

Ansseau M, Frenckell RV, Cerfontaine JL, et al: Blunted response of growth hormone to clonidine and apomorphine in endogenous depression. Br J Psychiatry 153:65–71, 1988

Badger TM, Lynch EA, Fox PH: Effects of fasting on luteinizing hormone dynamics in the male rat. J Nutr 6:788–797, 1985

Benedict FG: A Study of Prolonged Fasting, Vol 203. Washington, DC, Carnegie Institute Publication, 1915

Bennett SM, Williamson DA, Powers SK: Bulimia nervosa and resting metabolic rate. International Journal of Eating Disorders 8:417–424, 1989

Bergendahl M, Perheentupa A, Huhtaniemi I: Effect of short-term starvation on reproductive hormone gene expression, secretion and receptor levels in male rats. J Endocrinol 3:409–417, 1989

Boyar RM, Katz J, Finkelstein JW, et al: Immaturity of the 24-hour luteinizing hormone secretory pattern. N Engl J Med 291:861–865, 1974

Boyar RM, Hellman LD, Rottwaug H, et al: Cortisol secretion and metabolism in anorexia nervosa. N Engl J Med 296:190–193, 1977

Brambilla F, Cocchi D, Nabile P, et al: Anterior pituitary responsiveness to hypothalamic hormones in anorexia nervosa. Neuropsychiatry 7:225–237, 1981

Broocks A, Liu J, Pirke KM: Influence of hyperactivity on the metabolism of central monoaminergic neurotransmitters and reproductive function in the semistarved rat, in The Menstrual Cycle and Its Disorders. Edited by Pirke KM, Wuttke W, Schweiger U. Heidelberg, Springer, 1989, pp 88–98

Broocks A, Schweiger U, Pirke KM: Hyperactivity aggravates semistarvation-induced changes in corticosterone and triiodothyronine concentrations in plasma but not luteinizing hormone and testosterone levels. Physiol Behav 48:567–569, 1990a

Broocks A, Liu J, Pirke KM: Semistarved-induced hyperactivity compensates for decreased norepinephrine and dopamine turnover in the mediobasal hypothalamus of the rat. J Neural Transm 79:113–124, 1990b

Brown GM, Kirwan P, Garfinkel P, et al: Overnight patterning of prolactin and melatonin in anorexia nervosa. Paper presented at the 2nd International Symposium on Clinical Psychoneuroendocrinology in Reproduction, Venice, May 1979

Brownell KD, Greenwood MRC, Stellar E, et al: The effects of repeated cycles of weight loss and regain in rats. Physiol Behav 38:459–464, 1986

Brozek J, Wells S, Keys A: Medical aspects of semi-starvation in Leningrad (siege 1941–1942). American Review of Soviet Medicine 4:70–86, 1946

Butkus NE, Burman KD, Smallridge RC: Angiotensin-converting enzyme activity decreases during fasting. Horm Metab Res 2:76–79, 1987

Cabranes JA, Almoguera I, Santos JL, et al: Somatomedin-C and growth hormone levels in anorexia nervosa in relation to the puberal or post puberal stages. Prog Neuropsychopharmacol Biol Psychiatry 6:865–871, 1988

Cameron JL: Influence of nutrition on the hypothalamic-pituitary-gonadal axis in primates, in The Menstrual Cycle and Its Disorders. Edited by Pirke KM, Wuttke W, Schweiger U. Heidelberg, Springer, 1989, pp 66–78

Campbell GA, Kurcz M, Marshall S, et al: Effects of starvation in rats on serum of follicle stimulating hormone, luteinizing hormone, thyrotropin, growth hormone and prolactin: response to LH-releasing hormone and thyrotropin-releasing hormone. Endocrinology 100:580–587, 1977

Carroll BJ: The dexamethasone suppression test for melancholia. Br J Psychiatry 140:292–304, 1982

Casper RC, Frohman D: Delayed TSH response in anorexia nervosa following injection of thyrotropin-releasing hormone (TRH). Psychoneuroendocrinology 7:59–68, 1982

Charney DS, Henninger GR, Sternberg DE, et al: Adrenergic receptor sensitivity in depression: effects of clonidine in depressed patients and healthy subjects. Arch Gen Psychiatry 39:290–294, 1982

Checkley SA, Slade AP, Shur E: Growth hormone and other response to clonidine in patients with endogenous depression. Br J Psychiatry 138:51–55, 1981

Cooke JNC, James VHT, Landon J, et al: Adrenocortical function in chronic malnutrition. Br Med J 1:662–666, 1964

Devlin MJ, Walsh BT, Katz JL, et al: Hypothalamic-pituitary-gonadal function in anorexia nervosa and bulimia. Psychiatry Res 1:11–24, 1989

Doerr P, Fichter MM, Pirke KM, et al: Relationship between weight gain and hypothalamic pituitary adrenal function in patients with anorexia nervosa. J Steroid Biochem 13:529–537, 1980

Dubey AK, Cameron JL, Steiner RA, et al: Inhibition of gonadotropin secretion in castrated male rhesus monkeys (Macaca mulatta) induced by dietary restriction: analogy with the prepubertal hiatus of gonadotropin release. Endocrinology 118:518–525, 1986

Estour B, Pugeat M, Lang F, et al: Rapid escape of cortisol from suppression in response to i.v. dexamethasone in anorexia nervosa. Clin Endocrinol 1:45–52, 1990

Fichter MM: Magersucht und Bulimia. Empirische Untersuchungen zur Epidemiologie, Symptomatologie, Nosologie und zum Verlauf. Berlin, Springer-Verlag, 1985

Fichter MM, Pirke KM: Effect of experimental and pathological weight loss upon the hypothalamo-pituitary-adrenal axis. Psychoneuroendocrinology 11:295–305, 1986a

Fichter MM, Pirke KM: Effects of experimental starvation on thyroid axis disorder of eating behavior: a psychoneuroendocrine approach, in Advances of the Biosciences. Edited by Ferraria E, Brambilla F. Oxford, Pergamon, 1986b, pp 189–198

Fichter MM, Pirke KM: Disturbances of reproductive function in eating disorders, in The Menstrual Cycle and Its Disorders. Edited by Pirke KM, Wuttke W, Schweiger U. Berlin, Springer-Verlag, 1989, pp 179–188

Fichter MM, Pirke KM: Endocrine dysfunctions in bulimia (nervosa), in Bulimia Nervosa: Basic Research, Diagnosis and Therapy. Edited by Fichter MM. New York, Wiley, 1990a, pp 235–257

Fichter MM, Pirke KM: Psychobiology of human starvation, in Anorexia Nervosa. Edited by Remschmidt H, Schmidt MH. Stuttgart, Hogrefe & Huber Publishers, 1990b, pp 15–29

Fichter MM, Doerr P, Pirke KM, et al: Behavior, nutrition and endocrinology in anorexia nervosa: a longitudinal study in 24 patients. Acta Psychiatr Scand 66:429–444, 1982

Fichter MM, Pirke KM, Holsboer F: Weight loss causes neuroendocrine disturbances: experimental study in healthy starvation subjects. Psychiatry Res 17:61–72, 1986

Fichter MM, Pirke KM, Poellinger J, et al: Disturbances in the hypothalamic pituitary adrenal and other neuroendocrine axes in bulimia. Biol Psychiatry 1021–1037, 1990

Fourest-Fontecave S, Adamson U, Lins PE, et al: Mental alertness in response to hypoglycaemia in normal man: the effect of 12 hours and 72 hours of fasting. Diabete Metab 4:405–410, 1987

Gorozhanin VS, Lobkov VV: Hormonal and metabolic reactions in the human body during prolonged starvation. Kosm Biol Aviakosm Med 3:47–50, 1990

Gwirtsman HE, Kaye WH, George DT, et al: Central and peripheral ACTH and cortisol levels in anorexia nervosa and bulimia. Arch Gen Psychiatry 46:61–69, 1989

Halmi KA, Sherman BM: Gonadotropin response to LH-RH in anorexia nervosa. Arch Gen Psychiatry 32:875–878, 1975

Heufelder A, Warnhoff M, Pirke KM: Platelet alpha$_2$-adrenoceptor and adenylate cyclase in patients with anorexia nervosa and bulimia. J Clin Endocrinol Metab 6:1053–1060, 1985

Ho KY, Veldhuis JD, Johnson ML, et al: Fasting enhances growth hormone secretion and amplifies the complex rhythms of growth hormone secretion in man. J Clin Invest 4:968–975, 1988

Howland BE, Skinner KR: Effect of starvation on gonadotropin secretion in intact and castrated male rats. Can J Physiol Pharmacol 51:759–762, 1973

Jung RT, Rosenstock J, Wood SM, et al: Dopamine in the pituitary adaptation to starvation in man. Postgrad Med J 717:571–574, 1985

Kaye WH, Berrettini WH, Gwirtsman HE, et al: Contribution of CNS neuropeptide (NPY, CRH and beta-endorphin) alterations to psychophysiological abnormalities in anorexia nervosa. Psychopharmacol Bull 3:433–438, 1989

Kennedy SH, Garfinkel PE, Parienti V, et al: Changes in melatonin levels but not cortisol levels are associated with depression in patients with eating disorders. Arch Gen Psychiatry 46:73–78, 1989

Keys A, Brozek J, Henschel A, et al: The Biology of Human Starvation. Minneapolis, MN, University of Minneapolis Press, 1950

Kiyohara K, Tamai H, Karibe C, et al: Serum thyrotropin (TSH) response to thyrotropin-releasing hormone (TRH) in patients with anorexia nervosa and bulimia: influence of changes in body weight and eating disorders. Psychoneuroendocrinology 12:21–28, 1987

Kling S: Einflufß totaler Nahrungskarenz auf klinisch-chemische Befunde bei adipösen Patienten unter besonderer Berücksichtigung der Serumproteinveränderung. Unpublished doctoral dissertation, Medical Faculty, University of Munich, Munich, 1978

Komaki G, Tamai H, Kiyohara K, et al: Changes in the hypothalamic-pituitary-thyroid-axis during acute starvation in non-obese patients. Endocrinol Jpn 3:303–308, 1986

Komaki G, Tamai H, Mori T, et al: Changes in serum angiotensin-converting enzyme in acutely starved non-obese patients: a possible dissociation between angiotensin-converting enzyme and the thyroid state. Acta Endocrinol 118:45–50, 1988

Krieg JC, Pirke KM, Lauer C, et al: Endocrine, metabolic and cranial computed tomographic findings in anorexia nervosa. Biol Psychiatry 23:377–387, 1988

Krieg JC, Lauer C, Pirke KM: Structural brain abnormalities in patients with bulimia nervosa. Psychiatry Res 27:39–48, 1989

Küderling I, Dorsch G, Warnhoff M, et al: The actions of prostaglandin E2, naloxone and testosterone on starvation-induced suppression of luteinizing hormone-releasing hormone and luteinizing-hormone secretion. Neuroendocrinology 39:530–537, 1984

Kupfer DJ: Neurophysiological "markers"–EEG sleep measures. Psychiatry Res 18:467–475, 1984

Leibowitz SF: The role of serotonin in eating disorders. Drugs 39:33–48, 1990

Loosen PT, Wilson I, Prange AJ Jr: Endocrine and behavioral changes in depression after TRH: alteration by pretreatment with thyroid hormone. J Affective Disord 2:267–278, 1980

Mansell PI, Fellows IW, MacDonald IA. Enhanced thermogenic response to epinephrine after 48-h starvation in humans. Am J Physiol 258:R87–R93, 1990

Marshall JC, Fraspo TR: Amenorrhea in anorexia nervosa: assessment and treatment with clomiphene citrate. Br Med J 4:590–592, 1971

Metropolitan Life Insurance Company: Statistical Bulletin 40:1–9, 1959

Miyai K, Yamamoto T, Azukizawa M, et al: Serum thyroid hormones and thyrotropin in anorexia nervosa. J Clin Endocrinol Metab 40:334–338, 1975

Moshang T, Parks JS, Baker L, et al: Low serum triiodothyronine in patients with anorexia nervosa. J Clin Endocrinol Metab 40:470–473, 1975

Mrosovsky N: Animal models: anorexia yes, nervosa no, in The Psychobiology of Anorexia Nervosa. Edited by Pirke KM, Ploog D. Heidelberg, Springer-Verlag, 1984, pp 22–34

Mullen PE, Linsell CR, Parker D: Der Einfluß von Schlafentzug und Kalorienrestruktion auf biologische Merkmale der Depression. Lancet (German ed) 1:114–118, 1987

Norris PD, O'Malley BP, Palmer RL: The TRH-test in bulimia and anorexia nervosa: a controlled study. J Psychiatr Res 19:215–229, 1985

Palmblad L, Levi L, Burger A, et al: Effects of total energy withdrawal (fasting) on the level of growth hormone, thyrotropin, cortisol, adrenaline, noradrenaline, T4, T3 and rT3 in healthy males. Acta Med Scand 201:15–22, 1977

Philip E, Pirke KM: Effect of starvation on hypothalamic tyrosine hydroxylase activity in adult male rats. Brain Res 413:53–59, 1987

Pirke KM: Central neurotransmitter disturbances in bulimia (nervosa), in Bulimia Nervosa: Basic Research, Diagnosis and Therapy. Edited by Fichter MM. New York, Wiley, 1990, pp 223–234

Pirke KM, Spyra B: Influence of starvation on testosterone-luteinizing hormone feedback in the rat. Acta Endocrinol (Copenh) 96:413–421, 1981

Pirke KM, Spyra B: Catecholamine turnover in the brain and the regulation of luteinizing hormone and corticosterone in starved male rats. Acta Endocrinol (Copenh) 100:168–175, 1982

Pirke KM, Fichter MM, Lund R, et al: Twenty-four-hour sleep-wake pattern of plasma LH in patients with anorexia nervosa. Acta Endocrinol 92:193–204, 1979

Pirke KM, Spyra B, Warnhoff M, et al: Effect of starvation on central neurotransmitter systems and on endocrine regulation, in The Psychobiology of Anorexia Nervosa. Edited by Pirke KM, Ploog D. Heidelberg, Springer-Verlag, 1984, pp 46–57

Pirke KM, Fichter MM, Schweiger U, et al: Gonadotropin secretion pattern in bulimia nervosa. International Journal of Eating Disorders 6:655–661, 1987

Pirke KM, Dogs M, Fichter MM, et al: Gonadotropins, oestradiol and progesterone during the menstrual cycle in bulimia nervosa. Clin Endocrinol 29:265–270, 1988

Robinson S, Winnek HZ: Severe psychotic disturbances following crash diet weight loss. Arch Gen Psychiatry 29:559–562, 1973

Root AW, Russ RD: Short-term effects of castration and starvation upon pituitary and serum levels of luteinizing hormone and follicle stimulating hormone in male rats. Acta Endocrinol (Copenh) 70:665–675, 1972

Scheithauer BW, Kovacs KT, Jariwala LK, et al: Anorexia nervosa: an immunohistochemical study of the pituitary gland. Mayo Clin Proc 63:23–28, 1988

Schelp FP, Migasena P, Saovakontha S, et al: Serum protein fractions from children of differing nutritional status analysed by polyacrylamide gel electrophoresis and electroimmunoassay. Br J Nutr 35:211–222, 1976

Schelp FP, Migasena P, Pongpaew P, et al: Serum proteinase inhibitor and other serum proteins in protein-energy malnutrition. Br J Nutr 38:31–38, 1977

Schelp FP, Migasena P, Pongpaew P, et al: Are proteinase inhibitors a factor for the derangement of homeostasis in protein-energy malnutrition. Am J Clin Nutr 31:451–456, 1978

Schumann K, Haen E: Influence of food intake on the 24-h variations of plasma iron concentration in the rabbit. Chronobiol Int 5:59–64, 1988

Schweiger U, Warnhoff M, Pirke KM: Brain thyrosine availability and the depression of central nervous norepinephrine turnover in acute and chronic starvation in adult male rats. Brain Res 335:207–212, 1984

Schweiger U, Laessle R, Kittl S, et al: Macronutrient intake, plasma large neutral amino acids and mood during weight-reducing diets. J Neural Transm 67:77–86, 1986

Smith SR, Bledsoe T, Chhetri MK: Cortisol metabolism and the pituitary-adrenal axis in adults with protein-calorie malnutrition. J Clin Endocrinol Metab 40:43–52, 1975

Smoller JW, Wadden TA, Stunkard AJ: Dieting and depression: a critical review. J Psychosom Res 31:429–440, 1987

Srebnik HH: FSH and ICSH in pituitary and plasma of castrated protein-deficient rats. Biol Reprod 3:96–104, 1970

Tamai H, Mori K, Matsubayashi S, et al: Hypothalamic-pituitary-thyroidal dysfunctions in anorexia nervosa. Psychother Psychosom 46:127–131, 1986

Tanaka G, Nakahara Y, Nakazima Y: Japanese reference man 1988-IV: studies on the weight and size of internal organs of normal Japanese. Nippon Igaku Hoshasen Gakkai Zasshi 49:344–364, 1989

Tibaldi JM, Surks MI: Effects of nonthyroidal illness on thyroid function. Med Clin North Am 69:899–911, 1985

Treasure JL: The ultrasonographic features in anorexia nervosa and bulimia nervosa: a simplified method of monitoring hormonal states during weight gain. Psychosom Res 32:623–634, 1988

Vigersky RA, Loriaux DL, Andersen AE, et al: Anorexia nervosa: behavioral and hypothalamic aspects. Clinical Endocrinology and Metabolism 5:517–535, 1976a

Vigersky RA, Loriaux DL, Andersen AE, et al: Delayed pituitary hormone response to LRF and TRF in patients with anorexia nervosa and with secondary amenorrhea associated with simple weight loss. Journal of Clinical Metabolism 43:893–900, 1976b

Waldhauser F, Toifl K, Spona J, et al: Diminished prolactin response to thyrotropin and insulin in anorexia nervosa. J Clin Endocrinol Metab 59:538–541, 1984

Walsh BT, Katz JL, Levin J, et al: Adrenal activity in anorexia nervosa. Psychosom Med 40:499–506, 1978

Walsh BT, Lo ES, Cooper T, et al: The DST and plasma dexamethasone levels in bulimia. Arch Gen Psychiatry 44:799–800, 1987

Warren M, van de Wiele RL: Clinical metabolic features of anorexia nervosa. Am J Obstet Gynecol 117:435–449, 1973

Wurtman RJ, Hefit F, Melamed E: Precursor control of neurotransmitter synthesis. Pharmacol Rev 32:315–335, 1981

Zeisel SH: Dietary influences on neurotransmission. Adv Pediatr 33P:23–47, 1986

Chapter 11

Metabolic Changes

Madelyn H. Fernstrom, Ph.D.
Theodore E. Weltzin, M.D.
Walter H. Kaye, M.D.

———————

Numerous recent studies suggest that significant alterations in energy balance occur in patients who have recovered from eating disorders (Table 11–1). Patients with anorexia nervosa require more calories to maintain body weight (see, e.g., Kaye et al. 1986b; Newman et al. 1987), and patients with bulimia nervosa require fewer calories for maintenance of body weight (Gwirtsman et al. 1989). That is, following short-term recovery, patients with anorexia nervosa are apparently inefficient in their energy utilization, whereas patients with bulimia nervosa seem overly energy efficient. These data raise the possibility that weight maintenance could be more difficult, metabolically, for the recovered eating disorder patient, perhaps rendering these patients more likely to relapse.

Indeed, both anorexia nervosa and bulimia nervosa are disorders with high relapse rates, despite effective treatment. For patients with anorexia nervosa, relapse within 1 year of successful inpatient weight restoration is frequently observed (Hsu 1980; Hsu et al. 1979). Long-term outcome

Studies discussed in this chapter were supported by National Institute of Mental Health grant awards to M.H.F. (MH41644) and W.H.K. (MH42984). The assistance of Denise Fantazier with preparation of the chapter is appreciated.

studies of patients with bulimia nervosa suggest that a majority of these patients have some degree of relapse after either physiological or psychological treatment (Hsu and Sobkiewicz 1989; Keller et al. 1989; Pope and Hudson 1986). Such high relapse rates have often been attributed to psychological or psychosocial factors, although increasing evidence suggests that metabolic abnormalities could also be contributing factors.

In this chapter we review the evidence indicating the apparent differences in both energy intake and expenditure observed within different subgroups of eating disorder patients and between eating disorder patients and healthy control subjects. How such alterations in energy balance could ultimately influence weight maintenance is also discussed.

Energy Regulation in Recovered Eating Disorder Patients

Several distinguishing characteristics used to classify subgroups of eating disorder patients are of particular relevance in any discussion of energy regulation: amount of weight loss, type of pathological eating behavior, and psychopathological traits (Herzog and Copeland 1985). These characteristics can have a significant impact on energy regula-

Table 11–1.   Energy balance abnormalities in eating disorder patients: calorie intake and body-weight studies

Study	Finding
Beaumont et al. 1976 Garfinkel et al. 1980	Bulimic anorectic patients have greater premorbid weight than nonbulimic anorectic patients.
Stordy et al. 1977 Walker et al. 1979	Previously obese anorectic patients gain weight more rapidly than previously normal-weight anorectic patients.
Kaye et al. 1986b	Bulimic anorectic patients require fewer kcal/day to maintain weight than restricting anorectic patients.
Kaye et al. 1986a	Short-term weight-restored anorectic patients require more calories for weight maintenance than long-term weight-restored anorectic patients.
Newman et al. 1987	Subgroups of eating disorder patients show different caloric need for body-weight maintenance.
Gwirtsman et al. 1989	Normal-weight bulimic patients require fewer kcal/day to maintain body weight compared with control subjects.

tion, demonstrating the importance of subgroup comparisons for meaningful discussion of changes in energy balance. As described later in this chapter, these major comparative subgroups are patients with anorexia nervosa, restricting subtype; patients with anorexia nervosa, bulimic subtype; normal-weight bulimic patients; and normal-weight bulimic patients with a history of anorexia nervosa.

Anorexia Nervosa

Anorexia nervosa is a disease characterized by severe emaciation (American Psychiatric Association 1987), within which two types of ingestive behavior are observed. Restricting anorectic patients are those who lose weight solely by food restriction (dieting) and most closely mirror the diagnosis of anorexia nervosa. Bulimic anorectic patients are those who restrict food intake, but also demonstrate periods of bingeing and purging, thus fulfilling the criteria for both anorexia nervosa and bulimia nervosa. Interestingly, compared with restricting anorectic patients, the bulimic anorectic patients demonstrate greater incidence of premorbid and familial obesity, as well as an increase in behaviors associated with impulse disorders (Beaumont et al. 1976; Casper et al. 1980; Garfinkel et al. 1980; Strober et al. 1982).

Beginning about 15 years ago, several observations clearly suggested the presence of energy-balance differences within subgroups of anorectic patients. It was reported that bulimic anorectic patients demonstrated a greater premorbid weight than nonbulimic anorectic patients (Beaumont et al. 1976; Garfinkel et al. 1980). Next, other investigators (Stordy et al. 1977; Walker et al. 1979) noted that previously obese anorectic patients (presumably a bulimic anorectic group) gained weight more rapidly than anorectic patients who had previously been of normal weight (presumably a restricting anorectic group). Together, these data suggested an apparent greater need for calories in patients with restricting anorexia nervosa when compared with patients with bulimic anorexia nervosa.

Within the past several years, other investigators have conducted highly controlled studies examining the caloric need of different groups of patients with anorexia nervosa. The first of a series of studies was conducted by Kaye et al. (1986b) at the National Institute of Mental Health. Patients with anorexia nervosa were subdivided based on the presence or absence of bingeing behavior (restricting anorectic patients or bulimic anorectic patients). Restricting anorectic patients required 30%–50%

more calories than the bulimic anorectic patients to maintain a stable body weight. This difference in calorie intake was observed throughout the phases of illness and occurred when patients were underweight (<75% of average body weight) and after short-term (3–4 week) and long-term (>1 year) weight restoration. These differences could not be accounted for by major differences in physical activity. Of particular interest was the observation that although the short-term-recovered anorectic patients showed greater-than-normal caloric requirements for body-weight maintenance, such patients studied after long-term weight restoration (>6 months) showed normal calorie intake (Kaye et al. 1986a). Shortly thereafter, Newman et al. (1987) examined the caloric requirements for weight gain and maintenance in both anorectic subgroups (restricting and bulimic) and in bulimic patients (with and without a history of anorexia nervosa). As a total group, the bulimic patients required fewer calories to maintain normal body weight, although bulimic patients with a history of anorexia nervosa showed increased caloric need compared with bulimic patients without earlier anorexia nervosa. In contrast to the study by Kaye et al. (1986b), no differences were observed between the subgroups of anorectic patients, although this may be a reflection of the units used to express caloric requirements (Weltzin et al. 1991).

Bulimia Nervosa

Energy intake. As described earlier, bulimic symptoms among patients with anorexia nervosa clearly modify caloric requirements: bulimic anorectic patients show an apparent reduction in caloric requirement for weight maintenance compared with restricting anorectic patients (Kaye et al. 1986b), suggesting that bulimia nervosa is associated with reductions in caloric need. This question was rigorously investigated by Gwirtsman et al. (1989), who compared caloric requirements for weight maintenance of bulimic patients (with and without a prior history of anorexia nervosa) and healthy control subjects. To maintain body weight, bulimic patients ate significantly fewer calories per day compared with control subjects ($1,173 \pm 260$ versus $1,694 \pm 299$ kcal, $P < .001$). This difference was consistent whether data were expressed in kilocalories per kilogram, kilocalories per body mass index, kilocalories per body surface area, or kilocalories per lean body mass. Prior history of anorexia nervosa did not alter caloric need: when subgroups of bulimic patients were compared, they were indistinguishable. These differences in calorie consumption could not be accounted for by activity level, body weight, or clinical variables, including history of laxative abuse or obesity. Such results are consistent with increases in caloric efficiency in this group.

Energy expenditure.   Energy expenditure comprises three components: resting metabolic rate (RMR), thermogenesis, and physical activity. RMR accounts for approximately 75%–80% of the daily caloric output of an average individual, with thermogenesis and exercise accounting for the remainder (Garrow 1978). RMR is measured in the resting state following an overnight fast. Thermogenesis is defined as an energy output above RMR: a thermogenic response can be elicited by a number of physiological factors, including food intake, exposure to cold, and fasting. Food intake, exposure to cold, and exercise all produce positive thermogenic responses, whereas fasting produces a negative thermogenic response (Jequier 1984).

Metabolic efficiency studies in humans have focused almost exclusively on people who are obese or people who used to be obese: such studies propose that these individuals have more efficient calorie utilization than do normal-weight control subjects. For example, obese or formally obese subjects have a smaller thermogenic response to several stimuli, including a glucose load (Golay et al. 1982), a mixed meal (Schutz et al. 1984), and postprandial exercise (Segal and Gutin 1983). Additional studies addressed the effect of overfeeding on the promotion of energy inefficiency (less storage of calories) in normal-weight subjects. The following discussion focuses on metabolic efficiency changes in normal-weight bulimic subjects, with studies to date examining resting metabolic rate and thermogenesis.

Although not the focus of this discussion, it is important to point out that the metabolic efficiency of anorectic patients parallels much of what is observed in the malnourished or fasted state, that is, reductions in RMR at low weight (e.g., Donahoe et al. 1984; Keys et al. 1950). Of particular note was the observation that increased physical activity occurred in many restricting anorectic patients, which was translated to an increase in caloric need to regain body weight during hospitalization (Kaye et al. 1988) (Table 11–2). These data suggest that physical activity is particularly important to consider in treating patients with anorexia nervosa, during weight restoration and weight maintenance.

Resting metabolic rate.   Normal-weight bulimic women appear to require fewer calories per day to maintain average body weight when compared with healthy control subjects (Gwirtsman et al. 1989). These data suggest that reductions in daily calorie expenditure occur. Whether such alterations result from alterations in RMR, thermogenesis, or activity is the focus of recent studies.

RMR accounts for roughly three-quarters of daily energy expenditure (Garrow 1978). Several groups have observed significant reductions in RMR among normal-weight bulimic women (untreated) compared with healthy subjects (Altemus et al. 1992; Bennett et al. 1988; Devlin et al. 1990; Fernstrom et al. 1990). The collective results are reasonably consistent, ranging between 10% and 15%, although Bennett et al. (1988) noted RMR reductions only in the most severely ill patients. The magnitude of this reduction is sufficient to render body-weight maintenance in these patients difficult. These data clearly point out a disturbance in energy expenditure, yet the etiology of these changes is unknown. Devlin et al. (1990) measured numerous metabolic indices in their study of 22 bulimic women. They noted that thyrotropin levels were reduced significantly, although other thyroid measures—thyroxine (T_4), triiodothyronine (T_3), and reverse T_3—were normal. Fasting blood glucose was reduced, and insulin levels remained unchanged compared with control subjects. No group differences occurred in body fat mass, fat cell size, or lipoprotein lipase activity.

Whether reductions in RMR are a result of food abstinence (prolonged periods of bingeing and food restriction), promoting a state of semistarvation, or a result of an underlying metabolic aberration in the patient is unknown. Reductions in RMR are consistent with a food restriction, although the blood measurements of metabolic intermediates (Devlin et al. 1990) do not generally support this. Possibly, such measurements need to be taken under stimulated conditions, rather than resting conditions, to reveal a meaningful difference.

Table 11–2.   Calorie expenditure studies in the eating disorders

Study	Finding
Kaye et al. 1988	Activity contributes to increased caloric needs of anorectic patients during refeeding.
Bennett et al. 1988 Devlin et al. 1990 Fernstrom et al. 1990	Resting metabolic rate is reduced in normal-weight bulimic patients compared with healthy control subjects.
Fernstrom et al. 1990	Diet-induced thermogenesis is reduced in normal-weight bulimic patients compared with healthy control subjects.

Diet-induced thermogenesis (DIT).   Food consumption is a major stimulus to metabolic rate (Jequier 1983). This phenomenon has been termed "specific dynamic action of foods," "postprandial thermogenesis," "thermic effect of food," and "diet-induced thermogenesis" and reflects the energy cost of digesting, absorbing, and storing nutrients. DIT varies with the metabolic fate of the ingested nutrients (Flatt 1978) and type of substrate (Sharief and MacDonald 1982; Welle et al. 1981). When the thermogenic response increases above normal in response to food ingestion, this means the body is less efficient at storing calories; a decrease in the normal response indicates more efficient storage of food. The implication is that an individual showing a reduction in DIT has more calories available for storage in body tissues, thus increasing metabolic efficiency and body weight. Reductions in DIT have been demonstrated in obese patients (e.g., Bessard et al. 1983; Schwartz et al. 1983; Segal et al. 1990), although this is not a uniform finding (e.g., Felig et al. 1983; Welle and Campbell 1983).

In our most recent study (Fernstrom et al., submitted for publication), we investigated whether the DIT response to a mixed meal would be blunted in normal-weight bulimic patients compared with healthy subjects. Our liquid meal simulated a breakfast meal and represented about one-sixth of daily calorie intake. We found a profound blunting of DIT of about 50% over a 2-hour period. Translated into calories, this represents about 15 calories for this calorie load. Although a small number of calories alone, when repeated throughout the day for meals and snacks this reduction in DIT could readily promote weight gain.

This reduction in DIT is consistent with the observed reductions in RMR, although the origins of this effect are speculative. However, it seems likely that disturbances of the sympathetic nervous system are important in mediating this effect. Reductions in sympathetic nervous system activity (e.g., heart rate, blood pressure) are notable in the eating disorders, and some literature suggests that these sympathetic disturbances are associated with alterations in metabolic function (Landsburg and Young 1978). It is well known that the sympathetic nervous system is strongly tied to both DIT and metabolic substrate utilization (e.g., Acheson et al. 1983; Young and Landsburg 1979; Young et al. 1980). Furthermore, despite the fact that the extent to which metabolic rate and metabolic substrate utilization in bulimic patients result from abnormal eating patterns or a metabolic predisposition remains unclear, either could likely have an impact on the sympathetic nervous system.

However, reductions in RMR and DIT were not consistently or significantly correlated (Figure 11–1), although this is apparent for at least a portion of the group. This is not particularly surprising, however, because the DIT response is predominantly driven by the sympathetic nervous system, whereas RMR is influenced by numerous metabolic and hormonal factors.

Antidepressant Drugs, Metabolic Rate, and Body-Weight Change

With the increasing use of antidepressant medications in the treatment of patients with eating disorders, it is important to consider the possible metabolic consequences of these drugs. Weight gain during treatment with tricyclic antidepressants has frequently been reported both in un-

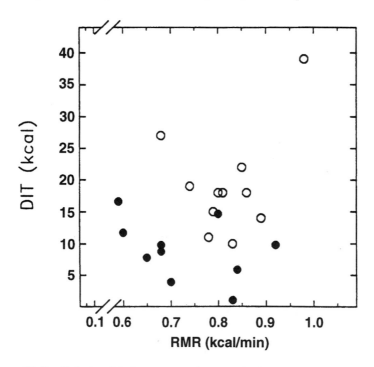

Figure 11–1. Relationship between resting metabolic rate (RMR) and diet-induced thermogenic (DIT) response among 10 normal-weight bulimic women *(filled circles)* and 11 control women *(open circles)*. The correlation ($r = .30$) was not statistically significant ($P < .09$).

controlled studies (e.g., Berken et al. 1984; Harris et al. 1986; Paykel et al. 1973) and in highly controlled studies (e.g., Fernstrom et al. 1986, 1988) (Table 11–3). Fernstrom et al. (1985) reported that depressed patients treated with tricyclic antidepressants (amitriptyline or imipramine) showed significant and metabolically meaningful reductions in RMR after 2–4 weeks of treatment (Figure 11–2). Translated into calories, a patient could gain a pound every 10–14 days in the absence of any change in food intake. These metabolic responses appear to be related to reductions in sympathetic nervous system activity, occurring after 2 weeks of treatment (Sethy et al. 1988), and do not appear to be related to changes in physical activity (e.g., the sedating effects of these medications). It is interesting to note that changes in appetite seem less important. For example, cravings for calorically dense (fat-rich) foods, with or without a sweet taste, do not appear to develop in the majority of treated patients (Fernstrom et al. 1987).

We have also initiated studies on the metabolic effects of nontricyclic medications on weight gain in depressed patients: we have already observed increases in RMR and weight loss in patients treated for 2 weeks with the serotonergic reuptake blocker fluvoxamine (e.g., Fernstrom et al. 1988). Moreover, with either drug group, clinical response was not related to the RMR change (all patients improved), nor were other fac-

Table 11–3. Weight change in patients treated with antidepressants for 1 month

Weight change (lb)	Amitriptyline (N = 18)		Nortriptyline (N = 18)		Desipramine (N = 24)		Zimelidine (N = 13)	
	n	%	n	%	n	%	n	%
Very rapid gain (>10)	5	28	2	11	4	17	0	0
Rapid gain (7–10)	8	44	2	11	3	12	0	0
Moderate gain (3–6)	3	17	8	44	7	29	1	8
No change (±2)	2	11	6	33	9	38	9	69
Moderate loss (3–6)	0	0	0	0	0	0	3	23
Rapid loss (7–10)	0	0	0	0	0	0	0	0
Very rapid loss (>10)	0	0	0	0	1	4	0	0

Note. Patients were weighed on a balance-beam scale in the clothes they wore to bed. Weight change represents the number of pounds gained or lost after 1 month of treatment.
Source. Reprinted from Fernstrom MH, Kupfer DJ: "Antidepressant-Induced Weight Gain: A Comparison Study of Four Medications." *Psychiatry Research* 26:265–271, 1988. Used with permission.

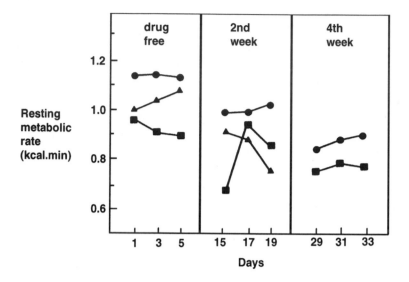

Figure 11–2. Effects of antidepressant treatment on resting metabolic rate in depressed patients. Data represent three separate measurements taken during each time period. Measurements were performed during the drug-free period (within the second of two drug-free weeks) and during the second and fourth weeks of treatment. Patient 1: *circle;* Patient 2: *triangle;* Patient 3: *square.*
Source. Reprinted from Fernstrom MH, Epstein LH, Spiker DG, et al: "Resting Metabolic Rate Is Reduced in Patients Treated With Antidepressants." *Biological Psychiatry* 20:688–692, 1985. Used with permission.

Table 11–4. Effect of fluoxetine (Prozac) on resting metabolic rate (RMR) in four hospitalized, short-term weight-stable patients

| Patient | Normal-weight bulimia nervosa (RMR in kcal/24 hr) | | |
	Admission no meds	Weight stable	Weight stable + Prozac
Patient A	1,152	ND	1,325
Patient B	729	ND	1,339
Patient C	1,138	1,354	1,800
Patient D	1,080	1,339	ND

Note. ND = no data.

tors, including degree of obesity or prior weight gain or loss during the depressive episode.

Clearly, such drugs could have an impact on the metabolic stability of recovering eating disorder patients. We recently observed in four bulimic patients an increase in daily caloric requirement after treatment with the serotonergic reuptake blocker fluoxetine (20–40 mg/day) (Table 11–4). Although very preliminary, these results suggest that such serotonergic agonists might consistently increase RMR, at least during short-term treatment. These kinds of results support the idea of very different metabolic effects of these mood-elevating drugs, an important consideration in the treatment of patients with eating disorders.

Conclusions

Differences in daily caloric need for recovered eating disorder patients have been well documented, both between patients and control subjects and within patient subgroups. Disturbances in calorie utilization (RMR, DIT, and activity) contribute to this energy-balance problem. In anorexia nervosa, increased activity contributes to increased caloric utilization. For normal-weight bulimic patients, both RMR and DIT are decreased, producing reductions in calorie utilization. Such declines in DIT most likely involve alterations in sympathetic nervous system activity. Whether such metabolic disturbances are related to years of abnormal eating (simulating semistarvation) or to a preexisting metabolic aberration is presently unknown. Either possibility could modify sympathetic tone. The observed alterations in energy expenditure among patients with eating disorders seem to be adequate to render body-weight maintenance more difficult and may be an important contributing factor to the high relapse rate reported in this group. Moreover, for the treatment of patients with eating disorders, the metabolic effects of these drugs are important to consider: tricyclic drugs tend to reduce RMR and promote weight gain, whereas nontricyclic drugs (e.g., serotonergic agonists like fluoxetine) tend to increase RMR and promote weight loss.

References

Acheson K, Jequier E, Wahren J: Influence of beta-adrenergic blockade on glucose induced thermogenesis in man. J Clin Invest 72:981–986, 1983

Altemus M, Hetherington M, Flood M, et al: Decrease in resting metabolic rate during abstinence from bulimic behavior. Am J Psychiatry 148:1071–1072, 1992

American Psychiatric Association: Diagnostic and Statistical Manual of Mental Disorders, 3rd Edition, Revised. Washington, DC, American Psychiatric Association, 1987

Beaumont PJV, George GCW, Smart DE: "Dieters" and "vomiters" in anorexia nervosa. Psychol Med 6:617–622, 1976

Bennett SM, Williamson DA, Powers SK: Bulimia nervosa and resting metabolic rate. International Journal of Eating Disorders 8:417–424, 1988

Berken G, Weinstein D, Stern W: Weight gain: a side effect of tricyclic antidepressants. J Affective Disord 7:133–138, 1984

Bessard T, Schutz Y, Jequier E: Energy expenditure and postprandial thermogenesis in obese women before and after weight loss. Am J Clin Nutr 38:680–693, 1983

Casper RC, Eckert ED, Halmi KA, et al: Bulimia: its incidence and clinical importance in patients with anorexia nervosa. Arch Gen Psychiatry 37:1030–1035, 1980

Devlin MJ, Walsh BT, Kral JG, et al: Metabolic abnormalities in bulimia nervosa. Arch Gen Psychiatry 47:144–148, 1990

Donahoe DP, Lin DH, Kirschenbaum DS, et al: Metabolic consequences of dieting and exercise in the treatment of obesity. J Consult Clin Psychol 52:827–836, 1984

Felig P, Cunningham J, Levitt M: Energy expenditure in obesity in fasting and postprandial state. Am J Physiol 244:E45–E51, 1983

Fernstrom MH, Kupfer DJ: Antidepressant-induced weight gain: a comparison study of four medications. Psychiatry Res 26:265–271, 1988

Fernstrom MH, Epstein LH, Spiker DG, et al: Resting metabolic rate is reduced in patients treated with antidepressants. Biol Psychiatry 20:688–692, 1985

Fernstrom MH, Krowinski R, Kupfer DJ: Chronic imipramine treatment and weight gain. Psychiatry Res 14:269–275, 1986

Fernstrom MH, Krowinski R, Kupfer DJ: Appetite and food preference in depression: effects of imipramine treatment. Biol Psychiatry 22:529–539, 1987

Fernstrom MH, Massoudi M, Kupfer DJ: Fluvoxamine and weight loss. Biol Psychiatry 24:941–960, 1988

Fernstrom MH, Weltzin TE, McConaha C, et al: Resting metabolic rate and diet-induced thermogenesis are reduced in patients with normal weight bulimia, in Abstracts of European Winter Conference on Brain Research Annual Meeting, 1990

Fernstrom MH, Weltzin TE, McConaha C, et al: Reductions in diet-induced thermogenesis in normal weight bulimia: relationship to energy efficiency and body weight maintenance. Biol Psychiatry (submitted for publication)

Flatt JP: The biochemistry of energy expenditure, in Recent Advances in Obesity Research, Vol 2. Edited by Bray G. London, Newman Publishing, 1978, pp 211–218

Garfinkel PE, Moldofsky H, Garner DM: The heterogeneity of anorexia nervosa. Arch Gen Psychiatry 37:1036–1040, 1980

Garrow JS: Energy Balance and Obesity in Man, 2nd Edition. Oxford, Elsevier–North Holland Press, 1978

Golay A, Schutz Y, Meyer HU, et al: Glucose-induced thermogenesis in nondiabetic and diabetic obese subjects. Diabetes 31:1023–1028, 1982

Gwirtsman HE, Kaye WH, Obarzanek E, et al: Decreased caloric intake in normal-weight patients with bulimia: comparison with female volunteers. Am J Clin Nutr 49:86–92, 1989

Harris B, Young J, Hughes B: Changes occurring in appetite and weight during short-term antidepressant treatment. Br J Psychiatry 145:645–648, 1986

Herzog DB, Copeland PM: Eating disorders. N Engl J Med 313:295–303, 1985

Hsu LKG: Outcome of anorexia nervosa: a review of the literature. Arch Gen Psychiatry 37:1041–1046, 1980

Hsu LKG, Sobkiewicz TA: Bulimia nervosa: a four- to six-year follow-up study. Psychol Med 19:1035–1038, 1989

Hsu LKG, Crisp AH, Harding B: Outcome of anorexia nervosa. Lancet 1:61–68, 1979

Jequier E: Thermogenic responses induced by nutrients in man: their importance in energy balance regulation, in Nutritional Adequacy, Nutrient Availability, and Needs. Edited by Mauron J. Basel, Bikhauser Verlag, 1983, pp 22–44

Jequier E: Energy expenditure in obesity. J Clin Endocrinol Metab 13:563–580, 1984

Kaye WH, Gwirtsman HE, George T, et al: Caloric consumption and activity levels in anorexia nervosa: a prolonged delay in normalization. International Journal of Eating Disorders 5:489–502, 1986a

Kaye WH, Gwirtsman HE, Obarzanek E, et al: Caloric intake necessary for weight maintenance in anorexia nervosa: non-bulimics require greater caloric intake than bulimics. Am J Clin Nutr 44:435–443, 1986b

Kaye WH, Gwirtsman HE, Obarzanek E, et al: Relative importance of caloric intake needed to gain weight and level of physical activity in anorexia nervosa. Am J Clin Nutr 47:987–994, 1988

Keller MB, Herzog DB, Lavori PW, et al: High rates of chronicity and rapidity of relapse in patients with bulimia nervosa and depression. Arch Gen Psychiatry 46:480–481, 1989

Keys A, Brozek J, Hanschel A, et al: The Biology of Human Starvation. Minneapolis, University of Minnesota Press, 1950

Landsburg L, Young JB: Fasting, feeding and regulation of the sympathetic nervous system. N Engl J Med 298:1295–1298, 1978

Newman NM, Halmi KA, Marchi P: Relationship of clinical factors to caloric requirements in subtypes of eating disorders. Biol Psychiatry 22:1253–1263, 1987

Paykel ES, Mueller PS, DeLaVergne PM: Amitriptyline, weight gain, and carbohydrate craving: a side effect. Br J Psychiatry 123:501–507, 1973

Pope HG, Hudson JI: Antidepressant drug therapy for bulimia: current status. J Clin Psychiatry 47:339–345, 1986

Schutz Y, Bessard T, Jequier E: Diet-induced thermogenesis measured over a whole day. Am J Clin Nutr 40:542–552, 1984

Schwartz RS, Hlater JB, Bierman E: Reduced thermic effect of feeding in obesity: role of norepinephrine. Metabolism 32:114–117, 1983

Segal KR, Gutin B: Thermic effects of food and exercise in lean and obese women. Metabolism 32:581–589, 1983

Segal KR, Edano A, Tomas MB: Thermic effect of a meal over 3 and 6 hours in lean and obese men. Metabolism 39:985–992, 1990

Sethy VH, Day JS, Cooper MM: Dose-dependent down-regulation of beta-receptors after chronic intravenous infusion of antidepressants. Prog Neuropsychopharmacol Biol Psychiatry 12:673–682, 1988

Sharief NN, MacDonald I: Differences in dietary induced thermogenesis with various carbohydrates in normal and overweight men. Am J Clin Nutr 35:267–272, 1982

Stordy BJ, Marks V, Kalucy RS, et al: Weight gain, thermic effect of glucose and resting metabolic rate during recovery from anorexia nervosa. Am J Clin Nutr 30:138–146, 1977

Strober M, Salkin B, Burroughs J, et al: Validity of the bulimia-restricter criteria in anorexia nervosa. J Nerv Ment Dis 170:345–351, 1982

Walker J, Roberts SI, Halmi KA, et al: Caloric requirements for weight gain in anorexia nervosa. Am J Clin Nutr 32:1396–1400, 1979

Welle SL, Campbell RG: Normal thermic effect of glucose in obese women. Am J Clin Nutr 37:87–92, 1983

Welle S, Lilavivat U, Campbell RG: Thermic effect of feeding in man: increased norepinephrine levels following glucose but not protein or fat consumption. Metabolism 30:953–958, 1981

Weltzin TE, Fernstrom MH, Hansen D, et al: Abnormal caloric requirements for weight maintenance in patients with anorexia and bulimia nervosa. Am J Psychiatry 148:1675–1682, 1991

Young JB, Landsburg L: Effect of diet and cold exposure on norepinephrine turnover in pancreas and liver. Am J Physiol 236:E524–E533, 1979

Young JB, Kore JW, Palloter JA, et al: Enhanced plasma norepinephrine response to upright posture and oral glucose administration in elderly human subjects. Metabolism 29:532–539, 1980

Section V

Family Studies

Chapter 12

Controlled Trials of Family Treatments in Anorexia Nervosa

Gerald F. M. Russell, M.D.
Christopher Dare, M.B.
Ivan Eisler, B.A.
P. Daniel F. Le Grange, Ph.D.

———————

Three main questions are explored in this chapter. First, under what conditions is family therapy beneficial to patients with anorexia nervosa? Second, what are the principal components of family therapy that render it effective under these conditions? Third, does the role of family therapy in reversing the course of anorexia nervosa throw light on family pathogenesis in this illness?

The conventional way of assessing a psychological treatment is to begin with the theoretical framework of the treatment. It is our view, however, that the theory of family therapy in anorexia nervosa requires reappraisal in light of empirical observations. We therefore reverse the usual order of presentation and begin with the data generated by controlled studies and then turn to an interpretation of their significance for the theory of family pathogenesis in anorexia nervosa.

The Patient's Family: Historical Introduction

We first glance back at the writings of our illustrious medical forbears, who, when they first described anorexia nervosa, made important observations on the families of their patients.

Charles Lasègue (1873) had surprisingly little to say about the management of the relatives of patients, but he was well aware of the need of physicians to extend their observations from the patients themselves to the patients' surroundings, and especially the patients' parents:

> In view of the undoubted psychological aspects [of the disorder], it would be equally regrettable to ignore or misinterpret the patient's psychological surroundings.
>
>   None should be surprised to note that I always consider the morbid state of the hysterical patient side by side with the preoccupations of her relatives. (p. 399)

We are indebted to Dr. Joseph Silverman (1989; see also Chapter 1 of this volume) for drawing our attention to Louis-Victor Marcé, whom he dubbed "anorexia nervosa's forgotten man." This is because in 1860, well before Lasègue and Gull, Marcé described young girls who avoided food to the point of extreme inanition and resisted the physician's attempts at refeeding. Marcé attributed the disorder to a severe hypochondriacal state in these girls leading to the delusion that they cannot or ought not to eat. Of particular interest to our topic is Marcé's (1860) observation:

> This hypochondrial delirium, then, cannot be advantageously countered so long as the subjects remain in the midst of their own family and their habitual circle. . . . It is therefore indispensable to change the habitation and surrounding circumstances, and to entrust the patients to the care of strangers. (pp. 17–18)

But it was William Gull (1874) who formed the clearest view of the management of the patient's parents:

> The inclination of the patient must be in no way consulted. In the earlier and less severe stages it is not unusual for the medical attendant to say, in reply to the anxious solicitude of the parents, "Let her do as she likes. Don't force food." Formerly I thought such advice admissible and proper, but larger experience has shown plainly the danger of allowing the starvation process to go on.

I have remarked that these wilful patients are often allowed to drift their own way into a state of extreme exhaustion, when it might have been prevented by placing them under different moral conditions. The patients should be fed at regular intervals, and surrounded by persons who would have moral control over them; *relatives and friends being generally the worst attendants* [emphasis added]. (pp. 310–311)

In the *Lancet,* the English physician Playfair (1888) chided William Gull over his choice of the term *anorexia nervosa,* preferring to describe the patients as examples of neurasthenia. In passing, however, he commented on the management of the disorder:

They must be removed entirely from their usual domestic surroundings, involving, as these almost always do, much that is unwholesome for the patient.

Absolute rest, massage, and abundant over-feeding, . . . are no doubt valuable adjuncts in the case, *but without isolation they will almost certainly fail* [emphasis added]. (p. 818)

These early observers are unanimous in expressing exasperation with the patients' families and in recommending that they should be excluded from the program of treatment. These therapeutic principles were expressed more than 100 years ago. We have progressed since then, and modern family therapy embodies a method of working with the relatives in a constructive manner so as to enroll their help in treating the sick family member. It may be noted in passing that, despite their criticism of relatives, none of these early clinical observers went so far as to blame the families for the patients' illnesses.

Controlled Trials of Family Therapy

Family therapy can be defined as a complex method of treatment based on a range of psychological interventions whose focus is the pattern of relationships within the family rather than just the individual patient.

Three controlled trials of family therapy have been undertaken at the Maudsley Hospital, London, since 1981 and are still currently in progress.

- *Study 1.* An evaluation of family therapy in anorexia nervosa and bulimia nervosa, now completed and including a preliminary 5-year follow-up.

- *Study 2.* A controlled trial of family therapy in older patients with anorexia nervosa. This study is still in progress but observations so far allow tentative conclusions regarding the indications for family therapy.
- *Study 3.* A controlled trial of two methods of family therapy in adolescent anorexia nervosa. Although the definitive trial is still in progress, the results of a preliminary pilot study are informative and will be presented in this chapter.

Evaluation of Family Therapy in Anorexia Nervosa and Bulimia Nervosa (Study 1)

Design of the Therapeutic Trial

The design of the therapeutic trial in Study 1 followed the traditional design of a controlled trial, involving a randomized allocation of patients to the treatment under study (family therapy) and a control treatment (a supportive individual therapy).

It was decided to commence the randomized trial itself after an initial period of intensive inpatient treatment directed at restoring the patients' nutritional state to an optimum level by applying well-developed methods of nursing care.

There were important advantages to this two-stage approach. First, the aims of the psychological treatments could be focused on maintaining and consolidating the gains already achieved by admission to the hospital, especially the weight gains. Second, the ethical problems were minimized because the patients were first restored to optimum weights before being randomly allocated to outpatient treatments, at least one of which (the control treatment) was relatively untried. The third stage of the design was to follow up the patients to assess their level of recovery. The first follow-up was carried out at the end of 1 year of outpatient psychological treatment, and the findings have already been reported (Russell et al. 1987). A more recent 5-year follow-up was carried out; although still incomplete, its results will be presented and compared with the 1-year follow-up.

The design was also refined so as to introduce greater homogeneity in the patient groups receiving treatment. The patients with anorexia nervosa were divided into subgroups according to two factors known to influence natural outcome: age at onset and duration of illness (Hsu et al. 1979; Morgan and Russell 1975; Ratnasuriya et al. 1991; Theander 1970). The patients with bulimia nervosa were placed in a separate subgroup. There were four subgroups of patients:

- *Subgroup 1.* Age at onset less than or equal to 18 years, and duration of illness less than 3 years ($n = 21$).
- *Subgroup 2.* Age at onset less than or equal to 18 years, and duration of illness more than 3 years ($n = 15$).
- *Subgroup 3.* Age at onset 19 years or older ($n = 21$).
- *Subgroup 4.* Patients with bulimia nervosa ($n = 23$).

Only after entry into the above subgroups were the patients randomly allocated to one of the two therapies.

It was not possible to have assessors kept "blind" to the form of treatment provided. To facilitate objective assessments, the patients were seen at follow-up by the research investigator who was not involved in the delivery of therapy. It was also thought necessary to allow for possible variations between therapists with regard to their personal effectiveness. This was achieved by having each of the four therapists conduct both treatments, and each treated approximately equal numbers of patients in family therapy and the control individual therapy.

One of the senior investigators (C.D.) served as the supervisor of the family therapy; the other (G.F.M.R.) supervised the control therapy. The supervisors formed the clear impression that all four therapists were equally committed to both forms of psychological treatment.

The Therapies

Family therapy.   The method of family therapy was that evolved by one of the authors (C.D.) in treating children and adolescents with anorexia nervosa at the Maudsley Hospital (Dare et al. 1990). The aim is to gain active cooperation from the family, achieved by presenting the problem of anorexia nervosa as one that requires all the family's resources for its conquest to help the starving youngster. Care is taken to exonerate the family from any blame for the illness. Thus, we take a neutral approach as to the causes of the illness, thereby minimizing guilt developing in family members, guilt that can disable and undermine the therapy's effectiveness. This neutral stance is also in accord with our scientific approach.

There are three stages to the therapy. In the first stage, the therapy is almost entirely focused on the eating disorder, and the first session usually includes a family meal. With younger patients, the therapist encourages the parents to take control of their child's eating. With older patients, the parents are asked to decide either to control their child's eating or to express consistently the attitude that her eating is none of their concern.

The second stage begins when the parents' management of the eating disorder results in a steady weight gain. The therapist advises the parents to accept as their chief task the return of their child to physical health. The aim is to achieve weight gain with minimum tension, after which a return to a more normal family life can be resumed and discussed.

The third stage can begin when the patient's weight is largely under control and responsibility for continued weight gain is returned to her. It now becomes possible to discuss more normal family concerns. For the patient under age 18, these concerns will include working toward increased personal autonomy and the need for the parents to reorganize their life together, after their children's prospective departure from home. With older patients, discussions are focused on their need to establish healthy young adult relationships with their parents, without requiring anorectic symptoms as a medium of communication.

This approach resembles that of Minuchin and his colleagues (Minuchin et al. 1975, 1978) and other writers from the Philadelphia Child Guidance Clinic (Sargent et al. 1985). There are differences, however. The design of the trial precluded the use of any individual or marital psychotherapy in the final stage of therapy. Moreover, the issues of food avoidance and weight loss remained the focus of treatment for a longer period. These issues led us to arouse anxiety deliberately in the parents, as we reminded them of the physical dangers of self-starvation in the adolescent. Efforts were made to avoid engendering guilt in the family; such efforts included giving deliberate praise and describing the family as loving and highly committed to one another.

The family therapy also included at times an exploration of the intergenerational organization of the family, so as to gain an understanding of the broader context in which the symptom occurred, as advocated by the Milan School (Selvini-Palazzoli et al. 1978). We used the method of drawing a family tree with the family to explore loyalty systems within the family. "Systemic interventions" might be made during periods of family resistance to treatment. For example, the loyalty systems were expressed as the family's "need" for the symptoms of anorexia nervosa.

Individual supportive therapy.   This treatment was not a formal psychoanalytic psychotherapy but was problem centered, educational, and supportive. It included elements of cognitive, interpretative, and strategic therapies. The therapist always focused on the patient's current weight during each session and responded with praise or dismay as was appropriate. If weight loss continued, the dangers of malnutrition were stressed and explanations were given in nutritional terms for the patient's preoccupations with food and symptoms of depression, irritability, and insomnia. Warnings that readmission would be necessary were incorporated in the "therapeutic threat" of the hospital. A session would also include an examination of interpersonal problems, whether these occurred in the family, at school, at work, or more generally within social life. The symptoms of food avoidance and weight loss were interpreted in terms of psychological processes.

The individual therapy was developed as a control treatment and was matched as closely as possible to the family therapy in its duration (hourly sessions) and its frequency. The therapy was also systematically supervised. The transference relationship was not explored or interpreted, but it was often observed that when improvement occurred, a greater therapeutic alliance was associated with a gradual gain in weight.

The patients.   Eighty patients, consecutively referred to our clinic, were enrolled in the trial: 57 patients had anorexia nervosa and fully satisfied DSM-III (American Psychiatric Association 1980) criteria; 23 patients had bulimia nervosa as originally described by Russell (1979) and would have satisfied the subsequent diagnostic criteria of DSM-III-R (American Psychiatric Association 1987).

The mean age of the patients on admission (and entry into the trial) was 21.8 years. Mean admission weight was 69.6% of average body weight (ABW). Mean weight when discharged from the hospital was 89.5% of ABW. Mean duration of their illness was 3.9 years. Of the 80 patients, 49 had previous hospital admissions. There was, therefore, a tendency for this population of patients to have suffered from severe illnesses. The randomized allocation resulted in 41 patients being entered into family therapy and 39 being entered into the control individual therapy.

Patient Assessments

The two principal assessments were the Morgan and Russell scales (Morgan and Hayward 1988) and changes in body weight.

Morgan and Russell scales.   These scales are part of a structured interview applied in several studies of the natural outcome of anorexia nervosa (Burns and Crisp 1984; Hsu et al. 1979; Morgan and Russell 1975; Ratnasuriya et al. 1991). Two sets of data are obtained. The first set concerns categories of general outcome, which is based on body weight and menstrual function:

- *Good outcome.*   Body weight is maintained within 15% of ABW according to actuarial tables (Diem and Lentner 1970), and menstrual cycles are regular.
- *Intermediate outcome.*   Body weight has risen to within 15% of ABW, but amenorrhea persists.
- *Poor outcome.*   Body weight is less than 15% below ABW, or bulimic symptoms have appeared.

The second set of data is a measure of general progress: the average outcome score. The patient's adjustment on each of five dimensions (nutritional status, menstrual function, mental state, psychosexual adjustment, and socioeconomic status) is scored on a 12-point scale. The average outcome score is derived as the mean of the scores on the five scales.

The Morgan and Russell scales were adapted to bulimia nervosa:

- *Good outcome.*   No bulimic symptoms, and weight is maintained within 15% of ABW.
- *Intermediate outcome.*   Bulimic symptoms occur less than once weekly, and weight is within 15% of ABW.
- *Poor outcome.*   Bulimic symptoms occur more than once weekly, or weight is less than 15% below ABW.

Body weight.   The maintenance of body weight is an accurate measure of the efficacy of the psychological treatment. Each patient's weight was recorded in kilograms and expressed as a percentage of ABW as recorded in the actuarial tables.

Results I: Comparison of Family Therapy and Individual Therapy at End of 1-Year Follow-Up

Effects of the two therapies as measured by categories of general outcome.   Table 12–1 shows the distributions of patients among the three categories of outcome (good, intermediate, and poor). The numbers of patients receiving each treatment are shown within the four clinical subgroups.

In Subgroup 1, the distribution of patients among the categories of general outcome favored family therapy. Of 10 patients in family therapy, 9 had a good or intermediate outcome compared to only 2 of 11 patients in individual therapy (Fisher's exact probability test: $P < .002$).

In Subgroups 2, 3, and 4, there were no significant differences in the distribution of patients among the categories of general outcome when family therapy was compared with individual therapy.

Effects of the two therapies as measured by the average outcome score. Only in Subgroup 1 was there a statistically significant difference in the improvement recorded on the average outcome score (optimum score = 12). Among the patients receiving family therapy, this score improved from 5.5 ± 1.3 (SD) on admission to 9.7 ± 2.0 at 1-year follow-up. Among the patients given individual therapy, the average outcome score improved only from 4.8 ± 1.4 to 5.7 ± 2.0 ($P < .01$, using t test).

Effects of the two therapies as measured by changes in body weight. In Subgroup 1, the patients receiving family therapy gained more weight

Table 12–1. Family therapy and individual therapy at 1-year follow-up ($N = 73$)

| Subgroup | General outcome category (n) | | | |
	Good	Intermediate	Poor	Total
Subgroup 1[a]				
Family	6	3	1	10
Individual	1	1	9	11
Subgroup 2				
Family	2	2	6	10
Individual	2	1	6	9
Subgroup 3				
Family	0	1	6	7
Individual	2	1	4	7
Subgroup 4				
Family	0	1	8	9
Individual	1	2	7	10

Note. Seven patients who refused outpatient therapy are excluded.
[a]Difference between good and combined intermediate and poor ratings: $P < .02$.
Difference between poor and combined good and intermediate ratings (both analyses by

(25.5%) compared with admission weight than those receiving individual therapy (15.5% weight gain) ($P < .01$).

In Subgroup 3, the effects of the two therapies were reversed. Individual therapy led to a greater weight gain (19.9%) than family therapy (5.5%) when comparing levels at 1 year of follow-up with those on admission ($P < .01$). In Subgroups 2 and 4, there were no significant differences in the weight gain resulting from the two therapies.

The effects of the two therapies are illustrated in Figures 12–1 and 12–2, which show the mean weights on admission, on discharge, and at 3-month intervals thereafter until the end of 1 year of therapy. In Subgroup 1 (Figure 12–1), the weights diverge after the patients are discharged from the hospital, with the greater weight loss occurring with individual therapy. Thereafter weight is gradually regained, much more

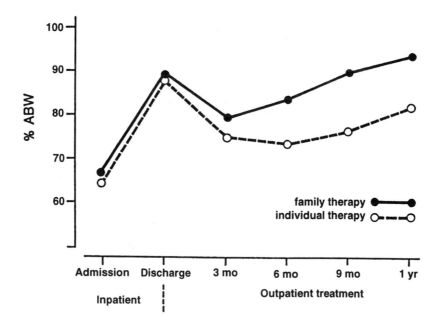

Figure 12–1. Weight charts for patients whose anorectic illness began when they were age 18 or younger and had lasted less than 3 years. Weights shown are the mean for the patients in each treatment group on admission, on discharge, and at 3-month intervals thereafter until the end of 1 year of therapy. ABW = average body weight.

steadily with family therapy than with individual therapy. The separation of the two weight curves showed the superiority of family therapy and was statistically significant at 6 months ($P < .03$), 9 months ($P < .005$), and 1 year ($P < .02$). In Subgroup 3 (Figure 12–2), the pattern was reversed. It was the patients receiving individual therapy whose weight loss was arrested before that of patients in family therapy. The separation of the two curves is statistically significant at 6 months ($P < .04$).

Results II: Comparison of Family Therapy and Individual Therapy at End of 5-Year Follow-Up

As of this writing, 67 patients have been followed up 5 years after entry into the trial.

Progress of the anorexia nervosa patients at 5 years.   Before comparing the long-term effects of the two therapies, data on the progress of the

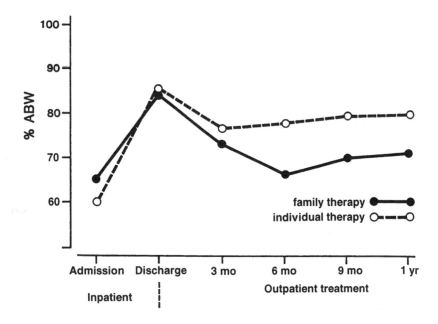

Figure 12–2.   Weight charts for patients whose anorectic illness began when they were age 19 or older. Weights shown are the mean for the patients in each treatment group on admission, on discharge, and at 3-month intervals thereafter until the end of 1 year of therapy. ABW = average body weight.

anorectic patients as a whole are presented, irrespective of the therapy received. Table 12–2 shows that the average outcome scores (on the Morgan and Russell scales) had continued to improve at the 5-year follow-up in comparison with those recorded on admission and at the 1-year follow-up. This improvement was most marked in Subgroup 1. Table 12–2 also shows that at the 5-year follow-up substantial gains in body weight had been achieved in each subgroup of patients, over and above those obtained at the 1-year follow-up.

Effects of the two therapies at 5-year follow-up as measured by categories of general outcome. Table 12–3 shows the distribution of patients among the good, intermediate, and poor categories of general outcome. The number of patients receiving family therapy or individual therapy are shown within each of the four clinical subgroups.

Subgroup 1, as in the earlier follow-up, shows the most important finding. At the 5-year follow-up, the distribution of patients among the three categories of general outcome again favors family therapy: 8 of 9 patients in family therapy had a good outcome compared to 3 of 8 in individual therapy (Fisher's exact probability test: $P < .05$). In Subgroups 2 and 3, there were no significant differences between family and individual therapy. In Subgroup 4, although neither treatment had produced striking long-term improvements, the individual therapy was significantly better than the family therapy.

Effects of the two therapies at 5-year follow-up as measured by average outcome scores (Morgan and Russell scales). Table 12–4 shows that statistically significant differences in the average outcome scores were obtained in Subgroup 1 and Subgroup 3. In Subgroup 1, there was a greater

Table 12–2. Patients with anorexia nervosa at 5-year follow-up: average outcome scores and weight (mean ± SD)

Subgroup	n	Average outcome scores (Morgan and Russell)			Weight (% ABW)		
		Admission	1-year follow-up	5-year follow-up	Admission	1-year follow-up	5-year follow-up
1	14	5.2 ± 1.4	7.6 ± 2.9	10.0 ± 1.6	66.0 ± 8.2	86.1 ± 13.8	99.3 ± 13.2
2	18	4.6 ± 1.4	6.6 ± 2.8	7.3 ± 2.7	66.0 ± 7.9	79.6 ± 12.6	90.4 ± 10.3
3	11	5.3 ± 1.4	7.1 ± 2.5	8.9 ± 1.3	63.1 ± 7.9	75.8 ± 11.0	93.9 ± 9.5

Note. ABW = average body weight.

improvement among the patients who had been in family therapy. This was reversed in Subgroup 3, the greater improvement being shown by patients who had received individual therapy.

Effects of the two therapies at 5-year follow-up as measured by changes in body weight.   Table 12–4 shows that even at 5-year follow-up the effects of therapy found at the 1-year follow-up were still evident. In Subgroup 1, the patients who had been in family therapy achieved a signifi-

Table 12–3.   Family therapy and individual therapy at 5-year follow-up $(N = 67)$

| | General outcome category (n) | | | |
Subgroup	Good	Intermediate	Poor	Total
Subgroup 1[a]				
Family	8	0	1	9
Individual	3	2	3	8
Subgroup 2				
Family	2	1	6	9
Individual	1	3	5	9
Subgroup 3				
Family	1	2	3	6
Individual	4	1	0	5
Subgroup 4[a]				
Family	0	4	7	11
Individual	4	2	4	10

[a]Difference between family and individual therapy: $P < .05$.

Table 12–4.   Patients with anorexia nervosa at 5-year follow-up: family therapy and individual therapy (mean ± SD)

| | | Average outcome scores (Morgan and Russell) | | Weight (% ABW) | |
Subgroup	n	Family therapy	Individual therapy	Family therapy	Individual therapy
Subgroup 1	14	10.7 ± 1.0	8.6 ± 2.2[b]	105.2 ± 11.2	89.9 ± 15.1[a]
Subgroup 2	18	7.0 ± 3.1	7.4 ± 2.3	87.4 ± 8.2	92.7 ± 12.3
Subgroup 3	11	7.2 ± 2.1	11.0 ± 0.5[c]	87.6 ± 12.8	101.3 ± 6.2[a]
Subgroup 4	21	7.4 ± 2.4	8.8 ± 2.9	94.2 ± 7.9	99.5 ± 8.0

Note.   ABW = average body weight.
[a]$P < .04$, [b]$P < .03$, [c]$P < .003$; by one-tailed t tests.

cantly higher weight (105.2% ABW) than those receiving individual therapy (89.9% ABW) ($t = 2.11$, 10 df, $P < .04$). In Subgroup 3, the effects of
the two therapies were reversed: individual therapy patients had reached
101.3% ABW, whereas family therapy patients weighed only 87.6% ABW
($t = 1.98$, 9 df, $P < .04$).

Figures 12–3 and 12–4 are extensions of Figures 12–1 and 12–2 to show
the mean body weights in Subgroups 1 and 3, respectively, at the end of
the 5-year follow-up. The same pattern shown at the end of 1 year persists
in the long term. In Subgroup 1 (Figure 12–3), patients in family therapy
retained significantly higher weights than those in individual therapy. In
Subgroup 3 (Figure 12–4), the respective benefits of the two therapies
were reversed: the superiority of individual therapy at 1 year was sustained
at 5 years.

Conclusions on the 5-year follow-up.   As expected, the anorectic patients, taken as a whole, had improved further by the time of the 5-year
follow-up compared with the 1-year follow-up. When the long-term ben-

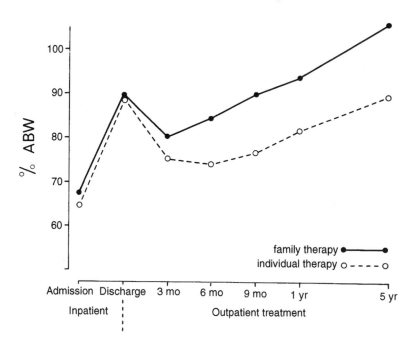

Figure 12–3.   Weight charts for patients shown in Figure 12–1 but extended to
include 5-year follow-up. Weights shown are the mean for the
patients in each treatment group. ABW = average body weight.

efits of the two therapies were compared, their relative effects found at 1 year were sustained at 5 years. Thus, the superior effects of family therapy were still apparent in the patients with the early age at onset and a relatively recent illness (Subgroup 1), whereas individual therapy had remained superior in the patients with an older age at onset (Subgroup 3).

Controlled Trial of Psychological Treatments in Older Anorectic Patients (Study 2)

Aims of the Second Controlled Trial

As it had previously been established that patients with an early onset and short duration of illness responded best to family therapy, it was decided to compare the benefits of three psychological treatments in older anorectic patients (ages 19 and over). Three treatments are being

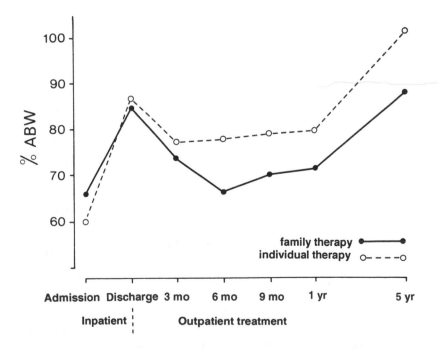

Figure 12–4.   Weight charts for patients shown in Figure 12–2 but extended to include 5-year follow-up. Weights shown are the mean for the patients in each treatment group. ABW = average body weight.

compared: 1) family therapy and 2) individual supportive therapy, as in the first study, and 3) "focal psychodynamic psychotherapy," devised by Malan (1963). This form of psychotherapy is derived from psychoanalytic theory and focuses on the "transference." This treatment was chosen in view of the commonly encountered therapeutic difficulties due to the patient's passive hostility and distrust toward the therapist (Bruch 1974; Garner and Bemis 1985).

Design of Study 2

The design of the second study is the same as the first. The patients receive a preliminary intensive inpatient treatment to elevate their weight to a level close to their premorbid weight. Before discharge, they are randomly allocated to one of the three outpatient treatments, which are matched in their intensity. The outpatient treatment is offered for 1 year, at which time the first follow-up assessment will be made. Each therapist will treat approximately equal numbers of patients in each of the three therapies. There are three supervisors, one for each therapy. The aim is to treat 100 patients; as of this writing 66 patients have been entered into the study.

Results

This second study is still in progress and no definitive results can yet be given. Nevertheless, we do present one preliminary result relevant to this chapter on family therapy. So far, 49 patients became engaged in one of three therapies and were fully assessed at the end of 1 year of treatment. The number of patients is still small, and no statistically significant differences have yet appeared for the series as a whole. However, an interesting finding is beginning to emerge when the series of patients is divided into two groups according to the age at onset of the illness: 1) 18 years and under and 2) 19 years and over.

There is a trend for patients with an early onset of illness to show better progress if they have been in family therapy than those receiving the individual therapies. Table 12–5 shows that among the patients with an early onset of illness, 7 of 12 had a good or intermediate outcome with family therapy, whereas only 5 of 18 patients receiving one of the individual therapies had such a good outcome (Fisher's exact probability test: $P = .08$). No conclusions can yet be drawn from the patients with a late age at onset.

It may therefore be tentatively concluded that an illness of early onset may remain associated with a good response to a family treatment even though the patients are no longer young when they receive it.

Controlled Trial of Two Forms of Family Treatment in Adolescents (Study 3)

Aims of the Third Controlled Trial

In Study 3, it was assumed that family therapy is effective in adolescent patients. The intention was to explore which components of family therapy are essential for success. Family therapy includes two crucial components: 1) altering the overall qualities of the "family as a system" and 2) improving the problem-solving skills of the family in dealing with the eating disorder.

The aim was to compare the efficacy of standard family therapy (which embodies both components) with family counseling (which relies mainly on the second component).

The Therapies

Family therapy.   This therapy has already been described. It depends on the treatment sessions including the whole family. It is thus possible to observe family interactions; interventions are made by the therapist to influence the pattern of family relationships.

Table 12–5.   Study 2: Comparison of three therapies, according to age at onset (general outcome categories): 1-year follow-up

Therapy	Age at onset ≤18 years			Age at onset ≥19 years		
	Good/ intermediate	Poor	Total	Good/ intermediate	Poor	Total
Family therapy	7	5	12	2	2	4
Focal psychotherapy	3	7	10	4	2	6
Individual supportive therapy	2	6	8	5	4	9

Family counseling.   In family counseling, both parents are seen together in regular sessions and are persuaded to attain strict control over their child's eating pattern so the child achieves sustained weight gain. The therapist again needs to convince the parents that they have the resources to undertake this task. They receive continued support and are exonerated from any blame.

The patient is seen separately by the same therapist, who counsels her about her diet and weight and adolescent problems of growing up, and who provides emotional support while her parents learn to manage her eating disorder.

Unlike family therapy, there is no possibility of direct intervention to change the family's functioning as a group. Of necessity, there is less confrontation in family counseling. As in the other trials, each therapist undertakes both forms of treatment.

Design of the Trial

Forty patients under age 18 have been recruited into the trial and randomly allocated to one of the family treatments. They are treated as outpatients for 1 year. The patients satisfied DSM-III-R criteria for anorexia nervosa, but the presence of bulimic symptoms and behavior did not exclude any. In the allocation of patients to the two therapies, the levels of expressed emotion were taken into account because they have been shown to predict poor engagement in family therapy (Szmukler et al. 1985).

The trial is not yet complete, and no results are available. The results of a pilot study are available, however (Le Grange 1989). The patient assessments included body weight and ratings on the Morgan and Russell scales. The family assessments included, among other measurements, measurements of expressed emotion (Szmukler et al. 1985; Vaughn and Leff 1976). In the pilot study, 18 patients (16 female, 2 male) were treated as outpatients, with the therapy lasting 32 weeks. Their mean age ($\pm$SD) was 15.3 ± 1.8 years, and the duration of illness averaged 1.1 ± 0.84 years. Their mean weight (expressed as ABW) was $77.9\% \pm 7.62\%$.

Results of the Pilot Study

Progress of the 18 patients irrespective of type of treatment.   The group of patients as a whole showed good progress, as shown by their weight gain and improved ratings on the Morgan and Russell scales. Their mean weight rose from 77.9% of ABW at entry to 92.2% of ABW by the end of the 32 weeks of treatment. The corresponding improvement in their mean average outcome scores was from 4.3 to 8.0.

Comparison of family therapy and family counseling.   Table 12–6 shows the improvements in average outcome scores and the gains in weight achieved by the end of 32 weeks of treatment, according to each form of therapy. The rise in the average outcome scores was similar for the two forms of therapy. The weight gain following family therapy (9.6% of ABW) was somewhat less than that following family counseling (13.1% of ABW; $P < .02$). This difference was no longer statistically significant, however, when patients with bulimic behaviors were excluded from the analysis.

Although family counseling appeared to give slightly better results than family therapy, we prefer to conclude at this stage that the two therapies give rise to similar benefits. This cautious conclusion is justified by the relatively small numbers of patients treated in the pilot study and the imperfect match between the two treatment groups as regards their initial weights and the presence of bulimic behaviors.

General response of family members to the two treatments.   An attempt was made to assess whether one form of treatment more often gives rise to conflict between family members than the other. One measure of expressed emotion is the number of critical comments made by a family member within a session. Most parents made very few critical comments at the initial assessment and at follow-up. There was a subgroup, however, whose initial expressed emotion scores were raised, and their response differed according to the form of therapy. When engaged in family ther-

Table 12–6.   Study 3 (pilot): Family therapy and family counseling: patients with anorexia nervosa under age 18 years ($N = 18$) (mean ± SD)

Therapy	Average outcome scores (Morgan and Russell)		Weight (% ABW)	
	At entry	End of treatment	At entry	End of treatment
Family therapy	3.8 ± 1.6	7.3 ± 2.0	75.9 ± 8.8	85.5 ± 10.9
Family counseling	4.8 ± 1.5	8.8 ± 1.4	80.5 ± 5.3	93.6 ± 6.9

Note. ABW = average body weight.

apy, five of seven parents continued to have high expressed emotion scores. While receiving family counseling, however, only one parent of four remained a high scorer.

A more direct assessment of the families' experience of the treatment was made at a 2-year follow-up, when the families were asked what they thought of the treatment. In both treatment groups the parents generally welcomed being told about the seriousness of the illness and the need on their part to take firm control of their child's eating. Somewhat surprisingly, most of the patients also said this aspect of the treatment was very difficult and unpleasant but necessary. The families who had received family therapy, however, more frequently reported that this control was achieved only at the cost of an intense struggle with their child, which they found distressing.

In conclusion, there is a preliminary suggestion that some families tolerate family counseling more readily than family therapy.

Discussion

In this review of controlled trials of family treatments at the Maudsley Hospital, the clearest finding is that family therapy is beneficial in a specific group of patients with anorexia nervosa. These are the patients in whom the illness began at 18 years or younger and had lasted less than 3 years. In the first trial, these criteria were thought to be simply synonymous with the patients being of a younger age when they received their therapy. The findings of the second trial suggest, however, that the relationship between responsiveness to family therapy and an illness of early onset may be a specific one. The most welcome finding is that the improved response to family therapy in comparison with the control treatment was sustained at the end of a 5-year follow-up. We believe this is the first time that a treatment has been shown to carry a long-term benefit in anorexia nervosa.

Some progress has also been made in the search for the specifically beneficial components of family therapy. The pilot study preceding the third controlled trial indicates that a crucial component is convincing the parents that they should take strict control of their ill child's eating pattern so that the child will achieve a sustained weight gain. This strategy was a key component of the two treatments being compared—family therapy and family counseling—both of which appear equally successful so far. A similar quest for specific effects of different therapies is being pursued by Robin et al. (1990), but their design may not permit the disentangling of two family approaches.

We now turn to the final question posed in the introduction to this chapter: Does the effectiveness of family therapy throw light on the question of family causation of anorexia nervosa? Several influential authors who have described their treatment for anorexia nervosa have drawn parallels with the presence of difficulties within the families of their patients (Bruch 1974, 1978; Crisp 1980; Selvini-Palazzoli et al. 1978). Minuchin et al. (1975) made their case most directly when they described their model of the "psychosomatic family" (including the families of anorexia nervosa patients):

> First the child is physiologically vulnerable; . . . second, the child's family has four transactional characteristics: enmeshment, overprotectiveness, rigidity and lack of conflict resolution. Third, the sick child plays an important role in the family's pattern of conflict avoidance; and this role is an important source of reinforcement for his symptoms. (p. 1032)

Not only are these modes of interaction excessively present, but they are also said to be detrimental.

> Family interactional patterns may trigger the onset or hamper the subsidence of the psychophysiologic process, or both. The resulting psychosomatic symptoms function as homeostatic mechanisms regulating family transactions. Therefore therapy must be directed towards changing the family processes that trigger and maintain the child's psychosomatic symptoms and toward changing the use of these symptoms within the family. (Minuchin et al. 1975, p. 1032)

Sargent et al. (1985) described this chain of interactions most specifically in anorexia nervosa. They believe this illness to be associated with characteristic dysfunctional patterns of family interaction. The family therapist is required to conceptualize the illness in relation to the organization and functioning of the entire family and plans therapeutic interventions to induce change in the family. We prefer to take the more cautious neutral approach that so far there is no evidence that families produce anorectic persons. There is an important practical reason for this stance. Family therapy can be very successful but it can also be hindered if families believe that they are in treatment because they are viewed as "the cause" of their child's illness.

The evidence in support of the family influencing the course of anorexia nervosa can be examined at three different levels. First, there is the level of compliance or responsiveness to treatment that is associated with certain family features. It has been found that early termination of treatment by the patient or her family was associated with high expressed emotion ratings within the family: defaulting from family therapy was more likely if the mother had frequently made critical comments (one index of expressed emotion) (Szmukler et al. 1985). Another example is the finding that a high parental expression of critical comments before treatment can be associated with a poor outcome at the end of the therapy (Le Grange 1989).

Most intriguing is our finding that family therapy is specifically effective in patients whose illness began at an early age. This was previously attributed to the greater ease of marshaling parental control over eating in younger patients (Russell et al. 1987). This interpretation will need revision if it is confirmed that the patient's age at the time of treatment is less important than the age at onset of the illness. An explanation considering the nature of the parent-child interaction during the adolescent start of the illness may then be called for.

The second level to be considered is the possible association of a pattern of family organization with anorexia nervosa and bulimia nervosa. An examination of this question by means of measures of expressed emotion and the Family Adaptability and Cohesion Evaluation Scales (FACES) (Olson et al. 1979) was undertaken by Le Grange et al. (in press). It was thought plausible that the low levels of criticism in these families, as measured by expressed emotion, might be equated with the lack of conflict resolution described by Minuchin et al. (1975). It was not possible, however, to find evidence of overprotectiveness with these measures. Despite the finding that, to the clinical observer, many of the families appeared close, a surprising finding from the FACES measure was that the family members themselves felt that they were not as close as they would have wished. It was concluded that these findings raised more questions about the theories of family transactions put forward by Minuchin et al. (1975, 1978) and Selvini-Palazzoli (1974) rather than simply confirming or rejecting them. There is thus a need for more precise hypotheses of family interactions in anorexia nervosa.

Finally, it should be stressed that even if a consistent family structure and functioning are identified in the families of patients with eating disorders, this does not necessarily identify them as causative factors. We are glad to conclude that Gull (1874) was wrong when he asserted that families could not be helpful in the treatment of anorexia nervosa.

Summary

The findings of three controlled trials of family therapy in anorexia nervosa are reported, as far as the available data permit:

1. Family therapy is effective in anorexia nervosa if the illness begins at a young age and is not yet chronic.
2. The benefits of family therapy are enduring in this group of patients, as shown by a 5-year follow-up.
3. The key component of family therapy is prevailing on the parents to take control of their child's eating, thereby ensuring a return to a normal weight.
4. These empirical findings do not support theoretical formulations that anorexia nervosa is due to a specific family organization, that is, there is no evidence that families cause anorexia nervosa. Certain family characteristics do influence compliance with and responsiveness to family therapy.

References

American Psychiatric Association: Diagnostic and Statistical Manual of Mental Disorders, 3rd Edition. Washington, DC, American Psychiatric Association, 1980

American Psychiatric Association: Diagnostic and Statistical Manual of Mental Disorders, 3rd Edition, Revised. Washington, DC, American Psychiatric Association, 1987

Bruch H: Eating Disorders: Obesity, Anorexia Nervosa and the Person Within. London, Routledge & Kegan Paul, 1974

Bruch H: The Golden Cage. New York, Basic Books, 1978

Burns T, Crisp AH: Outcome of anorexia nervosa in males. Br J Psychiatry 145:319–325, 1984

Crisp AH: Anorexia Nervosa: Let Me Be. London, Academic, 1980

Dare C, Eisler I, Russell GFM, et al: The clinical and theoretical impact of a controlled trial of family therapy in anorexia nervosa. Journal of Marital and Family Therapy 16:39–57, 1990

Diem K, Lentner C (eds): Geigy Scientific Tables, 7th Edition. Basel, JR Geigy, 1970

Garner DM, Bemis KM: Cognitive therapy for anorexia nervosa, in Handbook of Psychotherapy for Anorexia Nervosa and Bulimia. Edited by Garner DM, Garfinkel PE. New York, Guilford, 1985, pp 107–146

Gull WW: Anorexia nervosa (apepsia hysterica, anorexia hysterica). Transactions of the Clinical Society of London 7:22–28, 1874

Hsu LKG, Crisp AH, Harding B: Outcome of anorexia nervosa. Lancet 1:61–65, 1979

Lasègue C: De l'anorexia mentale. Archives Générales de Medecine 21:385–403, 1873

Le Grange PDF: Anorexia nervosa and family therapy: a study of changes in the individual and the family during the progress of body weight restoration. Unpublished doctoral thesis, University of London, London, 1989

Le Grange PDF, Eisler I, Dare E, et al: Evaluation of family treatments in adolescent anorexia nervosa: a pilot study. International Journal of Eating Disorders (in press)

Malan DH: A Study of Brief Psychotherapy. London, Tavistock, 1963

Marcé L-V: Note sur une forme de délire hypochondriaque consécutive aux dyspepsies et caractérisée principalement par le refus d'aliments. Annales Médico-psychologiques 6:15–28, 1860

Minuchin S, Baker BL, Rosman BL, et al: A conceptual model of psychosomatic illness in children: family organisation and family therapy. Arch Gen Psychiatry 32:1031–1038, 1975

Minuchin S, Rosman BL, Baker BL: Psychosomatic Families: Anorexia Nervosa in Context. Cambridge, MA, Harvard University Press, 1978

Morgan HG, Hayward AE: Clinical assessment of anorexia nervosa: the Morgan-Russell Outcome Assessment Schedule. Br J Psychiatry 152:367–371, 1988

Morgan HG, Russell GFM: Value of family background and clinical features as predictors of long-term outcome in anorexia nervosa: four-year follow-up study of 41 patients. Psychol Med 5:355–371, 1975

Olson DH, Sprenkle DH, Russell CS: Circumplex model of marital and family systems, I: cohesion and adaptability dimensions, family types and clinical applications. Fam Process 18:3–28, 1979

Playfair WS: Note on the so-called "Anorexia Nervosa." Lancet 1:817–818, 1888

Ratnasuriya RH, Eisler I, Szmukler GI, et al: Anorexia nervosa: outcome and prognostic factors after 20 years. Br J Psychiatry 158:495–502, 1991

Robin AL, Siegel P, Koepke T: Family versus individual therapy for anorexia and bulimia. Paper presented at the International Eating Disorder Conference, New York, April 1990

Russell GFM: Bulimia nervosa: an ominous variant of anorexia nervosa. Psychol Med 9:429–448, 1979

Russell GFM, Szmukler GI, Dare C, et al: An evaluation of family therapy in anorexia nervosa and bulimia nervosa. Arch Gen Psychiatry 44:1047–1056, 1987

Sargent J, Liebman R, Silver M: Family therapy in anorexia nervosa, in Handbook of Psychotherapy for Anorexia Nervosa and Bulimia. Edited by Garner DM, Garfinkel PE. New York, Guilford, 1985, pp 257–279

Selvini-Palazzoli M: Self-Starvation From the Intrapsychic to the Transpersonal Approach. London, Chaucer, 1974

Selvini-Palazzoli M, Boscolo L, Cecchin G, et al: Paradox and Counterparadox. New York, Jason Aronson, 1978

Silverman J: Louis-Victor Marcé, 1828–1864: anorexia nervosa's forgotten man. Psychol Med 19:833–835, 1989

Szmukler GI, Eisler I, Russell GFM, et al: Anorexia nervosa, parental "expressed emotion" and dropping out of treatment. Br J Psychiatry 147:265–271, 1985

Theander S: Anorexia nervosa: a psychiatric investigation of 94 female patients. Acta Psychiatr Scand Suppl 214:1–94, 1970

Vaughn CE, Leff JP: The measurement of expressed emotion in the families of psychiatric patients. British Journal of Social and Clinical Psychology 15:157–165, 1976

Chapter 13

Family Relationships

Laura Lynn Humphrey, Ph.D.

———————◦⊃●⊂◦———————

The field of eating disorders began to come of age during a broader movement toward multidimensional model building in psychology and psychiatry. The emergence of this integrative approach reflected a mutual respect for the reciprocal influences of biological, psychological, familial, and sociocultural factors (e.g., Garfinkel and Garner 1982; Johnson and Connors 1987; Williamson et al. 1989). Within this paradigmatic context, researchers and theoreticians in each specialized area have established some compelling evidence in support of the independent impact of each set of factors. The publication of this integrative volume gives testimony to the mainstream acceptance of such a multifactorial understanding of anorexia nervosa and bulimia nervosa. However, at this juncture, we know relatively little about the nature and mechanisms of reciprocal influence from an empirical perspective. This is not surprising when you consider that such complex and multifactorial research will, hopefully, develop out of a strong base of empirical evidence informing each domain, separately. That would seem to provide the most parsimonious and cost-effective strategy for clinical research in general, and eating disorders in particular.

Research progress in the family domain has paralleled these broader patterns almost exactly. Studies describing the nature of the differences between anorectic and bulimic daughters' perceptions of their families,

263

as compared with control subjects, have proliferated. Findings from these studies have been quite consistent with one another and with the theories that stimulate them. A few researchers have even examined parents' perceptions, differences among subtypes, and behavioral observations of the family's link to anorexia nervosa and bulimia nervosa. In this chapter, I critically review current research on the family's role in eating disorders with an explicit respect for the other important factors in the etiology and maintenance of anorexia nervosa and bulimia nervosa, and how they may have an impact on one another.

Theoretical Foundations

Theoretical formulations from both psychodynamic and family systems perspectives converge in describing the anorectic or bulimic daughter as having developmental arrests in separating from the family and consolidating a unique, individuated identity. These problems with separation and individuation are thought to result from family-wide disturbances in communication, role structure, affect modulation, and boundary diffusion. The earliest systemic conceptualization of anorexia nervosa was developed by Minuchin et al. (1978), who considered it to be similar to other psychosomatic disorders. They observed that the anorectic child's regressive state is needed by the family to preserve a tenuous homeostasis and harmony at a time of crisis. They described the family with an anorectic member as enmeshed, overprotective, and conflict-avoidant, and as co-opting the anorectic daughter in destructive alliances with one parent or another, as in triangulation or detouring. Independently, Palazzoli (1978) made some parallel observations regarding the families' emphasis on self-sacrifice, supreme loyalty, and preserving appearances despite underlying misery and desperation.

More recently, there have been some specific and well-elaborated theories of bulimia nervosa as well. Schwartz et al. (1985) concurred with Minuchin et al.'s (1978) view of anorexia nervosa but proposed that families of bulimic individuals are also more isolative, more conscious of appearances, and influenced greatly by cultural and filial values and customs through the generations. Schwartz et al. also explicated the richly symbolic meanings of food in families with a bulimic member. In her transgenerational model, Roberto (1986) elucidated family legacies and rituals involving weight, eating, attractiveness, achievement, and loyalty to the family above the self in families with a bulimic member.

Within a multigenerational family systems approach, Root et al. (1986) described all families of bulimic patients as having problems with individual and subsystem boundaries; an overemphasis on weight and appearances, which symbolizes deeper issues; and an uneven distribution of power in the families, reflecting the larger culture. They go on to delineate a typology of three subtypes of families of bulimic patients, which are thought to represent the majority of the population. Their "perfect," "overprotective," and "chaotic" types differ on dimensions of identity and self-image, boundary issues, expression of feelings, power dynamics, and ways of coping with grief and loss.

In an attempt to integrate object relations and family systems theories, Stern and I (Humphrey 1991; Humphrey and Stern 1988) characterized the families of both anorectic patients and bulimic patients as having transgenerational failures in the "holding environment" (Winnicott 1965), which lead to developmental adaptations through the generations. These adaptations are based on part-self and part-object relations and primitive defenses that require others to complete the sense of self. Such deficits and subsequent adaptations affect the quality and level of intrapsychic experience within the individual, as well as the interpersonal and systemic functioning of the family as a whole. We differentiated between anorectic and bulimic subtypes not so much on the basis of the underlying deficits, but more on the nature of the adaptations they employ. Families of anorectic patients more often idealize their daughter and themselves, whereas families of bulimic patients utilize projective identification to ward off their "bad" unwanted parts.

As in virtually all areas of clinical inquiry, the empirical research on familial contributions to eating disorders has lagged well behind the richly articulated and elaborated theories. Existing family research here, however, is more abundant, informative, and consistent with our conceptualizations of the disorders than in most other clinical groups, with the exception of schizophrenia and possibly chemical dependence. This is due in large measure to the early acceptance, within the field of eating disorders, of a multidimensional model of reciprocal influence to explain both the etiology and the ongoing maintenance of anorexia nervosa and bulimia nervosa. Although it would be premature at this point to test these models directly, we can begin to build the foundation of findings necessary to guide us in the more complex and encompassing task of model testing. Toward that goal, the extant research on family relationships and interaction patterns is reviewed from the perspective of daughters' self-reports, parents' ratings, behavioral observations, and differences within subtypes of eating disorders. Then I consider the methodological and paradigmatic limitations and advances that will either impede or further our progress toward the ultimate goals.

Research on Family Relationships and Interactions

Daughters' Perceptions

Most of the studies on family relationships in eating disorders have been based exclusively on anorectic or bulimic daughters' self-ratings of their families, without incorporating parental perceptions. Two of the earliest such projects found fairly consistent differences between bulimic patients and control subjects on the Family Environment Scale (FES) (Moos and Moos 1980) and the Family Adaptability and Cohesion Evaluation Scale (FACES) (Olson et al. 1978). Both Johnson and Flach (1985) and Ordman and Kirschenbaum (1986) found that bulimic patients experienced their families as less cohesive, expressive, and active in recreation as well as more conflictual on the FES than did control women. In addition, Johnson and Flach also reported less independence, organization, moral emphasis, and intellectual orientation, as well as greater achievement orientation, in the families of bulimic patients as compared with control women. Ordman and Kirschenbaum also employed the FACES in their study and found that bulimic patients saw their families as less cohesive and socially desirable than did control subjects.

Utilizing the Parent Bonding Instrument (Parker et al. 1979), Pole et al. (1988) also compared bulimic patients to control women. Their results showed that bulimic patients, but not the control group, remembered their mothers as less caring during their first 16 years of life, regardless of their status on depression. There were no significant differences for fathers or the variable "overprotectiveness." In a similar study, Palmer et al. (1988) employed the Parent Bonding Instrument but also included anorectic patients in their sample. Again, there were no differences on the protection score, but both anorectic patients and bulimic patients remembered their mothers as less caring (equally so), and bulimic patients saw their fathers this way as well.

Comparisons among subtypes of eating disorders represent an advance over studies that merely establish that bulimic children's perceptions of their parents are different from those of control women.

Comparative studies can help us to identify family factors that might be pathognomonic for anorexia nervosa or bulimia nervosa specifically. Utilizing the Family Assessment Measure (Skinner et al. 1983), Garner et al. (1985) compared anorectic, bulimic, and bulimic anorectic patients. They found that both bulimic anorectic patients and bulimic patients described their families as having more difficulty on every dimension (affective expression, affective involvement, control, communication, task accomplishment, role performance, and values and norms), whereas restricting anorectic patients did not.

In a study based on the Family Assessment Device (Epstein et al. 1983), Waller et al. (1989) compared anorectic patients, bulimic patients, and bulimic patients with no history of anorexia nervosa with control women. They also found that although patients in all subtypes of eating disorders reported more "unhealthy" family relationships than did their control counterparts, normal-weight bulimic patients were the most severely distressed.

Similarly, Humphrey (1986) compared the same three subtypes of eating disorders and found that those with bulimia nervosa and those with anorexia nervosa, bulimic subtype, were more like one another and different from classic restricting anorectic patients. Based on the Structural Analysis of Social Behavior (SASB) (Benjamin 1974), all three subgroups experienced their parents as more blaming, rejecting, and neglectful, but only those with bulimia nervosa and those with anorexia nervosa, bulimic subtype, also perceived a deficit in parental affection and empathy. These differences have not been found on every measure, however. Another study by Waller et al. (1990) contrasted women with anorexia nervosa, bulimia nervosa, or bulimia nervosa with no prior history of anorexia nervosa on the FACES II (Olson et al. 1982), an updated version of the original FACES. They found that patients in all of the eating disorder subtypes (in aggregate) perceived their families as less adaptive and cohesive than did control subjects, but there were no differences among subtypes.

Taken together, the findings from daughters' perceptions of their family relationships suggest that families of both anorectic patients and, especially, bulimic patients are more disturbed than are families where there is no eating disorder and, according to five of the six comparative studies, that there may be more severe or pervasive deficits experienced by bulimic patients than by classic restricting anorectic patients. More specifically, bulimic patients with and without anorexia nervosa perceive their families as more neglectful, rejecting, blaming, and conflictual and as less cohesive, expressive, caring, involved, adaptive, empathic, nurturant, and communicative and as less able to share activities. Although they did so less often than their bulimic counterparts, restricting anorectic patients did differ from control subjects in perceiving their mothers as less caring (Palmer et al. 1988) and their families as more unhealthy (Waller et al. 1989), blaming, neglectful, and rejecting (Humphrey 1986) and as less adaptive and cohesive. Let us now examine how convergent or divergent the daughters' perceptions are relative to their parents' perceptions.

Parents' and Daughters' Perceptions

In assessing family relationships, it seems critical to incorporate more members than just the daughter in distress. It is conceivable that the patients themselves have a unique perspective because of their disorder, or that some members more than others would have a tendency either to minimize or exaggerate the nature and severity of such problems. There have been about six such multiperspective studies on the perceived family relationships in anorexia nervosa and bulimia nervosa, virtually all of which have also contrasted the specific subtypes. Strober (1981) did the first of these studies and compared parents (only) of bulimic and restricting anorectic patients on the FES and the Short Marital Adjustment Test (Locke and Wallace 1959). He found that parents of bulimic anorectic children were more conflictual, disorganized, and dissatisfied with their marriages and were also less cohesive than were parents of the restricting counterparts.

Garfinkel et al. (1983), who also studied parents of anorectic children and compared them with controls, found no differences on a series of measures of personality and depression. However, utilizing the Family Assessment Measure, they did show that anorectic children and their mothers both viewed the family as having more problems with task accomplishment, role performance, communication, and affective expression than did families in which there was no member with an eating disorder. More recently, Stern et al. (1989) used the FES to compare patients with anorexia nervosa, bulimia nervosa with a history of anorexia nervosa, and pure bulimia nervosa (i.e., bulimia simplex), along with one parent each, with control subjects. Their results showed that although parents' ratings were generally more positive than were their daughters' ratings, they perceived the same deficits in family relationships that their daughters did. Generally, the restricting anorectic daughters and their parents experienced less expressiveness and active recreational orientation than did control subjects. The bulimic groups also reported less cohesion (both bulimic groups) and more conflict (bulimia nervosa with history of anorexia nervosa) and achievement expectations (bulimia simplex) as compared with the control group.

In a similar study based on a factor-analyzed version of the FACES, Kog et al. (1985) contrasted anorectic patients, bulimic patients, bulimic anorectic patients, patients with atypical eating disorders, and control subjects, and their parents, on the empirical factors of conflict, cohesion, and disorganization. Their results indicated that all of the patients with eating disorders reported greater conflict and disorganization than did the control group, and that only the bulimic anorectic patients scored higher on these two variables and lower on cohesion than did their restricting anorectic counterparts. There were no other differences among subtypes. They further reported that the overall differences between families of patients with eating disorders and control families were replicated during the adolescent years (ages 16–18), but not during the puberty (ages 12–15) or launching (> age 18) phases.

A study from our lab (L. L. Humphrey and R. E. Villejo, unpublished manuscript, August 1992) also compared patients in these subgroups of eating disorders and their parents on factor-analyzed versions of both the FACES and the FES, with consistent results. We found that fathers, mothers, and daughters from all three anorectic and bulimic subtypes (restricting anorectic, bulimic anorectic, and bulimic) concurred that their families were less expressively cohesive and more chaotically disengaged than were the control families. These findings were most consistent and robust for the families of bulimic anorectic patients, who also experienced less idyllic involvement and less flexible independence in their mutual relationships. As in most prior studies, the restricting anorectic patients were most distinct among the eating disorders groups, and this seems attributable largely to their more positive reports of family life. In fact, the anorectic children themselves reported no family distress except on the variable of chaotic disengagement, unlike their parents or bulimic peers.

In a related study based on the SASB questionnaires (Humphrey 1988), the findings for families of children with different subtypes of eating disorders were similar. Families with a bulimic anorectic child or a bulimic child were generally more like one another than they were like families of restricting anorectic children. Families with a bulimic anorectic child or with a bulimic child experienced more mutual blaming, rejection, and neglect toward each other, and less understanding, nurturance, and support than did control families. These two subtypes also differed from one another in two important respects as well. The mothers of bulimic children blamed their daughters for the problems between them and, unlike their daughters, denied that they contributed in any way themselves. This was not true for the mothers of bulimic anorectic children, who agreed with their daughters that both of them participated in the struggle. Similarly, both parents of bulimic children denied that there were any problems in their marriages, whereas the parents of bulimic anorectic children agreed that the husbands were more hostile on a number of dimensions than did the parents in the control families. In contrast to both bulimic children and bulimic anorectic children, restricting anorectic children and their parents were much more positive about their relationships and were similar to control subjects. The greatest source of subjective distress in these families came from mothers' and daughters' perceptions of the fathers. Both saw the fathers as more sulky, withdrawn, and avoidant relative to how the mothers and daughters in the control group perceived their fathers.

To summarize the findings based on daughters' and parents' perceptions of family relationships among subtypes of eating disorders, generally the three subgroups converge in their perspectives and the bulimic subtype and bulimic anorectic subtype are more similar to one another and less like the restricting anorectic subtype. One interesting exception to the finding that daughters, mothers, and fathers concur is that two studies (Garfinkel et al. 1983; Humphrey 1988) showed restricting anorectic children and their mothers to agree in their descriptions of the family, or at least of the father, as being more disturbed than did the children and their mothers in the control families, whereas fathers denied any such problems. Perhaps this reflects the kind of covert alliance that Minuchin et al. (1978) observed in triangulation of the anorectic child with one parent against the other, or a greater degree of denial overall in these families.

In terms of differences among subtypes, the bulimic and bulimic anorectic patients and their parents characterized their families as less understanding, affectionate, supportive, cohesive, expressive, idyllically involved, flexibly independent, and actively engaged in shared recreation, as well as more blaming, rejecting, neglectful, conflictual, disorganized, achievement oriented, dissatisfied with the marriage, and chaotically disengaged than did the restricting anorectic patients and their families. Parents and their restricting anorectic daughters were gen erally more positive about their relationships than bulimic children, but did sometimes report greater conflict, disorganization, disengagement, and sulking and withdrawing by fathers (mothers' and daughters' views only), along with less expressiveness and active involvement in recreational activities relative to control families. Overall, there is consistent evidence that families of individuals with eating disorders, especially families of bulimic children, do experience significant distress along a number of theoretically relevant dimensions and that there is a good degree of convergence in their perceptions. How their subjective reports compare with more objective, behavioral observations is considered next.

Behavioral Observations

Not surprisingly, there have only been a few experimental studies of observed interactions within families of anorectic or bulimic children. Such studies are very challenging, time consuming, and expensive to implement. Only very recently have the observational methodologies even become relevant and available within the field in general. I review both the methods themselves and the outcomes they produce as described in the existing literature on family interactions in eating disorders.

Kog and Vandereycken (1989) developed their own methodology to operationalize and study family perceptions and interactions in subtypes of eating disorders. They utilized their factor-analyzed version of the FACES and two semistructured tasks, jointly, to measure Minuchin et al.'s (1978) constructs of enmeshment, rigidity, overprotectiveness, and poor conflict resolution. The behavioral tasks involved either consensual decision making or conflict resolution and were scored for outcome using a unidimensional scale for each of the resulting variables: cohesion, adaptability, and conflict. They did not include ongoing behavioral observations of the nature and quality of the families' interpersonal communications as they discussed the issues. Their results showed that families of anorectic, bulimic anorectic, and bulimic children all had fewer disagreements between parents and children, and more rigidity in who joined with whom, than did families in which there was no eating disorder. They interpreted this as partial support for Minuchin et al.'s theory.

In a more process-oriented vein, a series of three studies have been based on Brown et al.'s (1972) construct of expressed emotion—that is, criticism and emotional overinvolvement—which was originally formulated for families with a schizophrenic member. First, Goldstein (1981) utilized verbatim transcripts of parental responses to the Thematic Apperception Test (Murray 1943) and videotaped interactions of families with anorectic patients and families of general psychiatric patients during a problem-solving task. Trained observers rated communication deviance (ambiguous or illogical statements), negative affective style (critical, intrusive, or guilt-inducing statements), and dependency insecurity in the family interactions and parental interviews. Families of anorectic patients differed from control families in the degree of dependency insecurity (solicitation of support and protection, tentativeness of response, and compliancy) as represented by a single score. In addition, whereas families of preschizophrenic patients showed greater frequencies of communication deviance and negative affective style, families of anorectic patients did not.

In a subsequent study, Szmukler et al. (1985) also investigated expressed emotion among parents of anorectic and bulimic inpatients. Observations were coded based on audiotapes of individual parent responses to the Camberwell Family Interview (Vaughn and Leff 1976). They found that both mothers and fathers of bulimic patients used a greater number of critical comments toward their daughters than did parents of the anorectic patients. Fathers of bulimic children were also more overinvolved emotionally, and the two factors together were associated with premature termination of treatment.

A more recent study by this group (Szmukler et al. 1987) compared findings from the individual parent interviews with those from videotaped interactions of a picnic lunch with 20 families of anorectic patients. The findings revealed that, of the four scales used, critical comments were highly correlated between the two settings, emotional overinvolvement showed a modest correlation, warmth was highly correlated for mothers only, and the number of positive comments was unrelated across the individual parent and family interviews. These findings suggest that the variables involved in measuring expressed emotion may well be influenced by the situation in which they are assessed, thus potentially undermining the validity of the construct itself, or at least a portion of it.

There is only one observational coding schema used in this area that truly captures the moment-to-moment, ongoing interpersonal process in these families (Humphrey 1987, 1989; Humphrey et al. 1986). It is based on Benjamin's (1974) model of SASB (Structural Analysis of Social Behavior) and also affords a multimethod assessment of self-ratings and others' ratings along with the observational system. The model and its applications are so rich that it deserves our attention here briefly.

The SASB is a circumplex model of interpersonal relationships and their intrapsychic representations. It consists of three circumplex surfaces, each of which corresponds to a different focus of attention: 1) focus on other *(top)*, 2) focus on self *(middle)*, and 3) intrapsychic *(bottom)*. Each surface or focus of the model comprises the same two primary, orthogonal dimensions of affiliation *(horizontal axis)* and interdependence *(vertical axis)*. Affiliation extends from attack on the left-hand side to attachment on the right. Interdependence ranges from freedom at the top to control or submission at the bottom. The cluster version of the model is depicted in Figure 13–1. It is intermediate in its degree of complexity and is the basis of the observational coding system. Individual points and clusters on one surface of the model have corresponding or complementary points on the other two surfaces.

Trained observers use the 24 cluster points of the model to describe ongoing interactions. Coders rate both the content (i.e., what is being talked about) and the process (all of the interpersonal nuances that color the transaction) of every interaction. Cluster codes can be used either singly or in combination to capture the sometimes complex and confusing interpersonal messages exchanged by family members. The system has broad-reaching applications and has been used to study psychotherapy process (Henry et al. 1986) as well as family interactions in schizophrenia (Humphrey and Benjamin 1986), eating disorders, and chemical dependence (D. L. Humes and L. L. Humphrey, unpublished manuscript, August 1992).

To illustrate the versatility and clinical richness of the SASB, consider how it would characterize a bulimic daughter's ambivalence about separation. One daughter in the clinic said to her parents about going away to college, "I can take care of myself," in a whiny, pleading tone of voice. In content, her statement would be coded as intrapsychic, cluster 4, self-nourishing and enhancing. However, in process, she is expressing her ambivalence between asserting and separating (self-1) by asserting her own opinion, and sulking and scurrying (self-6) in her defensive, reactive tone of voice and interpersonal stance. Three distinct codes were needed to capture fully the interpersonal meaning of her statement. Clearly, no other coding schema has this degree of richness and precision. Interestingly, a study by Hubschmid and Zemp (1989) showed that there were solid correlations between certain aspects of the expressed emotion construct and specific clusters from the SASB model, when applied to families with a schizophrenic member.

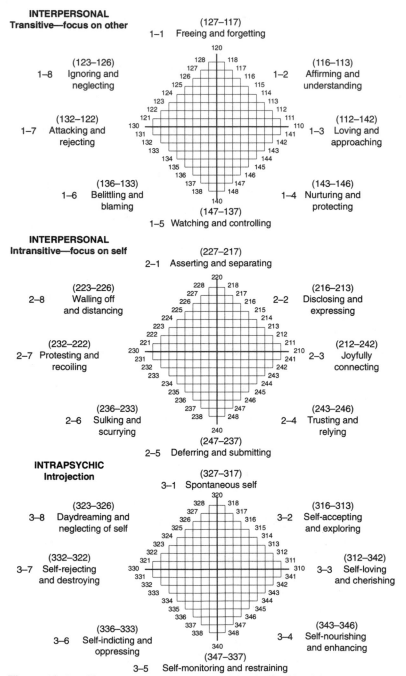

Figure 13–1. Cluster version of Structural Analysis of Social Behavior.
Copyright 1986, Lorna Smith Benjamin. Used with permission.

In our laboratory, we have used the SASB observational coding system and rating scales to assess family relationships and interaction patterns among subtypes of eating disorders. Fathers, mothers, and daughters are asked to discuss an aspect of the daughter's separation from the family, and these 10-minute transactions are videotaped for later coding. In the first such studies, we compared observational codes from the SASB system with those from another well-respected schema based on a more behavioral approach (Humphrey et al. 1986)—the Marital Interaction Coding Schema (Robin and Weiss 1980)—for families of bulimic anorectic children and for control families. The findings showed that the two systems were equally successful at predicting group status, and they jointly accounted for 50% of the total variance. Three variables from the SASB differentiated between the groups, including helping and trusting on the positive side, and ignoring and walling off and complex, contradictory communications on the negative side. Similarly, the Marital Interaction Coding Schema also discriminated between the bulimic anorectic families and the families of children without an eating disorder on the basis of positive and negative interpersonal messages.

A subsequent study (Humphrey 1989) compared the observed family interaction patterns among anorectic, bulimic anorectic, and bulimic triads and triads of families without an eating disorder, using the SASB approach. Parallel to the results from the rating scales, the parents of both the bulimic and the bulimic anorectic children were more hostile and controlling toward their daughters and less supportive and trusting than were families of children without an eating disorder. Bulimic daughters, in turn, were also more hostile and less trusting and approaching toward their parents. In families with an anorectic child, a different pattern emerged. The parents of anorectic children were both more affectionate and also more neglectful (both parents) and controlling (fathers only) relative to families of children without an eating disorder and families with a bulimic child. Their anorectic daughters were more submissive than daughters in any other group and were also less trusting and approaching than were teens without an eating disorder.

In addition, all three groups of families with eating disorders used more complex, confusing communications with one another than did the families of children without an eating disorder, and there were specific combinations of clusters for anorectic versus bulimic subtypes. Fathers of restricting anorectic daughters combined pseudoaffection and control (i.e., loving and controlling) and pseudohelp and negation (i.e., nurturing and ignoring) when speaking to their daughters. The anorectic daughters reacted with a predictably ambivalent response. They juxtaposed pseudo-self-disclosure with submission. On the other hand, fathers of bulimic daughters combined pseudounderstanding with taking control of their daughters (i.e., understanding and controlling); the bulimic daughters, in turn, responded with ambivalent self-assertion and sulky resentment.

These findings suggest that families of bulimic children are enmeshed in a hostile, rigid interaction pattern combining issues of attachment and autonomy. Families of anorectic children are not so overtly hostile and, instead, communicate a mixed message of loving affection with control or negation of the daughters' needs to separate. This pattern in families of anorectic children may help to explain why they do not consistently perceive their relationships as negative. They may be attending consciously only to the positive side of the message and denying the enmeshment and neglect of the daughter's separate self. The negative aspect of the interactions may be what is internalized and turned against the self, leaving only a false representation of self on the outside.

In a recent study, we used essentially the same research paradigm to study family relationships and interaction patterns in families with a daughter being treated for polydrug dependence (D. L. Humes and L. L. Humphrey, unpublished manuscript, August 1992). Although we have not yet been able to compare this population directly with anorectic patients and bulimic patients as we plan to, comparisons with control subjects prove interesting and distinctive. Specifically, parents of substance-abusing teens were both more hostile and more affirming toward their daughters than were control parents. They also used more mixed messages containing a hostile element. Surprisingly, the drug-abusing daughters themselves did not differ from teens without an eating disorder on any SASB cluster, unlike their anorectic and bulimic counterparts.

Still, the most compelling results emerged by comparing the observational ratings to the perceptions of the family members themselves. Whereas observers found the parents of the chemically dependent daughter to be more blaming, affirming, and contradictory in their interactions, the parents perceived themselves just as the parents of the control subjects did. Instead, the parents experienced the daughters as being the source of hostility and turmoil in the family, whereas the observers saw them as "normal." These results suggest to us that there may be some unconscious projective process operating in the families of drug-abusing children, in which the child is experienced as an extension of the "bad" parts of the parent. The findings from this study also highlight the ability of the SASB to capture complex and unique clinical phenomena among different populations as well as the value of a multimethod approach.

In aggregate, the results of the observational studies of families with eating disorders are consistent with daughters' and parents' perceptions. These mothers, fathers, and daughters generally agree that they are very dissatisfied and distressed, whereas control families are not. Bulimic and bulimic anorectic subtypes are also distinguished from the restricting anorectic subtype. Overall, the observational findings suggest that families of bulimic and bulimic anorectic daughters are more critical, rigid, emotionally overinvolved, blaming, pseudounderstanding, controlling, and ambivalent and antagonistically enmeshed in separation, as well as less supportive and trusting than are families of children without an eating disorder and families of anorectic children. In contrast, families with anorectic daughters are more dependent and insecure, rigid, pseudoaffectionate, pseudohelpful, pseudodisclosing, negating, and submissive and also less trusting than are families of children without an eating disorder and families of bulimic children.

There have also been two studies that suggest that interactions in families of anorectic children may be different from interactions in families of preschizophrenic children (Goldstein 1981) and that both families of anorectic children and families of bulimic children may be unique relative to families of polydrug-dependent adolescents (D. L. Humes and L. L. Humphrey, unpublished manuscript, August 1992). In addition, findings from the observational methods have been less equivocal than self-ratings in establishing that families of restricting anorectic children are actually disturbed. They also help to explain why self-ratings alone cannot capture the essence of the anorectic pathology because of the extent of anorectic patients' denial and idealization.

Implications and Recommendations

Given the current status of family research, how much do we really know about the contribution of disturbed family relationships and interactions to the development and maintenance of eating disorders? It is well established at this point that families of anorectic children, bulimic anorectic children, and bulimic children are not "normal." They show distinct and disturbed patterns of relationships, both through their perceptions and behavioral observations of their actual interactions. As clinical theory would predict (e.g., Humphrey and Stern 1988; Johnson and Connors 1987; Root et al. 1986), families of bulimic children and bulimic anorectic children are more similar to one another, and more consistent across methods, in their degree of hostility, chaos, and feelings of isolation, as well as in substantial deficits in nurturance and empathy. Families of children in these two subgroups also tend to experience greater subjective distress and behave toward one another in ways that are consistent with their perceptions—with one exception. The mothers of normal-weight bulimic children see their daughters' treatment of them as the only problem in the family; they fail to perceive their own contribution to the turmoil between them (which is considerable according to the observational data).

The families of restricting anorectic children appear to be quite different from their bulimic counterparts on a number of dimensions. Families of anorectic children less consistently experience or report much subjective dissatisfaction with the ways in which their families operate. There are a few exceptions to this pattern (e.g., Garfinkel et al. 1983; Humphrey 1989), but overall these families present themselves as being less unhappy and less poorly adjusted on self-ratings. Given the discrepancy with behavioral observations, in which they are seen as actually quite disturbed, the results based on self-reports alone would seem to reflect their phenomenology of denial and idealization, which have been considered a hallmark of anorexia nervosa in the clinical and theoretical literatures (e.g., Minuchin et al. 1978; Palazzoli 1978).

Findings from the observational studies suggest an interactional mechanism through which these complex relationships might occur. Parents of anorectic daughters communicate a mixed message of antithetical meanings. They are extremely affectionate, more so than even families of children without an eating disorder, at the same time as they control the daughter and negate her separateness (Humphrey 1989). It may be that the parents and daughter alike collude in attending consciously only to their mutual attachment and warmth, while denying or disavowing the more enmeshing and squelching aspects of their relationships. This would explain how the daughter becomes so entrapped in the family circle and fails to emerge with a truly individuated sense of herself.

Beyond these differences among subtypes of eating disorders, two preliminary studies suggest that such family processes could be unique to anorexia nervosa and bulimia nervosa per se. Families of preschizophrenic adolescents (Goldstein 1981) and polydrug-dependent adolescents

(D. L. Humes and L. L. Humphrey, unpublished manuscript, August 1992) do appear to relate to one another differently from families of bulimic patients and, especially, anorectic patients. These differences could be pathognomonic of each disorder and would be important to the field's broader understanding of the nature and mechanisms of familial contributions to psychopathology.

In light of the fact that the first controlled studies of family relationships were published little more than 10 years ago (Goldstein 1981; Strober 1981), there has been substantial progress in that time. However, we do need to address certain methodological limitations if we are to continue to move beyond our current level of knowledge. The vast majority of existing family research is based on self-report data alone, most often only from daughters' perspectives, using some version of the FES or the FACES. Given the potential distortions possible with self-report measures, and the discrepancies already established between self-ratings and behavioral observations for certain subgroups, it seems imperative for future researchers to at least include the parents in such studies. It would be much stronger still, of course, to use exclusively multimethod assessments including behavioral observations. This would enable us to examine the full phenomenology of parent-child and parent-parent relationships from both subjective and objective perspectives. Discrepancies across methods could even help us to operationalize subtle and complex clinical phenomena like projective identification in families.

In addition to multimethod assessments, we would also benefit from observational systems that incorporate both positive, "healthy" dimensions as well as negative, unhealthy ones. It is conceivable that certain clinical groups have "too much of a good thing"—such as the way that the parents of anorectic children seem to use excessive affection to keep their daughter dependent and undifferentiated. Observational measures are best when they provide microscopic, moment-to-moment descriptions of process in ongoing interactions. This seems much more precise and informative than schemata that afford only global frequencies of a few dimensions. Measuring elusive and complex constructs that are often at the heart of clinical theory will require that we move beyond global ratings of cohesion or adaptability in favor of more versatile and sophisticated methods.

Benjamin's SASB model and multimethod approach to assessment have already proven invaluable in capturing some of the complex, elusive, and "pseudo"-interpersonal processes operating in families of patients with eating disorders (e.g., Humphrey 1988, 1989). They seem well suited to the challenging task of measuring the mechanisms of separation, enmeshment, denial, projective identification, idealization, and power dispersion and even more purely systemic concepts like triangulation or detouring, which remain at the heart of our theoretical conceptualizations. Another advantage of the SASB's own structure is how it defines the nature of the relationship between autonomy and attachment as distinct elements that can either remain orthogonal or become blended in family relationships. Given our emphasis on both dimensions in eating disorders, this would be an important advantage in this field.

Another benefit that is implicit in the SASB model itself is its explicit linkage between interpersonal and intrapsychic processes. If we are to understand how anorectic and bulimic persons come to hate themselves and their bodies, we must be able to examine the connections between their family relationships and their self-representations (Sugarman 1991). The connections between family interaction patterns and intrapsychic experiences have never been investigated directly, but this would be quite feasible with the SASB multimethod approach.

It is also possible with SASB observations to examine these complex transactions sequentially, using probability statistics like Markov chains (Isaacson and Madsen 1976). For example, in an earlier study we compared parents of bulimic anorectic children and of children without an eating disorder on their moment-to-moment responses to their daughters' efforts to separate through self-assertions (Humphrey 1987). We found that especially mothers of the bulimic anorectic children responded to their daughters' self-assertive statements by moving to positions of control, whereas mothers of children who did not have an eating disorder responded with much less rigidity and squelching of their daughters. This kind of sequential approach to analyzing observed interactions between family members seems quite promising for testing our richly elaborate but elusive theories.

Beyond issues of measurement, future research will also progress more fruitfully if we incorporate some further methodological improvements. We need to establish whether the existing patterns of family distress are, in fact, specific etiologically to these disorders and not just secondary to the profound disruption of having a sick child. It would be very instructive, for example, to know whether the patterns we see are also found in families of medically ill children or of children with other related psychiatric problems (e.g., depression and drug abuse). It would also be important to know whether such patterns can be ameliorated with treatment of and improvement in the eating pathology itself. Although it would be a daunting challenge, it would be extremely convincing if we could establish that the observed patterns exist in families of pre-anorectic and pre-bulimic children, even before the clinical syndrome emerged. These populations are relatively accessible in this regard because we do know the likely ages at onset of eating disorders as well as certain predisposing factors (e.g., Garfinkel and Garner 1982; Johnson and Connors 1987).

Ultimately, it will be necessary to put the familial contributions to anorexia nervosa and bulimia nervosa in perspective, relative to other psychological, biological, and sociocultural factors. Clearly, they do seem important, but how do they compare with, and interact with, these elements—the potential impact of which has also been documented empirically? Do family relationships account for a significant proportion of the total variance in eating disorders, relative to a propensity toward depression or alcoholism, or a vulnerability toward dieting and an overemphasis on appearances? Some models do exist, both in eating disorders (Johnson and Connors 1987; Strober 1991; Williamson et al. 1989) and in other areas like depression (e.g., Keitner and Miller 1990), for explicating the reciprocal influences of these multifactorial contributions.

Multidimensional models by Johnson and Connors (1987) and Williamson et al. (1989) incorporate family factors as one of several types of interpersonal stressors that may initiate or exacerbate an episode of disturbed eating. According to their views, long-standing, deficient family relationships may either make a young person more vulnerable overall to experiences of dysregulation and poor self-concept or they may exert a more ongoing, moment-to-moment negative influence on the patient's capacity to modulate affect, behavior, and self-esteem.

Strober (1991) recently applied an organismic developmental approach to the conceptualization of anorexia nervosa and bulimia nervosa. His model emphasizes the complex interplay among environmental factors (particularly family relationships) and level of physiological activation, degree of harm avoidance, and reward dependence in the development and resilience of the self in patients with eating disorders. Most current models of anorexia nervosa and bulimia nervosa propose that these disorders are multidetermined and that family relationships and interactions play a significant role in their development and amelioration (Strober and Humphrey 1987). Whatever the mechanisms of transmission and reciprocal influence, future knowledge will progress only if we begin to test these interactive models directly and incorporate sophisticated and comprehensive assessments of family processes.

References

Benjamin LS: Structural analysis of social behavior. Psychol Rev 81:392–425, 1974

Brown GW, Birley JL, Wing JK: Influence of family life on the course of schizophrenic disorders: a replication. Br J Psychiatry 121:241–258, 1972

Epstein NB, Baldwin LM, Bishop DS: The McMaster Family Assessment Device. Journal of Marital and Family Therapy 9:171–180, 1983

Garfinkel PE, Garner DM: Anorexia Nervosa: A Multidimensional Perspective. New York, Brunner/Mazel, 1982

Garfinkel PE, Garner DM, Rose J, et al: A comparison of characteristics in families of patients with anorexia nervosa and normal controls. Psychol Med 13:821–828, 1983

Garner DM, Garfinkel PE, O'Shaughnessy M: The validity of the distinction between bulimia with and without anorexia nervosa. Am J Psychiatry 142:581–587, 1985

Goldstein MJ: Family factors associated with schizophrenia and anorexia nervosa. Journal of Youth and Adolescence 10:385–405, 1981

Henry WP, Schacht TE, Strupp HH: Structural analysis of social behavior: application to a study of interpersonal process in differential psychotherapeutic outcome. J Consult Clin Psychol 54:27–31, 1986

Hubschmid T, Zemp M: Interactions in high and low-EE families. Soc Psychiatry Psychiatr Epidemiol 24:113–119, 1989

Humphrey LL: Structural analysis of parent-child relationships in eating disorders. J Abnorm Psychol 95:395–402, 1986

Humphrey LL: A comparison of bulimic-anorexic and nondistressed families using structural analysis of social behavior. J Am Acad Child Adolesc Psychiatry 26:248–255, 1987

Humphrey LL: Relationships within subtypes of anorectic, bulimic, and normal families. J Am Acad Child Adolesc Psychiatry 27:544–551, 1988

Humphrey LL: Observed family interactions among subtypes of eating disorders using structural analysis of social behavior. J Consult Clin Psychol 57:206–214, 1989

Humphrey LL: Object relations and the family system: an integrative approach to understanding and treating eating disorders, in Psychodynamic Treatment of Anorexia Nervosa and Bulimia. Edited by Johnson C. New York, Guilford, 1991, pp 321–353

Humphrey LL, Benjamin LS: Using structural analysis of social behavior to assess critical but elusive family process. Am Psychol 41:979–989, 1986

Humphrey LL, Stern S: Object relations and the family system in bulimia: a theoretical integration. Journal of Marital and Family Therapy 14:337–350, 1988

Humphrey LL, Apple RF, Kirschenbaum DS: Differentiating bulimic-anorectic from normal families using interpersonal and behavioral observational systems. J Consult Clin Psychol 54:190–195, 1986

Isaacson DL, Madsen RW: Markov Chains Theory and Practice. New York, Wiley, 1976

Johnson C, Connors ME: The Etiology and Treatment of Bulimia Nervosa: A Biopsychosocial Perspective. New York, Basic Books, 1987

Johnson C, Flach A: Family characteristics of 105 patients with bulimia. Am J Psychiatry 142:1321–1324, 1985

Keitner GI, Miller IW: Family functioning in depression: an overview. Am J Psychiatry 147:1128–1137, 1990

Kog E, Vandereycken W: Family interaction in eating disordered patients and normal controls. International Journal of Eating Disorders 8:11–23, 1989

Kog E, Vertommen H, Degroote T: Family interaction research in anorexia nervosa: the use and misuse of a self-report questionnaire. International Journal of Family Psychiatry 6:227–243, 1985

Locke HJ, Wallace KM: Short marital adjustment and prediction tests: their reliability and validity. Marriage and Family Living 21:251–255, 1959

Minuchin S, Rosman BL, Baker L: Psychosomatic Families: Anorexia Nervosa in Context. Cambridge, MA, Harvard University Press, 1978

Moos R, Moos B: Family Environment Scale. Palo Alto, CA, Consulting Psychologists Press, 1980

Murray HA: The Thematic Apperception Test. Cambridge, MA, Harvard University Press, 1943

Olson DH, Bell R, Portner J: Family Adaptability and Cohesion Evaluation Scale. St. Paul, MN, Family Social Science Press, 1978

Olson DH, McCubbin HI, Barnes H, et al: Family Inventories. St. Paul, MN, Family Social Science Press, 1982

Ordman AM, Kirschenbaum DS: Bulimia: assessment of eating, psychological adjustment, and familial characteristics. International Journal of Eating Disorders 5:865–878, 1986

Palazzoli M: Self-Starvation: From Individual to Family Therapy in the Treatment of Anorexia Nervosa. New York, Jason Aronson, 1978

Palmer RL, Oppenheimer R, Marshall PD: Eating-disordered patients remember their parents: a study using the parental-bonding instrument. International Journal of Eating Disorders 7:101–106, 1988

Parker G, Tupling H, Brown LB: A parental bonding instrument. Br J Clin Psychol 52:1–10, 1979

Pole R, Waller DA, Stewart SM, et al: Parental caring vs. over-protection in bulimia. International Journal of Eating Disorders 7:601–606, 1988

Roberto LG: Bulimia: the transgenerational view. Journal of Marital and Family Therapy 12:231–240, 1986

Robin AL, Weiss JG: Criterion-related validity of behavioral and self-report measures of problem solving communication in distressed and nondistressed parent-adolescent dyads. Behavioral Assessment 2:339–352, 1980

Root MP, Fallon P, Friedrich WN: Bulimia: A Systems Approach to Treatment. New York, WW Norton, 1986

Schwartz RC, Barrett MJ, Saba G: Family therapy for bulimia, in Handbook of Psychotherapy for Anorexia Nervosa and Bulimia. Edited by Garner DM, Garfinkel PE. New York, Guilford, 1985

Skinner HA, Steinhauer PD, Santa-Barbara J: The Family Assessment Measure. Canadian Journal of Mental Health 2:91–105, 1983

Stern SL, Dixon KN, Jones D, et al: Family environment in anorexia nervosa and bulimia. International Journal of Eating Disorders 8:25–31, 1989

Strober M: The significance of bulimia in juvenile anorexia nervosa: an exploration of possible etiologic factors. International Journal of Eating Disorders 1:28–43, 1981

Strober M: Disorders of the self in anorexia nervosa: an organismic-developmental paradigm, in Psychodynamic Treatment of Anorexia Nervosa and Bulimia. Edited by Johnson C. New York, Guilford, 1991, pp 354–373

Strober M, Humphrey LL: Familial contributions to the etiology and course of anorexia nervosa and bulimia. J Consult Clin Psychol 55:654–659, 1987

Sugarman A: Bulimia: a displacement from psychological self to body self, in Psychodynamic Treatment of Anorexia Nervosa and Bulimia. Edited by Johnson C. New York, Guilford, 1991, pp 3–33

Szmukler GI, Eisler I, Russell GFM, et al: Anorexia nervosa, "parental expressed emotion" and dropping out of treatment. Br J Psychiatry 147:265–271, 1985

Szmukler GI, Berkowitz R, Eisler I, et al: Expressed emotion in individual and family settings: a comparative study. Br J Psychiatry 151:174–178, 1987

Vaughn CE, Leff JP: The influence of family and social factors on the course of psychiatric illness: a comparison of schizophrenic and neurotic patients. Br J Psychiatry 129:125–137, 1976

Waller G, Calam R, Slade P: Eating disorders and family interaction. Br J Clin Psychol 28:285–286, 1989

Waller G, Slade P, Calam R: Family adaptability and cohesion: relation to eating attitudes and disorders. International Journal of Eating Disorders 9:225–228, 1990

Williamson DA, Prather RC, Goreczney AJ, et al: A comprehensive model of bulimia nervosa: empirical evaluation, in Advances in Eating Disorders. Edited by Johnson WG. Greenwich, CT, JAI Press, 1989, pp 137–156

Winnicott DW: The Maturational Processes and the Facilitating Environment. New York, International Universities Press, 1965

Section VI

Treatment Studies

Chapter 14

Integration of Psychodynamic Concepts Into Psychotherapy

Regina C. Casper, M.D.

————————⟫●⟪————————

Both anorexia nervosa and bulimia nervosa form discrete
clinical disorders that are seri-
ous and protracted in their course and difficult to treat. The fairly homogeneous behavioral and somatic picture conceals a Pandora's box of
psychological manifestations that elude easy classification.

Observations and case studies (Bell 1985; Janet 1903; Morton 1694)
furnished the earliest psychological data base. As nosological theories
began to be formulated, theoretical concepts began to be applied to explain the psychological manifestations in anorexia nervosa (Benedek
1936; Bruch 1962; Freud 1954; Selvini-Palazzoli 1978). Comparatively little was published on bulimia nervosa (Ziolko and Schrader 1985) because the disorder was only recently classified as a diagnostic entity. When
treatment strategies became more effective and as the patients' participa-
tion in the treatment process improved, knowledge about different personal motives and conflicts increased. Yet even today, generalizations
about the psychodynamics derive from case observations and not from
hypothesis testing in well-defined patient samples.

Since no science of the mind comparable to physical science has been
devised that uses a common language and shares a framework for relating
complex psychological mechanisms, an attempt is made to use plain English and to avoid as much as possible technical terms associated with

particular psychological theories or concepts.

Throughout the centuries, there has been speculation about the meaning, the motivation, and the function of the puzzling symptoms we encounter in anorexia nervosa, with early recognition that a deliberate personal element plays a role. In this chapter I review some historical psychological concepts that have proven innovative and creative (Tables 14–1 and 14–2). Unfortunately, the sheer volume of this literature precludes mentioning all worthwhile contributions.

Following this review, I present some thoughts about one particular psychodynamic frequently observed in contemporary anorexia nervosa: the interactions between the patient and food and/or her body, which gradually evolve in the course of the psychological and physiological regression induced by the weight loss. This psychological constellation can typically be observed in contemporary adolescent patients with severe anorexia nervosa and even more so in patients with chronic anorexia nervosa. This self-body relationship is so unusual that one cannot help wondering whether the patient may not be reenacting and trying to master certain traumatic aspects of her past interpersonal experiences. Aside from willfulness, complicated psychological processes aided by organic defects seem to be at work. Neither are fully understood. Much of what is presented here is conjectural and requires confirmation in systematic studies.

The relationship between the psychic and somatic components of anorexia nervosa puzzles us on many accounts. Is it an emotional disease or a somatic disease? Is it principally a psychosomatic or somatopsychic disorder? How is the somatic process different from starvation? Is the emotional reaction different from social withdrawal or grief as a result of trauma or loss?

Table 14–1. Historical cases

Study	Concepts
Bell 1985, 13th–14th century	Personal motivation
	Sense of self-determination
	Resistance to eating
Morton 1694	Asceticism
Janet 1903	Shame or loathing of the body
Gull 1874	Morbid mental state
Lasègue 1873	Intellectual perversion
Freud 1954	Pubertal form of melancholia

Table 14–2.   Cases in the 20th century

Study	Concepts
Benedek 1936	Ego-syntonic dominant idea
Bruch 1962	Body image distortion
Bruch 1973	Perceptual deficits
Bruch 1980	Developmental deficits in self-awareness and initiative
Minuchin et al. 1975	Pathological family interactions
Selvini-Palazzoli 1978	Body takes on characteristics of the bad experiences with the mother
Crisp 1980	Defense against demands of puberty
Casper 1983	Cognitive overcontrol versus emotional dyscontrol
Goodsitt 1984	Disruption of the self
Strober 1990	Defective sense of self

There is evidence that the nature of the individual psychodynamics and the psychological disturbance influence the prognosis and outcome of eating disorders.

Psychodynamics in Anorexia Nervosa

Anorexia nervosa has been recognized as a fairly uniform clinical entity for centuries. The earliest descriptions of anorexia nervosa acknowledged the contribution of mental forces and the contribution of personal motivation. For instance, the Italian women saints in the 13th century studied by Bell (1985) developed anorexia nervosa as a result of religious fasting; all pursued their fasting regimen with willful determination. They refused to resume eating, even when admonished by their father confessors. The initial abstinence often served as personal sacrifice to attain higher spiritual goals, but religious beliefs seem to have been intermingled with other intentions since some of the young women fasted excessively to become unattractive and to avoid marriage for the purpose of devoting their lives to God.

The first of Morton's (1694) two cases, an 18-year-old girl, fell into a total suppression of her "monthly courses" from a "multitude of cares and passions of her mind." Since her appetite diminished, how do we know she did not suffer from a depression? Morton related that "she was wont by her studying at night and continued poring upon books to expose herself both day and night to the injuries of the air" (it was winter in England). This kind of asceticism as deliberate activity is uncommon in depression. In Janet's (1903) case of Nadine, an obsession of personal malcontent eventually extended to the body. This "l'obsession de la honte du corps"—obsessional shame and loathing for the feminine body—was traced by Janet to Nadine's fear of getting fat since she was age 4, when she was told by her parents that she was big for her age. Since Nadine fought intense hunger feelings and occasionally devoured sweets and, as Janet noted, since she did not become overactive in distinction to true hysterical anorexia, we would probably classify her today under the bulimic subtype of anorexia nervosa.

Freud (1954) mistakenly assumed true loss of appetite in anorexia nervosa. He considered anorexia nervosa an eating neurosis, a pubertal form of melancholia, and implicated sexual immaturity in its etiology. Gull (1874) referred to a "perversion of the ego," although Gull too assumed a "want of appetite," which he believed to be due to a "morbid mental state." Lasègue (1873) had little doubt about the psychological origin in hysterical anorexia when he called the patient's indifference to her emaciation an "intellectual perversion," aided he thought by unpleasant gastric physical sensations. Lasègue clearly noticed capriciousness; for example, one patient would not eat anything but a biscuit made by a particular Paris baker. Most early analytic writers followed Freud's lead and viewed food refusal as a means to mute unconscious oral or sexual wishes or conflicts or interpreted the refusal as a counterphobic measure to ward off wishes of oral impregnation (Waller et al. 1940).

Terese Benedek (1936), a psychoanalyst, proved to be an independent theoretician. She suggested from treating two patients that the forces driving the prohibition against food were crystallized in a new cognitive structure, akin to a dominant idea. One adolescent patient appeared obsessed with the conscious thought that she did not want to have a woman's body; another young woman appeared dominated by the idea not to become like her mother. These ideas preempted the patients' minds, but, unlike obsessive ideas, which are experienced as alien, these ideas were ego-syntonic and seemed to be an irremovable part of the ego. Benedek noted that, with the formation of these ideas, an alteration in the ego had taken place, which exerted a decisive influence on but one aspect of the patient's reality: eating and body size. Remarkably, in all other areas, these patients had no problems with reality testing. According to Benedek, these newly formed cognitive processes, considered inaccessible to reason and reality testing, represented a monosymptomatic psychosis.

Another analyst who decisively advanced our understanding of anorexia nervosa by describing the body-image distortion and other perceptual deficits was Hilde Bruch (1962, 1973). She refined her psycho-dynamic formulations over the years. She believed that serious developmental and perceptual defects in the ownership and control of the body contributed to the development of anorexia nervosa. Bruch (1980) later advanced an interpersonal theory, suggesting that in the early mother-child interaction, the child's needs and expression were not sufficiently encouraged, confirmed, and reinforced or that the mother's reaction to the child's cues were contradictory or inaccurate, which left the child feeling perplexed, ineffective, and helpless "under the influence of internal urges or external forces." These deficits in self-awareness and initiative became manifest only when the person was confronted with having to adapt to new situations, such as puberty or the prospect of adulthood, that required self-sufficiency and independence. The anorectic patient tried, Bruch believed, to compensate for this lack of inner structure and control by rigid discipline and control over her body size and food intake to attain a sense of structure and personal identity.

Selvini-Palazzoli (1978), who worked in Italy and was acquainted with Bruch's work, came to similar conclusions. Her concepts are formulated much more along classical psychoanalytic lines as she tried to link deficits in object relations to pathological body experiences. Selvini-Palazzoli argued that the infant's fundamental experiences are body experiences. In a comfortable relationship with the mother, the body will be a source of predominantly pleasurable sensations. In the case of a defective or disturbed emotional relationship, which presumably occurs in those disposed to anorexia nervosa, the body may feel alienated, imperfect, distressed, and out of control. In Selvini-Palazzoli's words, the bad aspects of the incorporated object (we would say the mother's handling of the child) become blended with the body experience; somehow the body takes on the characteristics of the bad object and is experienced as all powerful, threatening, growing, and indestructible. The memories of these experiences seem to remain more or less repressed until anorexia nervosa develops, and we might wonder whether the starvation process activates pathways to repression of these experiences, which are then acted out through the patient's behavior. Selvini-Palazzoli's formulation does address the clinical observation that the anorectic patient is not afraid of food intake per se but fears an instant increase in body size, which would be experienced as threatening.

Another contribution that has given some guidance to psychotherapeutic intervention takes the cognitive rigidity described by Benedek (1936) one step further. Garner and Bemis (1982) described the irrational ideas and beliefs of patients with anorexia nervosa; however, these authors deliberately avoided tracing these thoughts to personality variables or childhood experiences. Under the premise that a thin body is of utmost importance, the patient's thinking has adopted uncompromising features such as overgeneralization, all-or-none reasoning, and excessive use of personal assumptions, which the patient often knows to be arbitrary but is unwilling to concede. Garner and Bemis pointed to the similarities in the reasoning of depressive patients described by Beck et al. (1979).

With the ascent of self psychology (Kohut 1971), dynamic explanations have become rephrased in the language of self psychology. Goodsitt (1984) concerned himself with the disruption of the self in anorexia nervosa and viewed the symptoms as emergency measures against further disruption. Here again a developmental deficiency in self-regulation is thought to interfere in separation and individuation. The importance of self psychology lies less in its theoretical propositions, such as the different kinds of selfobject transferences (Wolf 1986), than in its opportunities for understanding the patient's communications through empathy instead of interpreting them functionally.

Strober (1990) similarly proposed that anorexia nervosa constitutes a disorder of the self; however, he brings research on early development, temperament, and personality traits into the equation, all seen as contributing to the quality of early experiences. Referring to the work on personality variables in anorexia nervosa (Casper 1990; Strober 1981), Strober (1990) suggested that particular traits, such as an extreme tendency toward harm avoidance, lowered reward dependence, and lowered novelty seeking, have colored the quality of early experiences and thus leave the future anorectic patient with a defective sense of self. This unpreparedness renders the adolescent girl vulnerable to the demands of puberty by reversing the physiological processes to a safe nonsexual self protected from social and sexual expectations. Ultimately, this view closely corresponds to Crisp's (1980) view that anorexia nervosa constitutes a defense against the maturational demands of adolescence.

In preadolescent young patients, fears of maturational changes of puberty and of sexuality not infrequently determine the food refusal leading to the weight loss and ultimately to anorexia nervosa. But rarely are sexual fears the only problem. In my experience, cases of anorexia nervosa in patients with maturity fears only are in the minority and are easy to reverse. The etiological importance attributed to sexual conflicts (Nemiah 1950) seems too simplistic when we see a hollow-faced, emaciated patient. Moreover, sexual conflict presupposes sexual feelings for which the hormonal condition, let alone the psychological interest, is lacking in the severely anorectic patient. Therefore, if the anorectic process becomes a matter of physical and spiritual survival, I agree with Bruch (1980) that sexual fears are secondary and arise out of more fundamental fears resulting from early developmental deficits. Thus, in the more severe cases that we mostly see as psychiatrists today, the psychological issues of anorexia nervosa go far beyond avoidance of adult sexuality. Their psychodynamics are more fruitfully conceived as a compensatory process to counterbalance a poor self-concept (Casper et al. 1981) and to reduce severe anxiety related to difficulties in psychological and social maladjustment through the creation of an ideal, acceptable bodily self at any cost, even that of physical demise.

Psychodynamics in Anorexia Nervosa— Bulimic Subtype and Bulimia Nervosa

The psychological issues in the bulimic subtype of anorexia nervosa seem to be state dependent. So long as the patient is underweight and successfully restricts her food intake, the issues resemble more closely those in patients with anorexia nervosa, restricting subtype. With weight gain, when the urge to eat cannot be curbed and binge eating develops, the issues are more similar to bulimia nervosa. The best documented case study of a patient with the bulimic subtype of anorexia nervosa is probably Binswanger's (1944) description of Ellen West, a pseudonym for a gifted young woman for whom depressive "shadows of doubt and dread" crystallized when she was age 21 into one fear: that of "getting fat." What interests us about this case is not that the patient almost certainly had a manic-depressive disorder (unrecognized I might add; Bleuler, who consulted on the case, diagnosed schizophrenia), but the clarity with which the patient described psychological manifestations of both anorexia nervosa and bulimia nervosa. The patient herself called her dread of getting fat a fixed idea, which she distinguished from the obsessional idea of having to think about eating all the time. At low weight, eating represented her "spiritual death." Weight gain from 92 to 165 pounds at medium height did not eliminate her torment. She renewed her dieting—"every meal is a torment accompanied by feelings of dread"—but then she had to fight a constant insatiable desire to eat; she became bulimic. Eventually she wrote:

I don't think that the dread of becoming fat is the real obsessive neurosis, but the constant desire for food. The pleasure of eating must have been the primary thing. Dread of becoming fat served as a break. Now that I see the pleasure of eating as the real obsessive idea, it has pounced upon me like a wild beast. I am defensively at its mercy. It pursues me constantly and is driving me to despair. (p. 253)

Bulimia nervosa has been documented since antiquity in various clinical expressions and under different names (Ziolko and Schrader 1985). The clinical syndrome as operationalized by Russell (1979) did not receive much attention until its recent rise in frequency about two decades ago; hence not much has been written about its psychodynamics (Casper 1983; Sours 1980). In a speculative article on the psychodynamics, Sugarman and Kurash (1982) suggested that bulimia nervosa "reflects an arrest at the early stage of transitional object development" (p. 58). The authors believe that bulimic patients fail to separate physically or cognitively from the "maternal object" and, hence, show a narcissistic fixation on their bodies. Food in bulimia is not seen as the issue; instead the bodily action of eating is considered essential in regaining a fleeting experience of the mother. The authors' case vignette actually suggests an intensely ambivalent mother-daughter relationship. Most other cases described in the literature struggle with issues and conflicts not much different from those seen in patients with affective or character disorders (Sours 1980; Swift and Stern 1982).

What then can the historical accounts teach us about the psychological side of eating disorders? First, the recognition of psychological or nervous or mental factors in anorexia nervosa early on is striking. Second, insight into psychodynamic issues was not gained until patients began talking or writing about their experiences. Last, over the past 30 years, there is convergence of opinion as a result of observations made during treatment that interpersonal factors contribute decisively to the psychological dysfunction.

Studies in Cognitive Style, Defenses, and Personality Features

Because it is often asked whether the psychological mechanisms in eating disorders can be experimentally confirmed, I will consider some of the studies that have attempted measurements.

The interpretation of studies that have assessed cognitive style or dynamic operations is complicated by findings of high correlations between cognitive distortions and affective pathology such as depression or dysphoria (Eckert et al. 1982; Laessle et al. 1988; Steiger et al. 1990; Steiner et al. 1991; Strauss and Ryan 1988). By and large, restricting and bulimic anorectic patients tend to show more cognitive dysfunction—they tend to overgeneralize or selectively abstract and to commit more cognitive errors—than normal-weight patients with bulimia nervosa and control subjects. All patients with eating disorders show fewer mature and more primitive defenses, and they employ primarily characterological and less neurotic-type defenses. Differences between restricting and bulimic anorexia nervosa based on eating behavior are well documented (Beumont et al. 1976; Casper 1990; Casper et al. 1980; Garfinkel et al. 1980; Haimes and Katz 1988; Strober 1980). The two subtypes seem to differ in manifest psychiatric symptomatology and in personality style. The bulimic anorectic patient tends to be more emotionally labile and given to impulsive behaviors than the restricting anorectic patient, who in temperament and personality tends to be more steady, deliberate, and conscientious. Of course, the described cognitive distortions, the psychological conflicts, and the personality style bear on the individual psychodynamics.

Anorexia Nervosa—
An Attachment Disorder

The psychological manifestations described here owe much to Benedek's (1936), Bruch's (1980), and Selvini-Palazzoli's (1978) writings. We should be reminded that anorexia nervosa is essentially a human condition, which at this point cannot be fully replicated in lower animals. This means that personal, social, and cultural factors play a disproportionate role. Nevertheless, the severely emaciated anorectic patient gives the impression of being barely human; how does this happen?

Starvation alone has been shown to have dehumanizing and demoralizing effects (Keys et al. 1950). What distinguishes anorexia nervosa from normal starvation is an even more profound emotional disengagement from relationships. Before we can try to understand how this happens, I need to provide some background information about the process.

Physiological and Psychological Adaptation to Weight Loss and Undernutrition

Fichter (Chapter 10, this volume) and Pirke et al. (Chapter 8, this volume) reviewed the numerous adaptive physiological adjustments to semistarvation, such as a reduction in basal metabolic rate, a reduction in heart rate and blood pressure, and a return of gonadal function to a prepubertal dormant status. This physiological regression is a function of the severity of the weight loss.

Simultaneously, adaptive psychological changes take place. Lack of sufficient food produces, as in any deprivation state, a preoccupation with food manifested in thinking, reading, and often dreaming about food. Semistarvation leads to self-absorption in other ways, including loss of interest in people and outside activities. But above and beyond these changes, the person who develops anorexia nervosa makes at some point a more or less conscious decision that the weight loss is something desirable. The reasons and personal motivations for this resolve vary from person to person and from culture to culture. However, clinical evidence suggests that additional, most likely physiologically or organically mediated factors promote this personal investment in the body-weight loss. Many patients report an outright energizing effect with starvation, much different from the lethargy and fatigue felt by normal starving individuals (Keys et al. 1950). Even if this phenomenon may be partly psychological in the sense that having a goal and purpose in life activates initiative, there seems to be a physical element, which some patients describe as a "charge of energy." Other patients simply say that they feel better than they have ever felt in their lives. Lasègue (1873) wrote the following about this feeling:

> . . . an inexhaustible optimism, against which supplications and menaces alike are of no avail: "I do not suffer and must then be well. . . ." So often have I heard this phrase repeated by patients, that now it has come to represent for me a symptom. (p. 151)

Reorganization of the Self Through Domination of the Body

The patient's identification with the weight-loss process has other consequences. As Benedek (1936) noted, the behavior is driven by one or more dominant, more or less fixed ideas varying in thought content from "I do not want to grow up," or "I must not be big (as my mother)," to "I must not be like others." Generally, these ideas are conscious. They are phrased in the negative, and their directive is oppositional, suggesting an aggressive component. The ideas generate a hierarchy of new goals and values with a transvaluation of all related values. For example, being hungry is considered good, and eating is "bad," or a previously honest girl will lie or cheat about what she ate. The new values entail new prohibitions that become fully integrated into the patient's intrapsychic processes and therefore cannot be lifted at will. Expressed differently, and easier to test experimentally, the weight-loss process, abetted by the patient's personal endorsement, powerfully recruits or entrains the reward and punishment system. Every transgression, eating even a small amount of food, is considered dangerous and invokes intense anxiety (Casper 1987a).

The more the patient invests in herself and her thinness, the more she detaches emotionally from previous relationships, from family, and from friends. During adolescence, a detachment from parents is expected. Normal adolescents reinvest in peer relations and friends, as well as in societal and cultural values. The future anorectic patient, having generally felt helpless and ineffective in relationships, puts, so to speak, all her eggs in one basket; she exclusively invests in her bony body as a representation of her self. Traumatic events, such as rejection by friends or loss of a friend or moving to a new home or to a new school, which renew memories of past painful experiences, lead to a reassessment of the value of close relationships and can contribute to ushering in this detachment. When the patient discovers that she can make herself feel better by controlling her body shape through losing weight, this discovery becomes a powerful reinforcer. Timid and conforming by disposition, patients derive a strong sense of self-directed identity from a situation in which they feel in control. Other personality characteristics—the patient's tendency toward self-discipline and her tendency to categoric uncompromising thinking—influence the way she takes control of her body.

The nature of each individual's life experiences and unresolved conflicts color the relationship to her new body. The patient's domination of her body looks to the observer like a reenactment of parental inflexibility and insensitivity, a sad caricature of what patients might have experienced from a mother who imposed her own wishes and ignored the child's reaction. Harsh discipline can be pursued with a vengeance: exercise in minutes or hours planned in detail, how little or when to eat, how to reduce sleep by staying up late or walking instead of sleeping in bed. The patient's body is treated as if it were a rebellious, willful object in need of control. Of course, any dieting attitude tends to treat the body like an object in need of limits. However, in anorexia nervosa there is a fundamental difference; aspects unacceptable to the patient—a low self-esteem, a fear of being nobody, feeling victimized—become attributed to and merge somehow with rejected aspects of the body. Conceptually then, the body becomes split into good and bad parts. Increased weight, under the connotation of too much flesh or fat, becomes linked to old bad experiences of ineffectiveness, humiliation, dysphoria, and ultimately to losing one's sense of self. Weight gain thus would represent a revival of past misery. The patient herself seems oblivious to and, I believe, truly unaware of this mistreatment of her body; to her, the behavior seems a small sacrifice, well worth the price of feeling in control, self-sufficient, and independent.

Remarkably, this wasted, reformed body is also a source of great pride. Patients with anorexia nervosa take care in their appearance. Some patients go so far as to parade their scantily dressed cadaverous figure to the horror of other patients on the ward. The patient seems totally unaware of the frightening aspects. This and a symptom called mirror gazing, in which patients admire their bony structure and caved-in abdomen in the privacy of their bathrooms, suggest that the patient visually perceives but fails to integrate and remains unaware of the life-threatening implications of her emaciation. Denial alone (Casper et al. 1979; Crisp and Kalucy 1974) cannot fully explain this defective integration of the bodily changes, which seems to have an organic component. All self-worth and self-confidence are derived from the emaciated body; this explains why some patients would rather die than gain weight. The exclusive emotional investment in the changed body means parents retain little control over their child and are "the worst attendents" (Gull 1868), unless they can be helped to relate to and understand their child's dilemma.

Psychodynamics in Bulimia Nervosa

Considered within the context of relationship theory, bulimia nervosa is psychodynamically much less complex than anorexia nervosa. The personality of the bulimic patient remains emotionally and socially engaged, albeit often in stormy and abusive relationships. Affective disorders are common in severe cases of bulimia nervosa. Most bulimic cases we see today are the result of unsuccessful dieting attempts motivated by the wish for a fashionable body shape. Bulimia nervosa begins as a struggle against hyperphagia triggered by restrained eating. What makes bulimia nervosa unique is that thoughts of food, the urge to eat, and dysphoric feelings are harnessed together in ways still poorly understood. I have previously suggested that the greater extroversion and relatedness of bulimic patients, their wish for attention, and their tendency toward multiple stormy, sometimes abusive, relationships to escape loneliness are mirrored in the way they eat (Casper 1983), in the cycle of possessing and rejecting. Such a hypothesis cannot be easily confirmed, because few patients can relate any thought content or fantasies during binge eating and vomiting. Because food cannot induce lasting relief for emotional distress, binge eating is ineffective as a mechanism for emotional control. Its only lasting result is weight gain. Medication is available for treating dysphoric affects and thus bulimia nervosa can be much more successfully treated with drugs. Of course, individual personality and character problems and the developmental immaturity require psychotherapy, family therapy, and group therapy.

Treatment

Nutrition

The treatment of anorexia nervosa and bulimia nervosa requires correction of malnutrition and normalization of weight along with help for the underlying developmental and personality problems with the assistance of the family. Because starvation effects are involved in producing the symptoms, refeeding alone improves the symptoms.

Psychotherapy

Treatment tries to free the patient from a psychological and physiological developmental impasse and a pathological solution. The proposed psychodynamics suggest a reciprocal relationship between the pathological body attachment and meaningful affective relationships with people. Such a hypothesis would have important prognostic and therapeutic implications. It suggests that the more the patient with anorexia nervosa has remained emotionally involved with her family or friends— in other words, as long as her social withdrawal remains partial—the less likely she is to become exclusively or irreversibly attached to her body, and hence the better her chances are for her to engage in therapy leading to full recovery.

Other influences that contribute to the pathological body attachment, such as personality factors, family psychopathology, the parents' attitudes and their emotional involvement (Main and Weston 1982), age, and a comorbid psychiatric or physical disorder, should not be overlooked; these, however, are not discussed here.

Posttraumatic Experience

Conversely, the more early and ongoing psychosocial traumata a patient has suffered, the more likely the patient is to show distrust and avoidance behavior and the less likely the patient is to have developed a secure attachment to people. On renewed disappointments, such patients withdraw more quickly from relationships; if they develop anorexia nervosa, they are at greater risk to develop a pathological attachment to their body shape and to remain fixated on their body.

The Therapeutic Alliance

The specific task of the psychological treatment, then, is to disengage the patient from her self-containment and fixation on her body and to help her reengage in human relationships. The patient will experience treatment as dangerous interference because treatment removes the only defensive solution available to her. Weight gain undoes the patient's independent accomplishment. It leaves her defenseless, reexposing her emptiness and depression, her emotional lability and tension, her feeling bad and ineffective, her lack of sense of self, and her fear of being nobody. Therefore, it is not surprising that patients should resist treatment so much. Because treatment in anorexia nervosa means refeeding and thus changing the patient's body shape against her will, insistence on weight gain recreates an interaction reminiscent of her early interpersonal experiences (Casper 1987b). By expecting the patient to gain weight, we disregard her individuality and her wishes and instead impose our own, invoking the danger that the patient feels once more violated and ignored. In fact, given the importance of the patient's bony structure for the patient's self-esteem and sense of competence, if we bring too much pressure to bear, the patient who feels we have taken away her only purpose in life may become depressed and acutely suicidal. Sometimes we are experienced as so threatening that the patient may become paranoid about us.

Dangers Inherent in Treatment

It is important to realize that by refeeding we run the risk of retraumatizing the patient. This risk can be diminished if we take a personal interest in the patient and thus behave differently from her previous caretakers. As we listen to the patient's grievances, and as we review her life history with her, we share our thoughts and understanding of her situation. Patients with anorexia nervosa are deeply distrustful and highly sensitive. They are excellent observers. The patient needs to sense that we are not merely interested in her physical survival, but equally interested in her personal suffering.

Psychotherapy focuses mainly on the reasons underlying the patient's faulty attachment to her body, on her failure of self-expression, and on her missing tools for organizing and expressing needs and dealing with others. From evaluating the family history and reviewing the past, we need to convey the hope that it would be possible for the patient to become an individual in her own right within her family were she to relinquish the excessive control over her body shape.

We have to know that, because a refeeding program interferes with a chosen goal and disrupts the ideas dominating her behavior, the patient is likely to experience confusion, a sense of emptiness, lost direction, and sometimes despair and suicidal ideation. We can support the patient's need for concrete cognitive control, for example by giving explicit information about any intervention, such as about meal times or the amount of food to be consumed. Gradually her repetitive, reverberating thinking will be replaced by memories and new ideas. Overall, the treatment approach is as flexible as possible within the context of consistent expectations and seeks to respond to the person's individual needs.

Psychotherapy of Bulimia Nervosa

If psychotherapy seeks to engage the emotionally withdrawn restricting anorectic patient and tries to mobilize her emotionally, then the patient with bulimia nervosa requires strengthening of her cognitive controls. She needs to learn to think before acting and needs help with tolerating her emotions by understanding their origin and organizing their expression. There is increasing evidence that bulimic patients have a history of violence and sexual abuse in childhood, even though the incidence seems to be similar in female patients with other psychiatric disorders (Bulik et al. 1989). The resulting dissociative states and their relationship to the bulimic behavior need to be a focus in treatment since, psychodynamically, the dissociated memories seem to contribute to the patient's sense of dyscontrol. In all other respects, the psychological issues resemble those seen in patients with other psychiatric conditions. In every case, a careful evaluation of each patient's premorbid and comorbid adjustment ought to precede the planning for psychotherapy and family therapy.

Conclusions

Anorexia nervosa is a classic example of a disorder in which the behavior initially guides the illness, until eventually the illness process takes hold of the behavior. In other words, in the full-blown picture, the patient shows an unrelenting need to engage in the behavior.

The dynamics I have described, the patient's pathological appropriation of and attachment to her changed body, appear to be specific to anorexia nervosa. They are typically seen in the postpubertal patient and show considerable differences in severity. The tenacity of the attachment seems to be a function of the patient's psychopathology, reflected in the quality of her interpersonal relationships. However, the pathological body attachment is not the only psychodynamic we observe in anorexia nervosa nor is it a psychodynamic that is necessary for anorexia nervosa. For instance, prepubertal patients may not display this pathological body attachment. What seems to be a recurring element in anorexia nervosa across cultures and centuries is the personal appropriation of and identification with the changed body contours.

Overall, the psychodynamics we observe in contemporary anorexia nervosa cases vary with the person's age, premorbid adjustment or pathology, personality, eating pattern or subtype, psychiatric symptomatology and comorbidity, physical health or illness, upbringing, family psychopathology, and strengths and talents (artistic or intellectual).

Anorexia nervosa affords a unique opportunity to examine the contribution of personality tendencies as risk factors to the development of a psychiatric disorder. Future research needs to address which biologic regulators or central nervous system sites may be involved in the defective body image integration and the illness-specific physiological response to partial starvation.

References

Beck AT, Rush AJ, Shaw BFD, et al: Cognitive Therapy of Depression. New York, Guilford, 1979

Bell RM: Holy Anorexia. Chicago, IL, University of Chicago Press, 1985

Benedek T: Dominant ideas and their relation to morbid cravings. Int J Psychoanal 17:40–56, 1936

Beumont PJV, George GCW, Smart DE: "Dieters" and "vomiters and purgers" in anorexia nervosa. Psychol Med 6:617–622, 1976

Binswanger L: Der Fall Ellen West. Schweiz Arch Neurol Psychiat 54:69–117, 1944 [Translated in Binswanger L: The case of Ellen West, in Existence. Edited by May R, Angel E, Ellenberger H. New York, Basic Books, 1958]

Bruch H: Perceptual and conceptual disturbances in anorexia nervosa. Psychosom Med 24:187–194, 1962

Bruch H: Eating Disorders. New York, Basic Books, 1973

Bruch H: Preconditions for the development of anorexia nervosa. Am J Psychoanal 40:169–172, 1980

Bulik CM, Sullivan PF, Rorty M: Childhood sexual abuse in women with bulimia. J Clin Psychiatry 50:460–464, 1989

Casper RC: Some provisional ideas concerning the psychologic structure in anorexia nervosa and bulimia, in Anorexia Nervosa: Recent Developments in Research. Edited by Darby PL, Garfinkel PE, Garner DM, et al. New York, Alan R Liss, 1983, pp 387–392

Casper RC: The psychopathology of anorexia nervosa: the pathological psychodynamic processes, in Handbook of Eating Disorders, Part 1. Edited by Beumont PJV, Burrows G, Casper RC. Amsterdam, Elsevier, 1987a

Casper RC: Psychotherapy in anorexia nervosa, in Handbook of Eating Disorders, Part 1. Edited by Beumont PJV, Burrows G, Casper RC. Amsterdam, Elsevier, 1987b

Casper RC: Personality features of women with good outcome from restricting anorexia nervosa. Psychosom Med 52:156–170, 1990

Casper RC, Halmi KA, Goldberg SC, et al: Disturbances in body image estimation as related to other characteristics and outcome in anorexia nervosa. Br J Psychiatry 134:60–66, 1979

Casper RC, Eckert ED, Halmi KA, et al: Bulimia: its incidence and clinical importance in patients with anorexia nervosa. Arch Gen Psychiatry 37:1030–1035, 1980

Casper RC, Offer D, Ostrov E: The self-image of adolescents with acute anorexia nervosa. J Pediatr 98:656–661, 1981

Crisp AH: Let Me Be. London, Academic Press, 1980

Crisp AH, Kalucy RS: Aspects of the perceptual disorder in anorexia nervosa. Br J Med Psychol 47:349–361, 1974

Eckert ED, Goldberg SC, Halmi KA, et al: Depression in anorexia nervosa. Psychol Med 12:115–122, 1982

Freud S: The Origins of Psychoanalysis: Letter to Wilhelm Fliess, Drafts and Notes: 1887–1902. Edited by Bonaparte M, Freud A, Kris E. Translated by Mosbacher E, Strachey J. New York, Basic Books, 1954

Garfinkel PE, Moldofsky H, Garner DM: The heterogeneity of anorexia nervosa: bulimia as a distinct subgroup. Arch Gen Psychiatry 37:1036–1040, 1980

Garner DM, Bemis KM: A cognitive-behavioral approach to anorexia nervosa. Cognitive Therapy and Research 6:123–150, 1982

Goodsitt A: Self psychology and the treatment of anorexia nervosa, in Handbook of Psychotherapy for Anorexia Nervosa and Bulimia. Edited by Garner DM, Garfinkel PE. New York, Guilford, 1984, pp 55–82

Gull WW: The address in medicine delivered before the annual meeting of the B.M.A. at Oxford. Lancet 2:171–176, 1868

Gull WW: Anorexia nervosa (apepsia hysterica, anorexia hysterica). Transactions of the Clinical Society of London 7:22–28, 1874

Haimes AL, Katz JL: Sexual and social maturity versus social conformity in restricting anorectic, bulimic and borderline women. International Journal of Eating Disorders 7:332–341, 1988

Janet P: Obsessions et la Psychasthenie, Vols 1 and 2. Paris, Felix Alcan, 1903

Keys A, Brozek J, Henschel A, et al: The Biology of Human Starvation. Minneapolis, University of Minnesota Press, 1950

Kohut H: The Analysis of the Self. New York, International Universities Press, 1971

Laessle RG, Kittl S, Fichter MM, et al: Cognitive correlates of depression in patients with eating disorders. International Journal of Eating Disorders 7:681–686, 1988

Lasègue D: De l'anorexie hysterique. Archives Generales de Medicine, 1873. [Reprinted in Evolution of Psychosomatic Concepts. Anorexia Nervosa: A Paradigm. Edited by Kaufman RM, Heiman M. New York, International Universities Press, 1964]

Main M, Weston DR: Avoidance of the attachment figure in infancy: descriptions and interpretations, in The Place of Attachment in Human Behavior. Edited by Parkes CM, Stevenson-Hinde J. London, Tavistock, 1982

Minuchin S, Baker L, Rosman BL, et al: A conceptual model of psychosomatic illness in children. Arch Gen Psychiatry 32:1031–1038, 1975

Morton R: Pthisiologica: Or a Treatise of Consumptions. London, Sam Smith & Benj Walford, 1694

Nemiah JC: Anorexia nervosa: a clinical psychiatric study. Medicine 29:225–268, 1950

Russell G: Bulimia nervosa: an ominous variant of anorexia nervosa. Psychol Med 9:429–448, 1979

Selvini-Palazzoli MP: Self-Starvation. New York, Jason Aronson, 1978

Sours JA: Starving to Death in a Sea of Objects. New York, Jason Aronson, 1980

Steiger H, Goldstein C, Mongrain M, et al: Description of eating-disordered women along cognitive and psychodynamic dimensions. International Journal of Eating Disorders 9:129–140, 1990

Steiner H, Smith C, Litt IF: The early care and feeding of patients with anorexia nervosa. Child Psychiatry Hum Dev 2:163–167, 1991

Strauss J, Ryan RM: Cognitive dysfunction in eating disorders. International Journal of Eating Disorders 7:19–27, 1988

Strober M: Personality and symptomatological features in young non-chronic anorexia nervosa patients. J Psychosom Res 24:353–359, 1980

Strober M: A comparative analysis of personality organization in juvenile anorexia nervosa. Journal of Youth and Adolescence 10:285–295, 1981

Strober M: Disorders of the self in anorexia nervosa: an organismic-developmental paradigm, in Psychodynamic Theory and Treatment for Eating Disorders. Edited by Johnson C. New York, Guilford, 1990, pp 354–373

Sugarman A, Kurash C: The body as a transitional object in bulimia. International Journal of Eating Disorders 1:57–67, 1982

Swift WJ, Stern S: The psychodynamic diversity of anorexia nervosa. International Journal of Eating Disorders 2:17–35, 1982

Waller JV, Kaufman MR, Deutsch F: Anorexia nervosa: a psychosomatic entity. Psychosom Med 2:3–16, 1940

Wolf ES: Selfobject transferences: an overview. Psychiatric Annals 16:491–493, 1986

Ziolko HU, Schrader HC: Bulimie. Fortschr Neurol Psychiatr 53:231–248, 1985

Chapter 15

Cognitive-Behavioral Therapy in Treatment of Bulimia Nervosa

James E. Mitchell, M.D.
Nancy C. Raymond, M.D.

—————

Recent research on the treatment of bulimia nervosa has focused primarily on the use of outpatient modalities. Economic as well as therapeutic considerations govern this choice. When treatment of bulimic patients is approached from a cognitive-behavioral perspective, the main goal is to encourage them to gain control over their bulimic behaviors and establish a healthier eating pattern. This is best accomplished in the natural environment, in which the new behaviors will have to be maintained; therefore, outpatient treatment is usually preferable. There are exceptions to this axiom. Severe medical complications may necessitate an inpatient stay for stabilization. Also, other complications of the disorder, such as suicidality or severe depression, may dictate an inpatient stay.

Currently, much research is being done to ascertain the most effective type or types of outpatient treatment for bulimia nervosa. Pharmacological strategies have been most extensively studied. These approaches are reviewed elsewhere (Walsh, Chapter 16, this volume). Since Lacey (1983) published the first controlled treatment study on psychotherapy of bulimia nervosa, most of the treatment studies have focused on the use of cognitive-behavioral techniques. In this chapter, we examine 19 controlled studies that have examined the efficacy of cognitive-behavioral therapy (CBT) in the treatment of bulimia nervosa. In some studies, CBT is compared with other types of therapy (Bossert et al. 1989; Connors et al. 1984; Fairburn et al. 1986, 1991; Freeman et al. 1988; Garner et al., in press; Hsu 1991; Kirkley et al. 1985). In other studies, waiting-list or minimal intervention controls have been used (Agras et al. 1989; Connors et al. 1984; Freeman et al. 1988; Laessle et al. 1987; Lee and Rush 1986; Leitenberg et al. 1988; Ordman and Kirschenbaum 1985; Wolchik et al. 1986). Two published studies explored the concomitant use of antidepressants as a part of the treatment (Agras et al. 1992; Mitchell et al. 1990). One study examined whether varying the intensity of CBT treatment affects outcome (Mitchell et al., unpublished manuscript, 1992). The components of the CBT programs have varied widely from study to study. In this chapter, we examine the components used in the various studies, the duration of treatment, and the outcomes of the studies.

Review of Methods

An overview of 19 controlled CBT treatment studies, including the nature of the comparison groups, the number of subjects, and the durations of treatment, is presented in Table 15–1. Six of the studies make use of "waiting-list controls"(Agras et al. 1989; Freeman et al. 1988; Laessle et al. 1987; Lee and Rush 1986; Leitenberg et al. 1988; Wolchik et al. 1986). Seven studies compared CBT with other types of psychotherapy. Some compared CBT to nondirective (Kirkley et al. 1985) or nonspecific (Bossert et al. 1989) or supportive (Freeman et al. 1988; Garner et al., in press) therapy. Others compared CBT to other manual-based therapies such as interpersonal therapy (IPT) (Fairburn et al. 1991). Hsu (1991) focused on a comparison to a nutritional education group. Two studies compared a purely cognitive approach with a behavioral approach that did not include cognitive restructuring (Yates and Sambrailo 1984; Wilson et al. 1986). Three studies examined whether the technique of exposure and response prevention (ERP) of vomiting is a beneficial adjunct to treatment (Agras et al. 1989; Leitenberg et al. 1988; Wilson et al. 1986). Eleven studies used a group therapy model (Connors et al. 1984; Hsu 1991; Kirkley et al. 1985; Laessle et al. 1987; Lee and Rush 1986; Mitchell et al. 1990; Mitchell et al., unpublished manuscript, 1992; Ordman and Kirschenbaum 1985; Wilson et al. 1986;

Table 15–1. Overview of controlled treatment studies

Study	Groups/individual[a]	Subjects completing (n)	Duration of sessions (weeks)	No. of sessions
CBT or BT only				
Connors et al. 1984	Psychoeducational group 1	10	9	12
	Psychoeducational group 2	10		
Ordman and Kirschenbaum 1985	Full CBT group	10	4–20	4–20
	Brief group	10		3
Lee and Rush 1986	CBT group	14	6	12
	Waiting-list controls			
Wolchik et al. 1986	CBT group + individual	11	7	7 group + 2 individual
	Waiting-list controls	7		
Laessle et al. 1987	BT group	8	16	24
	Waiting list			
Mitchell et al., unpublished manuscript, 1992	CBT groups[b]			
	High/high	29	10	20 (20 hours)[c]
	High/low	36	10	14 (22.5 hours)[c]
	Low/high	30	10	20 (45 hours)[c]
	Low/low	28	10	10 (22.5 hours)[c]
CBT versus other psychotherapies				
Kirkley et al. 1985	CBT groups	13	16	16 (90 minutes)
	Nondirective groups	91		
Fairburn et al. 1986	CBT individual	11	18	19
	Short-term focal psychotherapy individual	11		
Freeman et al. 1988	CBT individual	21	15	15 (1 hour)
	BT individual	25		
	Group therapy (supportive and educational)	19		
	Waiting-list controls	15		

(continued)

Table 15–1. Overview of controlled treatment studies *(continued)*

Study	Groups/individual[a]	Subjects completing (n)	Duration of sessions (weeks)	No. of sessions
CBT versus other psychotherapies *(continued)*				
Bossert et al. 1989	CBT individual—inpatient	8	3/week	Varied between patients
	Nonspecific psychotherapy individual—inpatient	6		
Fairburn et al. 1991	CBT individual	21	18	19 (40–50 minutes)
	IPT individual	22	18	19 (40–50 minutes)
	BT individual	19	18	19 (40–50 minutes)
Hsu 1991	Nutritional counseling group		14	
	Cognitive group		14	
	Nutritional and cognitive group		14	
	Support group		14	
Garner et al., in press	CBT individual	25	18	19 (45–60 minutes)
	Supportive and expressive individual therapy	24	18	19 (45–60 minutes)
CBT versus specific behavioral technique				
Yates and Sambrailo 1984	CBT groups (cognitive restructuring)	8	6	6 (90 minutes)
	CBT groups (specific behavioral instruction)	8		
Wilson et al. 1986	Cognitive restructuring groups	6	16	16 (90 minutes)
	Cognitive restructuring + ERP	6		
Leitenberg et al. 1988	ERP (clinic) individual	12	14	24 (2 hours)
	ERP (multiple settings) individual	12		
	CBT	11		
	Waiting-list controls	12		

Study	Treatment group	N	Number of sessions	Time per session
Agras et al. 1989	CBT individual	17	16	14 (1 hour)
	CBT + ERP individual	16		
	Self-monitoring individual	16		
	Waiting-list controls	18		
CBT and medication				
Mitchell et al. 1990	Imipramine only	45[d]	10	Weekly medication management
	Placebo only	29		
	Imipramine + CBT groups	48		
	Placebo + CBT groups	33		20 (1.5–3 hours)
	CBT individual + desipramine	40	15 CBT, 24 desipramine	15 (50 minutes)
Agras et al. 1992	CBT individual + desipramine	40	15 CBT, 16 desipramine	15 (50 minutes)
	Desipramine only	40	24	
	Desipramine only	40	16	
	CBT individual only	23	15	15 (50 minutes)

Note. CBT = cognitive-behavioral therapy; BT = behavior therapy; ERP = exposure and response prevention.
[a]All subjects are outpatient studies unless otherwise indicated.
[b]High/high = high emphasis on abstinence early in treatment and high intensity of treatment session; high/low = high emphasis and low intensity; low/high = low emphasis and high intensity; low/low = low emphasis and low intensity.
[c]Length of groups varies. Time represents total hours for all groups.
[d]All subjects with data after baseline.

Wolchik et al. 1986; Yates and Sambrailo 1984). All subjects in these studies were outpatients, with the exception of the subjects in the study by Bossert et al., who studied the effectiveness of CBT in inpatients seen in individual sessions.

The components of what is termed *CBT* vary from study to study. It is difficult to assess the details of most treatment programs because of the space limitations in journal publications. The components employed by the various authors are summarized in Table 15–2 and are described in more detail below. Nearly all studies utilize a psychoeducational component and a self-monitoring component, and it is clear in these reports that self-monitoring is an important part of the treatment. The psychoeducational component usually includes information on such factors as the sociocultural emphasis on thinness; set-point theory; the physical effects and medical complications of bingeing, purging, and laxative or diuretic abuse; and how dieting and fasting perpetuate binge-and-purge cycles. Self-monitoring may be as simple as a daily record of the times and durations of meals and bingeing and purging episodes, or it may be more complex, with emphasis on recording detailed descriptions of moods and circumstances surrounding binge-and-purge episodes.

Most of these CBT approaches encourage patients to modify their eating pattern, in particular stressing the importance of eating regular meals (Table 15–2), and nine of the studies actually describe a formal meal planning component (Fairburn et al. 1986; Freeman et al. 1988; Kirkley et al. 1985; Laessle et al. 1987; Lee and Rush 1986; Mitchell et al. 1990; Mitchell et al., unpublished manuscript, 1992; Ordman and Kirschenbaum 1985; Wolchick et al. 1986). Nine studies emphasize the reintroduction of feared or "high-risk" foods (Agras et al. 1989, 1992; Fairburn et al. 1986, 1991; Garner et al., in press; Kirkley et al. 1985; Leitenberg et al. 1988; Mitchell et al. 1990; Mitchell et al., unpublished manuscript, 1992), but the timing of this component varies among studies.

Cognitive restructuring is central to all of these CBT programs. Behavioral approaches that are also commonly employed include restricting exposure to cues that trigger a binge-and-purge episode, developing a strategy of alternative behaviors, and delaying the vomiting response to eating.

A debate has arisen in the literature regarding the use of ERP in the treatment of bulimia nervosa. The procedure, originally developed by Leitenberg and Rosen (1989), involves having the patient binge eat to the point of discomfort, and then preventing or delaying vomiting. The details of this debate are discussed later. Some studies include assertiveness

Table 15–2. Components in controlled psychotherapy trials

Study	Groups/individual	Education	Self-monitoring	Modify eating pattern	Meal plan	Practice feared foods	Cognitive restructuring	Cue restriction	Alter behavior	Delay vomiting	ERP	Assertiveness training	Relaxation training
CBT or BT only													
Connors et al. 1984	Psychoeducational group	+	+	+			+		+			+	+
Ordman and Kirschenbaum 1985	Full CBT group	+	+	+	+		+				+		
	Brief group	+	+		+					+			
Lee and Rush 1986	CBT	+	+				+		+				+
	Waiting-list controls												
Wolchik et al. 1986	CBT individual and group	+	+	+	+		+	+	+			+	+
	Waiting-list controls												
Laessle et al. 1987	BT group	+	+	+	+		+	+	+				+
	Waiting-list controls												
Mitchell et al., unpublished manuscript, 1992	CBT groups[a]												
	High/high	+	+	+	+	+	+	+	+			+	
	High/low	+	+	+	+	+	+	+	+			+	
	Low/high	+	+	+	+	+	+	+	+			+	
	Low/low	+	+	+	+	+	+	+	+			+	
CBT versus other therapies													
Kirkley et al. 1985	CBT groups	+	+	+	+	+	+	+	+	+		+	+
	Nondirective groups	+	+					+					

(continued)

Table 15–2.   Components in controlled psychotherapy trials *(continued)*

Study	Groups/individual	Education	Self-monitoring	Modify eating pattern	Meal plan	Practice feared foods	Cognitive restructuring	Cue restriction	Alter behavior	Delay vomiting	ERP	Assertiveness training	Relaxation training
CBT versus other therapies *(continued)*													
Fairburn et al. 1986	CBT individual	+	+	+	+	+	+	+	+				+
	Short-term focal psychotherapy individual	+	+		+								
Freeman et al. 1988	CBT individual	+	+				+						
	BT individual	+	+									+	+
	Group therapy (supportive)	+	+	+	+								
	Waiting-list controls												
Bossert et al. 1989	CBT individual		+						+		+		
	Nonspecific psychotherapy individual												
Fairburn et al. 1991	CBT individual	+	+	+		+	+	+					
	IPT individual												
	BT individual		+	+		+		+					
Hsu 1991	Nutritional counseling groups	+											
	Cognitive groups	+	+				+						
	Nutritional and cognitive group	+	+				+						
	Support group	+											
Garner et al., in press	CBT individual		+	+		+	+						
	Psychodynamic individual												

CBT versus specific behavioral technique

Yates and Sambrailo 1984
- CBT groups
- CBT groups (behavioral)

Wilson et al. 1986
- Cognitive restructuring groups
- Cognitive restructuring + ERP

Leitenberg et al. 1988
- ERP (clinic) individual
- ERP (multiple settings) individual
- CBT
- Waiting-list controls

Agras et al. 1989
- CBT individual
- CBT + ERP individual
- Self-monitoring
- Waiting-list controls

CBT and medications

Mitchell et al. 1990
- Imipramine only
- Placebo only
- Imipramine and CBT group
- Placebo and CBT group

Agras et al. 1992
- CBT individual + desipramine (24 weeks)
- CBT individual + desipramine (16 weeks)
- Desipramine only (24 weeks)
- Desipramine only (16 weeks)
- CBT individual only

Note. ERP = exposure and response prevention. CBT = cognitive-behavioral therapy. BT = behavior therapy. IPT = interpersonal therapy.
[a]High/high = high emphasis on abstinence early in treatment and high intensity of treatment session; high/low = high emphasis and low intensity; low/high = low emphasis and high intensity; low/low = low emphasis and low intensity.

training and relaxation training as components in the treatment program (see Table 15–2).

Outcome Measures and Results

Various measures have been used to assess outcome. Many authors reported the reduction in frequency of bingeing or purging as primary measures of improvement in bulimia nervosa (Table 15–3). In addition, several authors reported the rate of abstinence from bulimic symptoms as a measure of outcome at follow-up. Most authors also have looked at several related problems, such as the degree of depression and anxiety, using various psychometric measures. The Eating Disorders Inventory (Garner et al. 1983) and the Eating Attitude Test (Garner et al. 1982) also have commonly been used to evaluate eating behavior and psychological factors associated with bulimia nervosa. The Beck Depression Inventory (Beck et al. 1961) has been the most frequently used self-rating scale to assess depression (Agras et al. 1989; Fairburn et al. 1991; Garner et al., in press; Kirkley et al. 1985; Laessle et al. 1987; Lee and Rush 1986; Leitenberg et al. 1988; Mitchell et al. 1990; Mitchell et al., unpublished manuscript, 1992; Ordman and Kirschenbaum 1985; Wilson et al. 1986). The Hamilton Rating Scale for Depression (Hamilton 1967) has been used by others (Agras et al. 1989; Lee and Rush 1986; Mitchell et al. 1990; Mitchell et al., unpublished manuscript, 1992), and the Montgomery and Åsberg Depression Scale (Montgomery and Åsberg 1979) has also been used (Fairburn et al. 1986; Freeman et al. 1988). Anxiety and self-esteem have also been assessed using various instruments.

All of the studies cited in this review found significant improvement in the CBT treatment groups when they were compared with waiting-list control subjects or the patient's own baseline; as one would expect, no studies cited significant changes in the symptoms of waiting-list control subjects. The reduced frequency of binge eating varies from 40% to 97%, with most of the studies finding a 70%–80% decrease in the frequency. Decreased frequency in vomiting ranged from 40% to 95%, with most of the studies again reporting a 70%–80% decrease in frequency. At follow-up, 50%–83% of the subjects reported a reduced frequency of symptoms (reduction of symptoms of >50%). However, abstinence rates the last week of treatment and at follow-up are less impressive. In the studies that report abstinence rates, abstinence at the end of treatment varies from 0% to 76%. Of the four studies that report follow-up data (see Table 15–

Table 15–3. Outcomes in controlled treatment studies

Study	Groups/individual	Reduced frequency of bingeing pre- to posttreatment (%)	Reduced frequency of vomiting pre- to posttreatment (%)	Abstinent last week of treatment (%)	Length of follow-up	>50% reduction in binge eating frequency at follow-up (%)	Abstinent at follow-up (%)
CBT or BT only							
Connors et al. 1984	Psychoeducational group	70			10 weeks	55	15
Ordman and Kirschenbaum 1985	Full CBT group			20			
	Brief group			20			
Lee and Rush 1986	CBT	70	63	29	3–4 months	36	14
	Waiting-list controls						
Wolchik et al. 1986	Individual and group	58		9	10 weeks	64	9
	Waiting-list controls						
Laessle et al. 1987	BT group			38	3 months	75	75
	Waiting-list controls						
Mitchell et al., unpublished manuscript, 1992	CBT groups[a]						
	High/high	76.7	77.4	69.7			
	High/low	77.9	82.0	73.2			
	Low/high	87.5	77.4	70.6			
	Low/low	61.8	56.1	32.4			
CBT versus other therapies							
Kirkley et al. 1985	CBT groups	97	95		3 months	76[b]	38
	Nondirective groups	64	69			78[b]	11
Fairburn et al. 1986	CBT individual	87	93	27	1 year		55
	Short-term focal psychotherapy individual	82	88	36			55

(continued)

Table 15–3.   Outcomes in controlled treatment studies (*continued*)

Study	Groups/individual	Reduced frequency of bingeing pre- to posttreatment (%)	Reduced frequency of vomiting pre- to posttreatment (%)	Abstinent last week of treatment (%)	Length of follow-up	>50% reduction in binge eating frequency at follow-up (%)	Abstinent at follow-up (%)
CBT versus other therapies (*continued*)							
Freeman et al. 1988	CBT group and individual	79	86		1 year		
	Behavior group and individual	87	92				
	Group therapy (supportive) and individual	87	93				
	Waiting-list controls	35	–21				
Bossert et al. 1989	CBT individual						
	Nonspecific psychotherapy individual						
Fairburn et al. 1991	CBT individual	97	95	71		96[c]	
	IPT individual	89	66	62	12 months	94[c]	
	BT individual	91	95	62			
Garner et al., in press	CBT individual	73	82				
	Supportive and expressive individual therapy	69	62				
CBT versus specific behavioral technique							
Yates and Sambrailo 1984	CBT groups			0	6 weeks	50	0
	CBT groups (behavioral)			13		50	25
Wilson et al. 1986	Cognitive restructuring groups	51	69	33	6 months	75	25
	Cognitive restructuring + ERP	82	91	71		83	50

Study	Condition						
Leitenberg et al. 1988	ERP clinic individual		73	36	6 months	73	18
	ERP (multiple settings) individual		67	42		90	50
	CBT		40	8		67	33
	Waiting-list controls		-1				
Agras et al. 1989	CBT individual		75	56	6 months		59
	CBT + ERP individual		52	31			20
	Self-monitoring		63	24			18
	Waiting-list controls		14	5.8			
CBT versus medication							
Mitchell et al. 1990	Imipramine only	49		16			
	Placebo only	3					
	Imipramine + CBT group	92		56			
	Placebo + CBT group	89		45			
Agras et al. 1992	CBT individual + desipramine (24 weeks)	75[d]	85[d]	64[e]	32 weeks	70	
	CBT individual + desipramine (16 weeks)	72[d]	67[d]	64[e]	32 weeks		
	Desipramine only (24 weeks)	54[d]	54[d]	33[e]	32 weeks	42	
	Desipramine only (16 weeks)	23[d]	49[d]	33[e]	32 weeks		
	CBT individual only	68[d]	73[d]	48[e]	32 weeks	55	55

Note. CBT = cognitive-behavioral therapy. BT = behavior therapy. IPT = interpersonal therapy. ERP = exposure and response prevention.

[a]High/high = high emphasis on abstinence early in treatment and high intensity of treatment session; high/low = high emphasis and low intensity; low/high = low emphasis and high intensity; low/low = low emphasis and low intensity.

[b]Greater than 60% reduction in symptoms.

[c]Actual percentage of reduction in binge eating frequency.

[d]Percentage at Week 24.

[e]Percentage at Week 16.

3), the rates of abstinence were worse than at the end of treatment, with the exception of Agras et al. (1989), who reported slight improvement in percentage of abstinent subjects at follow-up.

The available literature suggests that CBT has some efficacy in the treatment of bulimia nervosa, but there is debate about whether other forms of therapy may be just as effective. Fairburn et al. (1986) and Freeman et al. (1988) did not find statistically significant differences between CBT and their active comparison treatments in reduction of bulimic episodes. However, Freeman et al. (1988) did report that there was a higher dropout rate in a supportive psychotherapy group. Kirkley et al. (1985) found that although both the CBT groups and the nondirective therapy groups had equal credibility ratings among participants, the CBT treatment resulted in greater reductions in bulimic behaviors than in the nondirective therapy group. They, like Freeman et al., found that the nondirective group had a higher dropout rate. Fairburn et al. (1991) compared the effectiveness of CBT to IPT and found that initially CBT and IPT both resulted in significant decreases in bulimic symptoms, but CBT was more powerful in modifying disturbed attitudes toward weight and shape. However, at 12-month follow-up (Fairburn et al., in press), the advantage of CBT over IPT disappeared, and the two treatments seemed to have approximately equal efficacy.

Mitchell et al. (unpublished manuscript, 1992) conducted a study designed to examine the efficacy of emphasizing abstinence from bulimic behaviors early during the course of CBT treatment and the efficacy of varying the high intensity of the treatments. Four groups were compared: the A-1 group (high emphasis on abstinence early in treatment and high intensity of treatment sessions), the A-2 group (high emphasis on abstinence early in treatment and low intensity of treatment), the B-1 group (low emphasis on abstinence during treatment and high intensity of treatment sessions), and the B-2 group (low emphasis on abstinence and low intensity of treatment). The study found that the B-2 group was less efficacious than the other three in inducing abstinence, but there was no statistically significant difference between the efficacy of A-1, A-2, and B-1 treatment conditions. Given the pressures for cost-effective treatment, a high emphasis on abstinence early in treatment and a less intensive treatment group may be the preferred choice according to the findings of this study.

Researchers also vary as to what they regard as the most important components of CBT and behavioral therapy based on their data. Both Yates and Sambrailo (1984) and Freeman et al. (1988) compared a cognitive approach to a behavioral approach. Yates and Sambrailo found that a somewhat higher percentage of patients improved significantly if behavioral techniques were added to CBT. However, Freeman et al. did not find that the cognitive component significantly improved the results obtained using behavioral therapy alone.

Another debate in the literature focuses on the addition of ERP techniques to a CBT regimen. Wilson et al. (1986) found that adding the ERP technique nonsignificantly improved the outcome for CBT treatment. Leitenberg and Rosen (1989) found greater improvement with the addition of ERP to CBT, but the results were not statistically significant. Agras et al. (1989), on the other hand, argued that the addition of ERP actually compromised the effectiveness of CBT in their treatment study, but Leitenberg and Rosen (1989) contended that problems in the way the technique was administered by Agras et al. (1989) caused the decrease in effectiveness of ERP. Differences in the time ERP was instituted during treatment and the length of the sessions may have affected outcome. Agras et al. also argued that self-monitoring is a central part of CBT. The group in their study that only self-monitored without any other therapy did better than the control group.

Two published studies have examined the relative efficacy of antidepressant medication (imipramine) and group CBT, and the combination, compared with placebo (Agras et al. 1992; Mitchell et al. 1990). Mitchell et al. (1990) concluded that CBT, either with a placebo medication or with imipramine, was more effective than placebo or imipramine alone on eating variables. Adding this antidepressant medication to CBT did improve outcome on mood and anxiety variables. In an article reviewing the 6-month follow-up data from this study, Pyle et al. (1990) concluded that initial treatment with CBT either alone or in combination with imipramine resulted in a lower relapse rate than initial treatment with imipramine alone. Agras et al. (1992) used a design in which medication (desipramine) was given for either 16 or 24 weeks alone or in combination with CBT for 15 weeks. CBT was also administered without medication for 15 weeks. The authors concluded that the use of CBT in combination with medication was the most effective treatment for bulimia nervosa and that the medication should be continued for at least 24 weeks.

Of the 19 studies reviewed here, 16 reported on changes in depressive symptoms over the course of treatment or follow-up periods. All of the authors reported significant improvement in depressive symptoms in all treatment groups in comparison with control subjects, self-monitoring

(Agras et al. 1989), or brief interventions (Ordman and Kirschenbaum 1985). Few intergroup comparisons were made between different cells in the same study, but when these comparisons were made, the different therapies were not found to result in significantly different degrees of improvement in depressive symptoms. One exception to this was the differences noted by Mitchell et al. (1990). Subjects given imipramine had a significantly greater improvement in depressive and anxious symptoms when compared with subjects receiving only CBT. In the study by Wilson et al. (1986), the subjects who were treated with CBT and ERP had a significantly lower depression subscale score on the Hopkins Symptom Checklist—90 (Derogatis et al. 1974) when compared with subjects treated with CBT only.

Three studies (Freeman et al. 1988; Garner et al., in press; Mitchell et al., unpublished manuscript, 1992) provided detailed results of the changes in the various subscales of the Eating Disorders Inventory, a tool to assess various aspects of psychopathology frequently found in patients with eating disorders. The subscales include drive for thinness, bulimia, body dissatisfaction, ineffectiveness, perfectionism, interpersonal distrust, interoceptive awareness, and maturity fears. Freeman et al. (1988) presented data that showed which subscales varied from the baseline measurement. The group therapy cell significantly improved on all subscales except bulimia, perfectionism, and interpersonal distrust. The CBT group improved on all subscales except perfectionism, interpersonal distrust, and maturity fears. The behavior therapy group significantly improved on all subscales except maturity fears. Mitchell et al. (unpublished manuscript, 1992) reported significant improvement in all areas except perfectionism, interoceptive awareness, and maturity fears. Garner et al. (in press) found that subjects in the CBT group had significantly greater improvement on the bulimia subscale than subjects in the ITP group.

Review of Cognitive-Behavioral Techniques

Psychoeducational Techniques

An important part of this approach is to provide patients with information about bulimia nervosa. This may include information about the physical and emotional consequences of the disorder and basic information about nutrition, metabolism, and the physiological changes associated with bulimic behaviors. It is also necessary to discuss the variety of abnormal eating-related behaviors in which these patients may engage, including use of laxatives, diuretics, diet pills, and less commonly rumination and enema misuse.

Self-Monitoring

An important early step in treatment of bulimia nervosa is to have patients self-monitor their eating behavior. Many patients are surprised at the frequency of the bulimic episodes when they first start self-monitoring. A food diary can also be useful in examining eating patterns in general. It has been demonstrated that simply having patients self-monitor will to some extent improve eating behavior (Agras et al. 1989).

Nutritional Counseling

Education about nutrition should be implemented early in the course of treatment. Patients should be instructed that the goal of the treatment is not simply to eliminate bingeing and vomiting episodes, but to develop a pattern of eating regular balanced meals. Many patients are initially quite resistant to this, but most patients will eventually be compliant if the therapist assumes a firm, directive approach. Some programs find it useful to have patients plan meals a day in advance so that they do not eat reactively, but instead eat what they should be eating based on their meal plan.

Cues, Responses, and Consequences

In using a CBT approach, it is important for patients to delineate cues involved in their eating behavior (social, situational, mental, and physiological) and the consequences, both short term and long term. The response set can be broken down into three parts: thoughts, behaviors, and feelings. It is useful for patients to begin to separate these three elements to understand better their own response sets. Certain styles of thinking are often commonly seen in patients with eating disorders, including overgeneralization, "catastrophizing," dichotomous thinking, and overreliance on the opinion of others.

It is important for patients to understand that both positive and negative consequences result from bulimic behaviors. Many of the short-term consequences are positive (avoiding stressful situations, handling anger), whereas the longer-term consequences (depression, medical instability, lack of control over one's life) tend to be negative. It is important for patients to learn to focus more on these long-term consequences of the behavior. One technique that is useful in teaching patients to gain control is to break the relationship between the cue and the response (stimulus control). This may include delaying bingeing episodes in response to a cue, avoidance of stimulus cues, and the development of behavioral alternatives. Consequences of behavior can also be rearranged so that appropriate behaviors will be reinforced and inappropriate behaviors not rewarded.

Restructuring Thoughts

Central to the CBT approach is the emphasis on understanding one's own cognitions about shape, weight, and other problems. After the thoughts are delineated, then they can be challenged directly using a Socratic approach. Thoughts can be questioned by examining their content, or they can be challenged prospectively by setting up experiments in which to evaluate them.

Relapse Prevention

CBT approaches generally incorporate relapse prevention techniques, such as exposure to high-risk foods and situations and the development of appropriate supports. It is also important for patients to learn to differentiate relapse from "slips" or lapses, because the latter may not necessarily portend ongoing problems.

Body Image

Body image is one of the problems most resistant to treatment. CBT techniques can be used to challenge the specific negative thoughts about body size and shape.

Other Elements

Commonly incorporated additional elements include social skills training, assertiveness training, stress management techniques, and problem-solving techniques. Relaxation techniques and the prescription of exercise are also included in some programs.

Treatment Recommendations

Based on this review of the controlled studies examining the use of CBT in the treatment of bulimia nervosa, the following conclusions can be drawn.

First, CBT is superior to waiting-list controls, and as effective or more effective when compared with other types of psychotherapy. However, the abstinence or remission rates in most studies are disappointingly low.

Second, psychoeducational techniques and self-monitoring are widely used methods and should be considered an important part of any treatment program for bulimia nervosa. The study by Agras et al. (1989) clearly supported the importance of self-monitoring; this technique alone leads to significant improvement.

Third, there are significant differences in the various CBT treatment protocols, both as to components of the program and in the ways the programs are run. It has not yet been determined what techniques are critical for an effective program or what form the process should take (e.g., the duration of treatment, the frequency of visits, the length of each session, or the size of the group).

Although these studies indicate that CBT is useful for improving the symptoms of bulimia nervosa, the ultimate goal of treatment must be curing the disorder. In the case of this disorder, a cure could best be measured by complete abstinence from bingeing and purging behaviors. The results of the current studies show we have much to learn about the treatment of bulimia nervosa if this is our goal. Should treatment programs include the expectation of and early interruption of the bulimic behaviors? What factors influence whether an individual patient will be able to obtain or maintain abstinence? Which persons would benefit from medication therapy only or medication in combination with psychotherapy? What really are the critical components of the treatment program? Clearly, there are many reasons for further research.

References

Agras WS, Schneider JA, Arnow B, et al: Cognitive-behavioral and response-prevention treatments for bulimia nervosa. J Consult Clin Psychol 57:215–221, 1989

Agras WS, Rossiter EM, Arnow B, et al: Pharmacologic and cognitive-behavioral treatment for bulimia nervosa: a controlled comparison. Am J Psychiatry 149:82–87, 1992

Beck A, Ward CH, Mendelson M, et al: An inventory for measuring depression. Arch Gen Psychiatry 4:561–571, 1961

Bossert S, Schnabel E, Krieg JC: Effects and limitations of cognitive behavior therapy in bulimia inpatients. Psychother Psychosom 51:77–82, 1989

Connors ME, Johnson CL, Stuckey MK: Treatment of bulimia with brief psychoeducational group therapy. Am J Psychiatry 141:1512–1516, 1984

Derogatis LR, Lipman RS, Rickels K, et al: The Hopkins Symptom Checklist (HSCL): a self-report symptom inventory. Behav Sci 19:1–15, 1974

Fairburn CG, Kirk J, O'Connor M, et al: A comparison of two psychological treatments for bulimia nervosa. Behav Res Ther 24:629–643, 1986

Fairburn CG, Jones R, Peveler RC, et al: Three psychological treatments for bulimia nervosa. Arch Gen Psychiatry 48:463–469, 1991

Fairburn CG, Jones R, Peveler RC, et al: Psychotherapy and bulimia nervosa: the longer-term effects of interpersonal psychotherapy, behaviour therapy and cognitive behaviour therapy. Arch Gen Psychiatry (in press)

Freeman CPL, Barry F, Dunkeld-Turnbull J, et al: Controlled trial of psychotherapy for bulimia nervosa. BMJ 296:521–525, 1988

Garner DM, Olmsted MP, Bohr Y, et al: The Eating Attitude Test: psychometric features and clinical correlates. Psychol Med 12:871–878, 1982

Garner DM, Olmsted MP, Polivy J: Development and validation of a multidimensional eating disorder inventory for anorexia nervosa and bulimia. International Journal of Eating Disorders 2:15–34, 1983

Garner DM, Rockert W, Davis R, et al: A comparison between cognitive-behavioral and supportive-expressive therapy for bulimia nervosa. Am J Psychiatry (in press)

Hamilton M: Development of a rating scale for primary depressive illness. British Journal of Social and Clinical Psychology 6:278–296, 1967

Hsu LKG: Four treatments of bulimic nervosa. Paper presented at the Seattle Symposium on Eating Disorders, Seattle, WA, December 1991

Kirkley BG, Schneider JA, Agras WS, et al: Comparison of two group treatments for bulimia. J Consult Clin Psychol 53:43–48, 1985

Lacey JH: Bulimia nervosa, binge eating, and psychogenic vomiting: a controlled treatment study and long term outcome. BMJ 286:1609–1613, 1983

Laessle RG, Waadt S, Pirke SJ: A structured behaviorally oriented group treatment for bulimia nervosa. Psychother Psychosom 48:141–145, 1987

Lee NF, Rush AJ: Cognitive-behavioral group therapy for bulimia. International Journal of Eating Disorders 5:599–615, 1986

Leitenberg H, Rosen JC: Cognitive-behavioral therapy with and without exposure plus response prevention in treatment of bulimia nervosa: comment on Agras, Schneider, Arnow, Raeburn, and Telch. J Consult Clin Psychol 57:776–777, 1989

Leitenberg H, Rosen JC, Gross J, et al: Exposure plus response-prevention treatment of bulimia nervosa. J Consult Clin Psychol 56:535–541, 1988

Mitchell JE, Pyle RL, Eckert ED, et al: A comparison study of antidepressants and structured intensive group psychotherapy in the treatment of bulimia nervosa. Arch Gen Psychiatry 47:149–157, 1990

Mitchell JE, Pyle RL, Eckert ED, et al: Cognitive behavioral group psychotherapy of bulimia nervosa: importance of logistical variables. Unpublished manuscript, June 1992

Montgomery SA, Åsberg M: A new depression scale designed to be sensitive to change. Br J Psychiatry 134:382–389, 1979

Ordman AM, Kirschenbaum DS: Cognitive-behavioral therapy for bulimia: an initial outcome study. J Consult Clin Psychol 53:305–313, 1985

Pyle RL, Mitchell JE, Eckert ED, et al: Maintenance treatment and 6-month outcome for bulimic patients who respond to initial treatment. Am J Psychiatry 147:871–875, 1990

Wilson GT, Rossiter E, Kleifield EI, et al: Cognitive-behavioral treatment of bulimia nervosa: a controlled evaluation. Behav Res Ther 277–288, 1986

Wolchik SA, Weiss L, Katzman MA: An empirically validated, short-term psychoeducational group treatment program for bulimia. International Journal of Eating Disorders 5:21–34, 1986

Yates AJ, Sambrailo F: Bulimia nervosa: a descriptive and therapeutic study. Behav Res Ther 503–517, 1984

Chapter 16

Pharmacological Treatment

B. Timothy Walsh, M.D.

⟹⟶⟵

A wide variety of techniques have been explored in efforts to treat anorexia nervosa and bulimia nervosa, including the use of medication. In recent years, such pharmacological treatment strategies have been examined in controlled trials, and evidence has accumulated suggesting that medication can provide significant clinical benefit, particularly in the case of bulimia nervosa. In this chapter, I review information gathered from controlled studies regarding the utility of medication in the treatment of eating disorders.

Anorexia Nervosa

In the last 50 years, psychiatry has witnessed impressive advances in the development of pharmacological treatments for many major psychiatric illnesses. Significant and at times life-saving assistance is available through the use of medication for patients with schizophrenia, manic-depressive illness, major depression, and anxiety disorders, among other psychiatric disorders. However, anorexia nervosa, although clearly described more than 100 years ago, remains relatively refractory to pharmacological intervention.

Antipsychotic Medication

The first systematic attempts to intervene with medication in the treatment of anorexia nervosa were described by Dally and Sargant (1960, 1966) in England. They prescribed large doses of chlorpromazine (up to 1,600 mg/day), often in combination with insulin, and compared the outcome of 30 inpatients treated with this method with the outcome of 27 patients treated at the same hospital in the previous 20 years without the use of chlorpromazine. The patients treated with chlorpromazine gained weight faster and were discharged sooner than those treated without medication. However, the use of chlorpromazine was associated with significant side effects, including the occurrence of grand mal seizures in 5 patients. Also, bulimia nervosa developed in 45% of the group treated with chlorpromazine, compared to only 12% of the comparison group. On follow-up, the chlorpromazine-treated patients fared no better than those treated without medication.

Only two placebo-controlled trials have examined the potential utility of antipsychotic medication in anorexia nervosa. Vandereycken and Pierloot (1982), noting the hypothesis of Barry and Klawans (1976) that some features of anorexia nervosa might be manifestations of increased central dopaminergic activity, carried out a controlled trial of pimozide (4 or 6 mg/day) using a crossover design. In this trial, 18 women with anorexia nervosa were included; 8 were treated with pimozide for 3 weeks and then switched to placebo for 3 weeks, and 9 received the opposite sequence. In addition to the medication treatment, all patients were treated on an inpatient unit with a structured behavioral program. There was a trend for patients to have a higher mean daily weight gain on pimozide than on placebo ($P = .07$). Staff ratings of patients' attitudes and behavior showed small and inconsistent differences between drug and placebo.

Vandereycken (1984) subsequently published a controlled trial of another neuroleptic, sulpiride. In this study, nine female inpatients with anorexia nervosa were treated with sulpiride (300–400 mg/day) for 3 weeks and then were given placebo for 3 weeks, and nine received the opposite sequence. There were no statistically significant effects of sulpiride on either the mean daily weight change or the behavioral and attitudinal characteristics of the patients.

Because of the lack of clear efficacy of neuroleptics in these studies and the potency of these agents in producing side effects, interest in the utility of neuroleptics in anorexia nervosa has waned, and this class of medication is now not commonly used. However, some experienced clinicians believe that, in rare cases, the use of antipsychotic medication may be of benefit.

Antidepressant Medication

Several studies have examined the effectiveness of tricyclic antidepressant medication in anorexia nervosa. These investigations were prompted mainly by two observations. First, depressive symptoms are frequently observed during the course of anorexia nervosa. Second, some patients with depressive illness, when treated with tricyclic antidepressants, experience significant weight gain, and it was thought that this side effect might be of clinical utility in anorexia nervosa.

In the first controlled trial of a tricyclic antidepressant in anorexia nervosa, Lacey and Crisp (1980) compared clomipramine (50 mg/day) with placebo in 16 inpatients. They could find no evidence of an increased rate of weight gain in the active medication group. In view of the recent suggestions of a link between anorexia nervosa and obsessive-compulsive disorder and of the documented efficacy of clomipramine in the treatment of obsessive-compulsive disorder, clomipramine is a theoretically appealing agent for the treatment of anorexia nervosa. Unfortunately, the low dose of clomipramine used in the study by Lacey and Crisp leaves its potential utility unresolved.

The effectiveness of amitriptyline in the treatment of anorexia nervosa has been assessed in two controlled studies. The first study was conducted by Biederman et al. (1985), who examined amitriptyline (at an average dose of 2.8 mg/kg/day) and placebo in a mixed group of 25 inpatients and outpatients at two centers. Over 5 weeks, there was no evidence of a difference between the drug-treated and placebo groups in rate of weight gain or improvement in any symptomatic measure.

A larger controlled trial of amitriptyline was conducted by Halmi et al. (1986), who compared amitriptyline (at a maximum dose of 160 mg/day) both with placebo and with the serotonin antagonist cyproheptadine. In this trial, 72 inpatients with anorexia nervosa were treated at two centers. Although there were some suggestions that amitriptyline was associated with a reduction in the number of days required to reach target weight among the patients who were able to achieve that goal, most of the analyses comparing amitriptyline with placebo did not demonstrate a significant advantage of amitriptyline. There was also no evidence for a significant effect of amitriptyline on mood.

In summary, the few studies of antidepressant medication in anorexia nervosa do not suggest a major role for tricyclic antidepressants in the treatment of this syndrome. Unfortunately, this conclusion rests on very few controlled trials. It is also of note that, in all of these studies, the question being addressed was not whether antidepressant medication alone had any efficacy in anorexia nervosa, but whether antidepressant medication increased the effectiveness of established treatment programs. Several investigators have suggested that fluoxetine may be of utility, not in the acute treatment of patients with anorexia nervosa, but in the maintenance of change (Weltzin et al. 1990). It will be interesting to see whether such suggestions can be substantiated by controlled trials.

Cyproheptadine

A third model for the use of medication in the treatment of anorexia nervosa involves the serotonin antagonist cyproheptadine. The use of this agent was noted to be associated with weight gain in the treatment of children with asthma. In addition, preclinical studies suggest that serotonin plays an important role in the control of eating behavior (Blundell and Hill 1987; Liebowitz et al. 1987). Experimental manipulations that increase the availability of hypothalamic serotonin generally lead to a decrease in food consumption. Conversely, depletion of serotonin is associated with increased food intake. These data provide a theoretical rationale for the use of cyproheptadine in anorexia nervosa.

The first controlled trial of cyproheptadine in anorexia nervosa was reported by Vigersky and Loriaux (1977). This study examined the use of cyproheptadine (12 mg/day) in 24 outpatients with anorexia nervosa over 8 weeks. Of 13 patients receiving cyproheptadine, 4 (31%) gained weight, compared to 2 of 11 patients (18%) receiving placebo; this difference was not statistically significant.

A second study was reported by Goldberg et al. (1979). Cyproheptadine (maximum dose 32 mg/day) and placebo were compared in a multicenter trial in which patients were also assigned to receive either behavior therapy or no behavior therapy. Overall, there was no significant difference between the cyproheptadine-treated and placebo groups in weight gain, but a post hoc analysis suggested that some patients with more severe forms of the illness benefited from cyproheptadine.

In Halmi et al.'s (1986) study, described previously, cyproheptadine was compared with both amitriptyline and placebo. Limited evidence indicated a clear benefit from cyproheptadine. However, when patients were divided into bulimic and nonbulimic groups, there was a differential drug effect. Cyproheptadine significantly increased treatment efficiency in nonbulimic patients, but impaired treatment efficiency in bulimic patients, when compared with the amitriptyline-treated and placebo groups. These data suggest that cyproheptadine may be of use in the treatment of some patients with anorexia nervosa who do not binge eat. They also add to other evidence indicating that there are important distinctions between bulimic and nonbulimic patients with anorexia nervosa.

Lithium

Gross et al. (1981) conducted a controlled trial of lithium carbonate in anorexia nervosa. These investigators were interested in whether the known association between lithium treatment and weight gain might be usefully applied to the care of patients with anorexia nervosa. In a 4-week trial, they examined weight gain in eight women treated with lithium carbonate and eight women given a placebo and found indications of a significant drug-placebo difference in the final 2 weeks. This study suggested that lithium carbonate might augment weight gain in patients with anorexia nervosa, but it has not been followed by trials of longer duration in larger samples.

Tetrahydrocannabinol

Gross et al. (1983) also carried out a controlled trial of delta-9-tetrahydrocannabinol to test the idea that the appetite-stimulating effects of this prominent psychoactive component of marijuana might be of benefit in anorexia nervosa. In a crossover trial that employed diazepam as an active placebo, 11 inpatients were examined. Tetrahydrocannabinol was not efficacious in promoting weight gain and was associated with severe dysphoric reactions in 3 patients.

Bulimia Nervosa

Progress toward the development of effective pharmacological treatment for bulimia nervosa has been much more rapid than for anorexia nervosa. Treatment studies of bulimia nervosa are more easily accomplished because of the greater prevalence of bulimia nervosa and the fact that bulimia nervosa can, for the most part, be treated on an outpatient basis, whereas many patients with anorexia nervosa require hospitalization.

A variety of conceptual models have prompted medication trials in bulimia nervosa. Some of the earliest work was based on the notion that patients with this illness had a form of seizure disorder (Green and Rau 1974), leading to controlled trials of phenytoin (Wermuth et al. 1977) and carbamazepine (Kaplan et al. 1983). Two studies explored the possible utility of the appetite suppressant fenfluramine (Blouin et al. 1988; Russell et al. 1988). Because of the involvement of serotonin in the control of food intake, the efficacy of precursor loading, using tryptophan, has been examined (Krahn and Mitchell 1985). Because animal studies have suggested that opiate antagonists can modify stress-induced eating, the utility of naltrexone has also been explored (Jonas and Gold 1986; Mitchell et al. 1989). Although the results of the trials of fenfluramine were encouraging to some degree, most of the data regarding the other agents were either negative or inconclusive.

Antidepressant Medication

Pharmacological trials using antidepressant medications have been much more successful. The starting point for these trials was the observation made by a number of clinicians in the early 1980s that many patients with bulimia nervosa exhibited significant mood disturbance. Questions concerning the etiological relationship between mood disturbance and bulimia nervosa have generated considerable controversy and have still not been entirely resolved (Devlin and Walsh 1989). But the observation that many patients with bulimia nervosa also experience mood disturbances prompted clinicians to investigate the potential utility of antidepressant medications in the treatment of this eating disorder. The initial open trials by Pope and Hudson (1982) and by our own group (Walsh et al. 1982) were published in 1982 and were followed, in relatively short order, by a large number of double-blind, placebo-controlled trials (Table 16–1).

Several observations can be made about these trials. First, virtually all classes of antidepressants have been examined. Second, the length of the trials is brief, usually 6 or 8 weeks. Therefore, data about the efficacy of medication from controlled trials are confined to relatively short intervals. Third, the overwhelming majority of individuals in these trials consisted of women of normal body weight who regularly employed

Table 16–1. Summary of controlled antidepressant trials in bulimia nervosa

Study	N	Design	Medication	% change in binge frequency[a]		% remission	
				Drug	Placebo	Drug	Placebo
Pope et al. 1983	19	Parallel	Imipramine	−70.0	0.0	NR	NR
Sabine et al. 1983	36	Parallel	Mianserin	NR	NR	NR	NR
Mitchell and Groat 1984	32	Parallel	Amitriptyline	−72.1	−51.8	NR	NR
Hughes et al. 1986	22	Parallel	Desipramine	−91.0	19.0	NR	NR
Barlow et al. 1988	24	Crossover	Desipramine	−46.8	−2.4	4.2	NR
Agras et al. 1987	20	Parallel	Imipramine	−72.4	−43.1	30.0	10.0
Blouin et al. 1988	10	Crossover	Desipramine	−40.0	NR	10.0	NR
Horne et al. 1988	81	Parallel	Bupropion	−67.0	−1.9	29.7	NR
Walsh et al. 1988	50	Parallel	Phenelzine	−64.2	−5.5	34.8	3.7
Kennedy et al. 1988	18	Crossover	Isocarboxazid	−35.0	5.0	33.3	NR
Pope et al. 1989	42	Parallel	Trazodone	−31.0	21.0	10.0	0.0
Mitchell et al. 1990	74[b]	Parallel	Imipramine	−49.3	−2.5	16.0	NR
Enas et al. 1989	387	Parallel	Fluoxetine (60 mg)	−65[c]	−30[c]	27[c]	14[c]
			Fluoxetine (20 mg)	−40[c]		14[c]	
Freeman et al. 1989	40	Parallel	Fluoxetine	−51.4	−16.8	NR	NR
Walsh et al. 1991	78	Parallel	Desipramine	−47.0	7.0	12.5	7.9

Note. NR = not reported.
[a]Mean of individual subject's percentage of reduction in binge frequency is given where available, otherwise percentage reduction in group mean binge frequency is given. [b]This study also examined the effects of group psychotherapy. These 74 patients received only imipramine or placebo. [c]Approximate figures.
Source. Adapted from Walsh BT: "Fluoxetine in the Treatment of Bulimia Nervosa." *Journal of Psychosomatic Research* 35 (suppl 1): 33–40, 1991. Used with permission. Copyright 1991 Pergamon Press PLC.

self-induced vomiting or laxatives to compensate for the eating binges. It is not clear that the results of these medication trials can be confidently extrapolated to other populations, for example, overweight individuals who binge eat or individuals who binge but do not purge.

As shown in Table 16–1, the results of these controlled trials are impressively consistent. In virtually all studies, the reduction in binge frequency is significantly greater among patients assigned to the active treatment group than among patients assigned to placebo. These studies leave no question about the fact that antidepressant medication is superior to placebo in the short-term treatment of bulimia nervosa.

It would be of interest to know whether one medication or class of medications is more efficacious in the treatment of this syndrome. As yet, no study directly comparing one antidepressant to another has been reported. In the absence of such studies, comparisons between different antidepressants using data from the studies presented in Table 16–1 are risky. For example, there are substantial differences among studies in the response to placebo, emphasizing the difficulty of interpreting differences in response across studies. Nonetheless, there do not appear to be major differences in the rates of response to the various antidepressants.

The doses used in these treatment studies have generally been similar to those employed for the treatment of depression, and, with one exception, no dose-response studies have been conducted. The exception is the large trial of fluoxetine (Enas et al. 1989), in which one group was given placebo, one group was treated with fluoxetine at a dose of 20 mg/day, and one group was treated with fluoxetine at a dose of 60 mg/day. This study found that the 60-mg/day dose was superior to both placebo and the 20-mg/day dose, and that the 20-mg/day dose was not clearly superior to placebo. As fluoxetine at a dose of 20 mg/day has been demonstrated to be effective for the treatment of depression, this result challenges the common assumption that the effective dose of antidepressant medication for the treatment of bulimia is the same as that for the treatment of depression.

It is interesting and surprising, at least in light of the original rationale for the use of antidepressant medication for bulimia nervosa, that the pretreatment presence of depression has not proven to be a good predictor of response to medication (Agras et al. 1987; Hughes et al. 1986; Walsh et al. 1988). Both depressed and nondepressed patients appear about equally responsive to antidepressant medication. This observation clearly poses an important and as yet unanswered question about the mechanism of action of antidepressants in bulimia nervosa.

Although the studies reviewed here leave little doubt about the short-term efficacy of antidepressants compared with placebo, important questions about the precise place of medication in the treatment of bulimia nervosa remain unanswered. One major question involves the long-term outcome of antidepressant treatment. Pope et al. (1985) described a 2-year follow-up of patients treated initially in their controlled trial of imipramine. Most patients remained improved at follow-up; the majority had required alterations of their antidepressant regimen, however, and most had had to remain on medication to maintain their response.

In a study recently completed by our group (Walsh et al. 1991), we found that almost half the patients who had initially responded to desipramine relapsed over the succeeding 4 months despite continued medication. In addition, medication treatment, although more effective than placebo, is not sufficient to induce remission for most patients, who therefore may remain quite symptomatic even at the conclusion of a course of antidepressant therapy.

In short, concerns about the overall response rate on antidepressant medication, about the maintenance of improvement on medication, and about the need for long-term medication treatment raise questions about the role of antidepressants in the treatment of bulimia nervosa. Furthermore, as is described elsewhere (Casper, Chapter 14, this volume; Mitchell and Raymond, Chapter 15, this volume), structured forms of psychotherapy, particularly those using cognitive and behavioral strategies, have been reported to produce impressive and sustained improvement.

Investigators have begun to compare pharmacological interventions with psychotherapeutic interventions. In the first such study, Mitchell et al. (1990) found that an intensive group therapy program was superior to treatment with imipramine. In a second study, Agras et al. (1992) compared individual cognitive-behavioral treatment with treatment with desipramine and with treatment with the combination of desipramine and psychotherapy; cognitive-behavioral treatment was clearly superior to medication alone. Concerns can be raised about both of these studies. The group intervention employed by Mitchell et al. (1990) was particularly intensive, for example, requiring patients to attend 3-hour treatment sessions five nights during the first week, and it is not clear that the results of this form of intensive treatment can be readily extrapolated to less intensive treatment methods. In the study by Agras et al. (1992), the average dosage of desipramine was modest (167 mg/day 6 weeks into treatment), as was the mean serum level (131 ng/ml), leaving open the possibility that additional benefit might have been obtained at higher dosages. In addition, in neither of the studies was a second pharmacological intervention systematically tried if the initial medication trial produced inadequate symptomatic change.

Nonetheless, the data currently available suggest that a single course of a single antidepressant agent in the absence of psychotherapy should not be considered an adequate or first-choice treatment for bulimia nervosa. Future studies are required to provide better guidelines for when medication is best employed in the treatment of bulimia nervosa. For example, it may be useful to assess the efficacy of sequential medication regimens and of combinations of medication and psychotherapy.

References

Agras WS, Dorian B, Kirkley BG, et al: Imipramine in the treatment of bulimia: a double-blind controlled study. International Journal of Eating Disorders 6:29–38, 1987

Agras WS, Rossiter EM, Arnow B, et al: Pharmacologic and cognitive-behavioral treatment for bulimia nervosa: a controlled comparison. Am J Psychiatry 1:82–87, 1992

Barlow J, Blouin J, Blouin A, et al: Treatment of bulimia with desipramine: a double-blind crossover study. Can J Psychiatry 330:129–133, 1988

Barry VC, Klawans HL: On the role of dopamine in the pathophysiology of anorexia nervosa. J Neural Transm 38:107–122, 1976

Biederman J, Herzog DB, Rivinus TM, et al: Amitriptyline in the treatment of anorexia nervosa: a double-blind, placebo-controlled study. J Clin Psychopharmacol 5:10–16, 1985

Blouin AG, Blouin JH, Perez EL, et al: Treatment of bulimia with fenfluramine and desipramine. J Clin Psychopharmacol 8:261–269, 1988

Blundell JE, Hill AJ: Serotoninergic modulation of the pattern of eating and the profile of hunger-satiety in humans. Int J Obes 11 (suppl 3):141–155, 1987

Dally P, Sargant W: A new treatment of anorexia nervosa. BMJ 1:1770–1773, 1960

Dally P, Sargant W: Treatment and outcome of anorexia nervosa. BMJ 2:793–795, 1966

Devlin MJ, Walsh BT: Eating disorders and depression. Psychiatric Annals 19:473–476, 1989

Enas GG, Pope HG, Levine LR: Fluoxetine in bulimia nervosa: double blind study, in New Research Abstracts of the American Psychiatric Association. Washington, DC, American Psychiatric Association, 1989

Freeman CPL, Davies F, Morris J, et al: A double-blind controlled trial of fluoxetine versus placebo for bulimia nervosa. Unpublished manuscript, 1989

Goldberg SC, Halmi KA, Eckert ED, et al: Cyproheptadine in anorexia nervosa. Br J Psychiatry 134:67–70, 1979

Green RS, Rau JH: Treatment of compulsive eating disturbances with anticonvulsant medication. Am J Psychiatry 131:428–432, 1974

Gross HA, Ebert MH, Faden VB, et al: A double-blind controlled trial of lithium carbonate in primary anorexia nervosa. J Clin Psychopharmacol 1:376–381, 1981

Gross HA, Ebert MH, Faden VB, et al: A double-blind trial of delta-9-tetrahydrocannabinol in primary anorexia nervosa. J Clin Psychopharmacol 3:165–171, 1983

Halmi KA, Eckert ED, LaDu TJ, et al: Anorexia nervosa: treatment efficacy of cyproheptadine and amitriptyline. Arch Gen Psychiatry 43:177–181, 1986

Horne RL, Ferguson JM, Pope HG, et al: Treatment of bulimia with bupropion: a multicenter controlled trial. J Clin Psychiatry 49:262–266, 1988

Hughes PL, Wells LA, Cunningham CJ, et al: Treating bulimia with desipramine: a double-blind, placebo-controlled study. Arch Gen Psychiatry 43:182–186, 1986

Jonas JM, Gold MS: Naltrexone reverses bulimic symptoms (letter). Lancet 1:807, 1986

Kaplan AS, Garfinkel PE, Darby PL, et al: Carbamazepine in the treatment of bulimia. Am J Psychiatry 140:1225–1226, 1983

Kennedy SH, Piran N, Warsh JJ, et al: A trial of isocarboxazid in the treatment of bulimia nervosa. J Clin Psychopharmacol 8:391–396, 1988

Krahn D, Mitchell J: Use of L-tryptophan in treating bulimia. Am J Psychiatry 142:1130, 1985

Lacey JH, Crisp AH: Hunger, food intake and weight: the impact of clomipramine on a refeeding anorexia nervosa population. Postgrad Med J 56 (suppl 1):79–85, 1980

Liebowitz SF, Weiss GF, Shor-Posner G: Medial hypothalamic serotonin in the control of eating behavior. Int J Obes 11 (suppl 3):110–123, 1987

Mitchell JE, Groat R: A placebo-controlled, double-blind trial of amitriptyline in bulimia. J Clin Psychopharmacol 4:186–193, 1984

Mitchell JE, Christenson G, Jennings J, et al: A placebo-controlled, double-blind crossover study of naltrexone hydrochloride in outpatients with normal weight bulimia. J Clin Psychopharmacol 9:94–97, 1989

Mitchell JE, Pyle RL, Eckert ED, et al: A comparison study of antidepressants and structured group psychotherapy in the treatment of bulimia nervosa. Arch Gen Psychiatry 47:149–157, 1990

Pope HG Jr, Hudson JI: Treatment of bulimia with antidepressants. Psychopharmacology 78:176–179, 1982

Pope HG Jr, Hudson JI, Jonas JM, et al: Bulimia treated with imipramine: a placebo-controlled, double-blind study. Am J Psychiatry 140:554–558, 1983

Pope HG, Hudson JI, Jonas JM, et al: Antidepressant treatment of bulimia: a two-year follow-up study. J Clin Psychopharmacol 5:320–327, 1985

Pope HG Jr, Keck PE Jr, McElroy SL, et al: A placebo-controlled study of trazodone in bulimia nervosa. J Clin Psychopharmacol 9:254–259, 1989

Russell GFM, Checkley SA, Feldman J, et al: A controlled trial of d-fenfluramine in bulimia nervosa. Clin Neuropharmacol 11 (suppl 1):S146–S159, 1988

Sabine EJ, Yonance A, Farrington AJ, et al: Bulimia nervosa: a placebo controlled double-blind therapeutic trial of mianserin. Br J Clin Pharmacol 15:195S–202, 1983

Vandereycken W: Neuroleptics in the short-term treatment of anorexia nervosa: a double-blind placebo-controlled study with sulpiride. Br J Psychiatry 144:288–292, 1984

Vandereycken W, Pierloot R: Pimozide combined with behavior therapy in the short-term treatment of anorexia nervosa. Acta Psychiatr Scand 66:445–450, 1982

Vigersky RA, Loriaux DL: The effect of cyproheptadine in anorexia nervosa: a double-blind trial, in Anorexia Nervosa. Edited by Vigersky RA. New York, Raven, 1977, pp 349–356

Walsh BT: Fluoxetine in the treatment of bulimia nervosa. J Psychosom Res 35 (suppl 1):33–40, 1991

Walsh BT, Stewart JW, Wright L, et al: Treatment of bulimia with monoamine oxidase inhibitors. Am J Psychiatry 139:1629–1630, 1982

Walsh BT, Gladis M, Roose SP, et al: Phenelzine vs placebo in 50 patients with bulimia. Arch Gen Psychiatry 45:471–475, 1988

Walsh BT, Hadigan CM, Devlin MJ, et al: Long-term outcome of antidepressant treatment for bulimia nervosa. Am J Psychiatry 148:1206–1212, 1991

Weltzin TE, Hsu LKG, Kaye WH: An open trial of fluoxetine in anorexia nervosa: maintenance of body weight and reduction of obsessional symptoms (abstract). Paper presented at the Fourth International Conference on Eating Disorders, New York, April 1990

Wermuth BM, Davis KL, Hollister LE, et al: Phenytoin treatment of the binge-eating syndrome. Am J Psychiatry 134:1249–1253, 1977

Index

*Page numbers printed in **boldface** type refer to tables or figures.*

—————— ⟶●⟶ ——————

A

—————— ⟶●⟶ ——————

Abuse, laxative, in bulimia
nervosa, 45–46

Adolescents, family therapy in,
controlled trial of, 253–256,
255

Affective disorders
bulimia nervosa and, 52
eating disorders and, 67–71,
69, 70

Age, as factor in eating disorders,
22

Alcoholism, eating disorders and,
71

Alpha$_2$-adrenergic functioning, in
eating disorders, 202–205,
204

Alpha$_2$ agonists, and running
activity, 157–158

Amenorrhea
in anorexia nervosa, 41,
159–161, **161**
cause of, 159

Amitriptyline
for anorexia nervosa, 331
for bulimia nervosa, **335**

Anorexia nervosa. *See also* Eating
disorders
in adolescents, family therapy
in, controlled trial of,
253–256, **255**
affective disorders and, 52,
67–71, **69**
age as factor in, 22
amenorrhea in, 41, 159–161,
161
antidepressant drug effects in,
228–231, **229, 230**
attitudes toward food in, 84–88
behavior designed to produce
marked weight loss in, 38–39
beta-endorphin in, **174,** 175
biological factors in, 25
body image disturbance in, 40
brain changes in, **101,** 106
bulimic subtype, 41–42
alcoholism and, 71
defined, 223
described, 171
psychodynamics in, 293
causes of, **101,** 105, 178
classification and diagnosis of,
37–55
clinical features of, **51**
continuum of, 54–55

endocrine changes in,
193–213, **200–201**
energy expenditure in, 225,
226
energy intake in, 224–225
family relationships and,
263–281
behavioral observations of,
271–277, **274**
daughters' perceptions of,
266–268
implications of, 277–281
parents' and daughters'
perceptions of, 268–271
recommendations
concerning, 277–281
research on, 266–277
studies of, 62–66, **65**
family therapy in
assessment scales in,
243–244
design of the therapeutic
trial, 240–241
evaluation of, 240–251
method of, 241–243
patient selection in, 243
fear of becoming fat in, 46–47
first-degree relatives of, risk of
major affective disorders
among, 68, **70,** 71
fluoxetine for, 104
follow-up studies of, 125–144.
See also Follow-up studies, of
eating disorders
hunger perceptions in, 80–84
hypothalamic-pituitary-adrenal
axis effects of, 208–210, **210**
hypothalamic-pituitary-gonadal
axis effects of, 205–208, **207**

hypothalamic-pituitary-thyroid
axis effects of, 198–202,
200–202
incidence of, 62
insulin in, 162–163
intermittent dieting in, 162
Johns Hopkins Eating
Disorders Program,
1975–1990, 94–121
lack of purging in, 45–46
luteinizing hormone in, 162,
163
male-to-female ratio in, 97
medication manipulation in, 46
menstrual cycle disturbances
in, 160, 162–165, **163, 164**
metabolic changes in, 224–228
neuroendocrine and
reproductive function in,
151–165
neuropeptide abnormalities
in, 169–185
norepinephrine in, 163–164
normal-weight
cholecystokinin in, 182
neuropeptide abnormalities
in, 179–183
opioids in, 183
peptide YY in, 180–182, **182**
pseudoatrophy of the brain
in, 211
obesity in, 45–46
outcome studies, 139–143, **141,
142**
overeating in, powerful and
intractable urges involving,
42–44
perceptual capacities in,
84–88

D

F

Failure to trace, rate of, 125–126
Family environment, as factor in
    eating disorders, 61–74
    studies of, 62–66, **65**
Family-genetic factors, in eating
    disorders, 61–74
Family relationships
    anorexia nervosa and, 263–281
    bulimia nervosa and, 263–281
    eating disorders and, 263–281
        behavioral observations of,
            271–277, **274**
        daughters' perceptions of,
            266–268
        implications of, 277–281
        parents' and daughters'
            perceptions of, 268–271
        recommendations
            concerning, 277–281
        research on, 266–277
        theories of, 264–266
Family therapy
    in anorexia nervosa, 237–259
        for adolescents, controlled
            trial of, 253–256, **255**
        assessment scales in,
            243–244
        controlled trials, 239–256
        evaluation of, 240–241
        individual therapy versus,
            244–251, **245–251**
        method of, 241–243
        patient selection in, 243
    in bulimia nervosa
        assessment scales in, 243

design of the therapeutic
    trial, 240–241
evaluation of, 240–241
method of, 241–243
patient selection in, 243
defined, 239
in eating disorders, **101,**
    104–105
Fasting, endocrine changes due
    to, 193–213
Fat, morbid fear of becoming
    in anorexia nervosa, 39–41
    in bulimia nervosa, 46–47
Financing, of Johns Hopkins
    Eating Disorders Program,
    1975–1990, 111–115, **112,**
    114
Fluoxetine
    for bulimia nervosa, **335**
    for eating disorders, 104
    effect on resting metabolic
        rate, **230**
Follow-up studies
    of anorexia nervosa, 128–139,
        128–131, 133, 135, 136, 138,
        139
    of bulimia nervosa, 139–143,
        141, 142
    of eating disorders, 125–144
        failure to trace in, 125–126
        idiosyncratic data
            presentation, 127
        inadequate duration of,
            126–127
        indirect methods in, 127
        insufficient outcome
            information in, 126
        undefined diagnostic
            criteria in, 126

N

S

T